D0824738

The Complete Family Guide to Schizophrenia

The Complete Family Guide to Schizophrenia

Helping Your Loved One Get the Most Out of Life

Kim T. Mueser, PhD, and Susan Gingerich, MSW

Foreword by Harriet P. Lefley

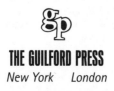

THE GUILFORD PRESS
New York   London

© 2006 The Guilford Press
A Division of Guilford Publications, Inc.
72 Spring Street, New York, NY 10012
www.guilford.com

The information in this volume is not intended as a substitute for consultation
with health care professionals. Each individual's health concerns should be
evaluated by a qualified professional.

Printed in the United States of America

This book is printed on acid-free paper.

Last digit is print number: 9 8 7 6 5 4 3 2 1

Library of Congress Cataloging-in-Publication Data

Mueser, Kim Tornvall.
     The complete family guide to schizophrenia: helping your loved one get the most
out of life / Kim T. Mueser, Susan Gingerich.
          p.   cm.
     Includes index.
     ISBN-10: 1-59385-180-4 ISBN-13: 978-1-59385-180-4 (pbk.: alk. paper)
     ISBN-10: 1-59385-273-8 ISBN-13: 978-1-59385-273-3 (hardcover: alk. paper)
     1. Schizophrenia. 2. Schizophrenics—Family relationships. 3. Mentally ill—Family
relationships.   I. Gingerich, Susan. II. Title.
     RC514.M84 2006
     616.89′8—dc22
                                                                              2005031492

To my wife, Susan McGurk
—K. T. M.

To my husband, Ted Chinburg
—S. G.

And to the individuals and families
with whom we have worked over the past 20 years.
We are honored that you invited us to be part of your lives.
—K. T. M. and S. G.

Contents

PART I

An Overview of Schizophrenia

PART II

Special Issues for Family Members

PART III

Preventing Relapses

PART IV

Creating a Supportive Environment

PART V

Coping with Specific Problems

PART VI

Improving Quality of Life

Foreword

Schizophrenia can be a baffling and difficult disease. Symptoms such as delusions and hallucinations can lead to destructive behavior. Apathy and withdrawal deprive once vital people of the joys of living and their families of the full companionship of those whom they love. Problems with attention and thinking often make ordinary communication a genuine challenge. Despite promising new treatments, many people with schizophrenia still lead unfulfilled lives.

It does not have to be this way. Many people with schizophrenia live with their families, and even for those who don't, caring families are natural, lifetime support systems. Lacking knowledge and support, however, family members are typically bewildered about how best to fill this role. A few mental health systems offer programs that provide state-of-the-art information and illness management techniques, but attempts to involve or educate families are still far from standard practice. To fill this need, advocacy groups and a few isolated mental health facilities have developed educational programs, such as the Family-to-Family program of the National Alliance on Mental Illness, Journey of Hope, Pebbles in the Pond, and other time-limited courses intended to help families understand and cope with major psychiatric disorders. However, these programs are just not enough for families that have to deal with special issues or crises on a day-to-day basis.

If you are helping a relative with schizophrenia, you'll find that *The Complete Family Guide to Schizophrenia* fills this gap. It is a handbook that provides a comprehensive overview of schizophrenia and answers many of the questions you are likely to ask. But it also offers an array of tools for resolving special problems that may arise during the course of the illness. Here you will find the most up-to-date view of schizophrenia and its causes as well as a multitude of strategies and techniques for coping on a daily basis and with special situations. You'll also learn to respect the strengths of your loved one in handling the demands and vicissitudes of the illness. The discussion of special issues faced by parents, siblings, spouses or partners, and children takes into account the unique emotional aspects of different kinship relationships. Because kinship roles are usually age-linked to the course and stages of the illness, you will also get some understanding of how schizophrenia is experienced by your relative, yourself, and others during different periods in the family life cycle.

It is noteworthy that a whole chapter (Chapter 3) in this book talks about recovery. This message of hope—a boon for families—is in keeping with ongoing research findings and the new recovery orientation in mental health services. People with schizophrenia vary widely in the degree to which they are impaired functionally and cognitively. With appropriate treatments, many people with schizophrenia are able to lead productive, satisfying lives without necessarily being symptom-free. The old predictions of progressive deterioration and a dead-end life are now thankfully obsolete. Early interventions enable young, first-episode patients to take jobs, finish high school or college, and avoid the developmental lags that interrupted the task-learning years of earlier generations as they transitioned into adulthood. Some people diagnosed with schizophrenia may even attain PhD and MD degrees.

Knowledge immeasurably reinforces the capacity for coping with the demands of this illness and for promoting recovery. In addition to basic, state-of-the-art information on schizophrenia, this book provides a rich lode of information on community resources, financial entitlements, useful organizations, and the like. These materials aid substantially in illness management, resource acquisition, and networking. Extensive information on medications, planning guides and worksheets for special situations, as well as checklists for signs of stress and relapse, preventive and response strategies, problem-solving techniques, and coping methods can all be found.

Using these tools in any household or clinical or residential facility can create a greater sense of mastery in individuals dealing with the illness and foster a more tranquil, accepting environment. The strategies in this book are attuned to the special sensitivities of those with schizophrenia and are stress-relieving for their caregivers. Family members have significant roles to play in supporting the recovery of their relative and in learning how to lead their own lives free of worry and pain. This handbook offers substantial help toward attaining these two important and clearly intertwined goals.

HARRIET P. LEFLEY, PhD
Department of Psychiatry and Behavioral Sciences
University of Miami School of Medicine

Preface

Schizophrenia is a major mental illness that can have a broad effect on the day-to-day functioning of those who have it—in school and work, in social relationships, and in the ability to take care of themselves. But it can also have a significant impact on the whole family, requiring substantial time, energy, and money to help the family member, and increasing stress and tension on a daily basis. As a relative or other loved one of someone with schizophrenia, you may be called on to provide support, to arrange for treatment, and to find ways of coping with common symptoms and other problems with the illness. Today, families are truly on the front line of the management of schizophrenia.

In the past, families usually had little or no role in the care of their loved one. However, the medical profession's understanding of schizophrenia and how to treat it has evolved tremendously over the past century. For many years doctors thought that palliative care, often in an institution, was the best that could be offered. But over the ensuing years, the discovery of effective medications and the development of rehabilitation approaches have enabled most people with schizophrenia to be treated in the community, with their families playing a major role in helping them cope with the illness. As knowledge about the nature of schizophrenia and its treatment has continued to grow, people with the illness and their families have further expanded their horizons. No longer satisfied with just coping, families and professionals have become united by a new vision of *recovery* and are now dedicated to helping people with schizophrenia grow past the devastating effects of their illness to develop rewarding and worthwhile lives. This book is aimed at helping families work with a loved one to develop and pursue such a vision of recovery.

How to Use This Book

Never before have the prospects for those with schizophrenia been so bright. But recovery, as you'll learn in this book, is an ongoing process rather than a single destination. Recovery means something different for every individual and every family. For this reason, we've structured this book so that you can turn to it again and again over the years to come, depending on the point you've reached in the recovery path and the needs of the family and the person with schizophrenia at the time.

If your relative has just been diagnosed or is in the process of being evaluated for schizophrenia, you'll probably save a lot of time and much trial and error if you read the whole book now and use the worksheets to come up with a plan for managing the illness and sustaining a vision of recovery. Parts I–III, at least, can help you create a solid foundation for helping your relative and, at the same time, protect your family from the vagaries of the illness. Once you have that foundation in place, you may feel you have more time to flesh out a recovery plan, using the strategies and information in Parts IV and VI. We strongly urge you to read these sections as soon as possible, though, because establishing a supportive environment and helping your relative achieve a fulfilling life are really not the "extras" that they may appear to be; both have something of a domino effect on the successful management of the entire disorder and produce benefits much greater than you might expect.

You'll undoubtedly find yourself turning to certain parts of this book repeatedly over time—to the individual chapters in Part V when you encounter a problem you may not have faced in the past, to the chapters in Parts II and IV when family dynamics shift and you need to polish your communication or problem-solving skills, to Part III when a new medication side effect arises or you need to learn a new method for relieving stress. Because this book is designed to be read in sequence and also referred to as needed, we have included a list of resources that apply to the specific subject matter at the end of each chapter. Whether it's an audiotape for learning relaxation techniques, an institute that can help with substance abuse, a support group for siblings, more detail on a specific topic from other books, or a social skills training program, you'll want to know how to find it when the need arises. The table of contents and index will remind you where you'll find the material on the problems you're trying to solve, and the resources at the end of each chapter will ensure that you lose no time in finding any additional help or information that you still need. We've listed the major organizations and information sources that address a variety of needs and subjects related to schizophrenia at the back of the book as well.

*   *   *

To help a relative with schizophrenia, you need basic information about the nature of the illness, principles of treatment, coping strategies for dealing with common problems, and suggestions for working together to achieve individual and shared recovery goals. You also need to know how to collaborate with mental health professionals, who have the knowledge, resources, and skills critical to treating the illness. Effective teamwork between you, your relative, and mental health professionals is important to helping the person manage the illness and live a fulfilling life.

The six sections in this book form a complete family guide for managing schizophrenia and helping a relative pursue personal recovery goals. Part I provides information about schizophrenia and its diagnosis, the meaning and hope of recovery, and the principles of treatment. It will tell you how to assess your relative's needs and what resources may be available in your community for addressing those needs. Whether you are a parent, a sibling, a son or daughter, or the partner of someone with schizophrenia, you'll benefit from reading this section.

Part II describes the experience with a loved one who has schizophrenia from the perspective of different relationships. You may find help with the specific issues involved in being a parent, sibling, partner, or son or daughter, or you might consult different chapters to get a better understanding of what one of your other family members may be experiencing with the relative who has schizophrenia. In Chapter 9 you'll find a discussion of what it is like to have a parent with the disorder and how you and your family can help if your relative with this illness *is* a parent.

Many years of rigorous research on the treatment of schizophrenia have shown that families can do a lot to prevent relapses in, and rehospitalizations of, a loved one with schizophrenia. If you are involved in your relative's daily or weekly life, Part III will help you develop specific plans to manage medications, reduce stress, recognize the early warning signs of a relapse, and prevent and respond to crises. Even if you have less contact with your loved one, you will benefit from reading these chapters.

Creating a supportive environment, solving problems together, and enjoying close relationships are important goals for all families, and they are even more critical when a relative has schizophrenia. Part IV provides guidelines for creating a positive home environment and maintaining mutually rewarding relationships. These chapters will be useful to you if you have ongoing contact, whether your loved one with schizophrenia lives at home or not.

Schizophrenia often presents a confusing array of symptoms, from the psychosis that most people associate with the illness to less familiar symptoms such as apathy and problems with thinking, depression, anxiety, and drug and alcohol abuse. Each chapter in Part V describes the nature of each group of symptoms, gives guidance for determining whether your relative experiences problems related to these symptoms, and suggests practical strategies for coping with them. The best way to use this section of the book is to consult the chapters that address the symptoms that pose the greatest difficulty for your loved one.

Part VI describes strategies for helping your relative reach for the horizons of recovery and improve his or her quality of life by discovering meaningful social relationships, success at work and school, independent living skills, and leisure and recreational activities. A separate chapter suggests ways to overcome the social stigma that is unfortunately still attached to mental illness. This section concludes with a chapter about planning for the future—a common concern for many families.

As one individual with mental illness told us: "Having strategies for coping with mental illness is extremely important. It's hard to enjoy your life if you are constantly having symptoms. However, believing in yourself, having hope that things will continue to get better, and looking forward to your future are also vital in overcoming mental illness. Our hopes and dreams are not delusions. Our hopes and dreams are what makes us human." It is our hope that you will find guidance in the following pages that will help you and your relative go beyond coping to achieve the personally meaningful goals that are the hallmark of recovery.

Acknowledgments

This book would not have been possible without the assistance, input, and inspiration of many people. Among our colleagues and members of the family and consumer community, we are especially grateful to the following people: Tim Ackerson, Jean Addington, Xavier Amador, Kerry Arnold, Julie Agresta, Susan Balder, Christine Barrowclough, Dan Beck, Debbie R. Becker, Alan S. Bellack, Max Birchwood, Gary Bond, Ken Braiterman, Amy Brodkey, Mary Brunette, Fred Bryant, Cori Cather, Donna Clancy, Richard Clancy, Dennis Combs, Pat Corrigan, Anne Crocker, Harry Cunningham, Ed Diksa, Robert E. Drake, Ian R. H. Falloon, David Fowler, Philippe Garety, Shirley M. Glynn, Joel Goldberg, Sylvia Gratz, Gillian Haddock, Michele Hamilton, Marvin Herz, the late David Hilton, Stefan Hofmann, Henry Jackson, Richard Jossiasen, David Kavanagh, Samuel M. Keith, David Kime, David Kingdon, Elizabeth Kuipers, Eric Latimer, Tania Lecomte, Harriet Lefley, Douglas L. Levinson, Robert P. Liberman, Elspeth Macdonald, Edie Mannion, William R. McFarlane, Christine McGill, Duncan McLean, Shery Meade, Marilyn Meisel, Anthony Menditto, Bodie Morey, Anthony Morrison, Sharon Scott Mulder, Doug Noordsy, Ken Park, David Penn, Roger Peters, Eric Pfeiffer, Maggie Pfeiffer, Helene Provencher, Neil Rector, Carole K. Rosenthal, Nina R. Schooler, George M. Simpson, James Smith, Nick Tarrier, Mary Ann Test, Graham Thornicroft, and Douglas Turkington.

We are also indebted to the thousands of individuals with schizophrenia and their families whom we have met over the years. We deeply admire the great strength and courage they show in coping with the illness and have learned so much from their love, resourcefulness, and determination.

Special thanks also goes to our editor at The Guilford Press, Kitty Moore, for her support and patience throughout our writing, and to Linda LaRose and Glenda Madden for their vital assistance in preparing this book for publication. On a final note, we are deeply indebted to Chris Benton, whose valuable insights, feedback, and suggestions improved our message immeasurably and truly captured the spirit of this book.

PART I

An Overview of Schizophrenia

CHAPTER 1

Schizophrenia: The Basics

Schizophrenia is a major psychiatric illness that can have a profound impact on the lives of individuals, their family members, and friends. As family members, you are in a unique position to help your relative with schizophrenia. You care deeply for your relative and know him better than any professional.[1] You probably have more contact with him and are in better touch with his moods, feelings, and needs than anyone else. Being aware of changes, for better or worse, before others are places you on the "front line" of treatment, often at a high cost to yourselves. The behavior of people with schizophrenia can be unpredictable, even frightening, at times. It may be difficult to find friends who understand the stress and emotions you're experiencing.

By learning more about schizophrenia and how to cope with common problems, you can reduce the strain of the illness on your family. In this chapter we review facts about schizophrenia that will help you understand your relative's illness and develop realistic goals for the future. Our discussion here is an introduction to schizophrenia and not a comprehensive review of everything known about the illness. For those interested in learning more about the nature and course of schizophrenia, we suggest additional readings at the end of the chapter.

What Is Schizophrenia?

Schizophrenia is a complex and confusing illness for people with the illness, family members, and mental health professionals alike. One reason for much of the misunderstanding about the illness is that the terms *schizophrenia* and *schizophrenic* have many different uses in everyday language, the popular media, and the medical community.

---

[1]For ease of reading, we alternate between masculine and feminine pronouns throughout this book.

In everyday language, the word *schizophrenic* is often used to mean "contradictory." For example, a person who says one thing and then does another might be described conversationally as "schizophrenic." In the news, a nation with a friendly foreign policy toward one country and an unfriendly foreign policy toward another, similar country might be described as having a "schizophrenic" foreign policy.

When it *is* used to refer to illness, the word *schizophrenic* is often used broadly by the popular media to mean psychosis (including symptoms such as hallucinations or delusions) in general or even any severe psychiatric illness. Mental health professionals know that schizophrenia is a specific medical illness that varies in severity. Not all people with psychotic symptoms have schizophrenia, and people with schizophrenia are not always psychotic. Similarly, not all people with schizophrenia are severely ill, nor do all people with severe mental illness have schizophrenia.

Used as a medical term, *schizophrenia* refers to a specific illness characterized by problems in social functioning, self-care skills, and difficulty distinguishing what's real from what's not real. There is strong evidence that schizophrenia has biological origins; that it is caused by an imbalance in chemicals in the brain. Medication plays an important role in treating the illness by correcting this imbalance. However, there is also evidence that environmental stress contributes to the severity of the illness, with high levels of stress resulting in more frequent symptoms.

The interplay between biology and the environment provides unique opportunities to help your relative by reducing stress and actively supporting the positive steps she takes toward better functioning.

Common Myths about Schizophrenia

Almost everyone in Western society has heard of schizophrenia, but inaccurate depictions of the illness and misuse of the term have perpetuated a number of misconceptions about it. To understand schizophrenia thoroughly, you have to dispense with these myths.

• *Myth 1: People with schizophrenia have a "split personality."* A split personality is a rare psychiatric illness (called *multiple personality disorder* or *dissociative identity disorder*) in which two or more personalities exist within the same person. Many people became acquainted with the disorder through the movie *The Three Faces of Eve* and the book *Sybil* (by Flora Rheta Schreiber) and the movie based on it. People with schizophrenia do *not* have a split personality. Sometimes the behavior of people with schizophrenia varies or is erratic due to fluctuations in symptoms such as paranoia, depression, or anxiety. However, this does not mean that the person has more than one personality.

- *Myth 2: People with schizophrenia are highly prone to violence*. Despite high-profile coverage of violent crimes committed by those with psychiatric disorders, violence in people with schizophrenia is more often the exception than the rule. Rather than becoming more violent when their symptoms worsen, most people with schizophrenia withdraw, preferring to spend time alone.

- *Myth 3: Families cause schizophrenia*. Mental health professionals once commonly believed that families caused schizophrenia. Although a few professionals still hold on to this outdated belief, most now understand that schizophrenia is a biological illness that is *not* caused by families. Rather, families can play a vital role in helping their loved ones develop and pursue personal visions of recovery.

- *Myth 4: Drugs and alcohol can cause schizophrenia*. Drugs such as marijuana, LSD, heroin, cocaine ("crack"), PCP ("angel dust"), ecstasy, and amphetamines ("speed") can cause symptoms that closely resemble schizophrenia. For example, drugs such as LSD and PCP can cause hallucinations, marijuana can lead to anxiety attacks and feelings of panic and unreality, and cocaine and amphetamines can cause frightening delusions. Similarly, alcohol abuse and withdrawal can result in many of these symptoms. Most people who experience schizophrenia-like symptoms while using drugs or alcohol stop having these symptoms soon after their substance abuse ceases. However, recent research *has* found that use of cannabis (such as smoking marijuana) during adolescence and early adulthood is related to an increased chance of developing schizophrenia. Scientists are debating whether using cannabis may trigger the onset of schizophrenia in vulnerable individuals or whether people who are more prone to developing the illness or are in the early stages of it are more likely to use cannabis. Regardless of the role of cannabis, the vast majority of people who abuse drugs and alcohol never develop schizophrenia.

An Overview of Schizophrenia

History of the Concept

The modern concept of schizophrenia as a psychiatric illness has developed mainly over the past 100 years. Although many different individuals have contributed to our current understanding, the work of two pioneers stands out above all others: Emil Kraepelin (1855–1926) and Eugen Bleuler (1857–1939). Kraepelin is credited with first describing the symptoms of schizophrenia as due to a single illness. Kraepelin called schizophrenia *dementia praecox*, a Latin term referring to the early onset of the illness (*praecox*) and deterioration in intellectual functioning (*dementia*). He identified the characteristic symptoms of schizophrenia as hallucinations, delusions, impaired attention span, and social withdrawal.

Bleuler focused more on the nature of symptoms of schizophrenia and less on its course than did Kraepelin. Bleuler believed that the illness did not necessarily have an early age of onset or result in a gradual deterioration in mental functioning. He rejected the term *dementia praecox* and proposed the word *schizophrenia* to describe what he saw as the essential feature of the illness: a split (*schizo*) in the mind (*phren*) between perception and reality—rather than a split between different personalities. However, he agreed with Kraepelin's description of many of the basic symptoms of the illness.

Diagnosis

There is no laboratory test, such as a blood test, X-ray, CT scan, or MRI, that can be used to diagnose schizophrenia. A diagnosis must be based on a careful interview conducted by a trained professional. In addition, a physical exam must be performed to rule out physical problems that could cause similar symptoms. For example, if the person has a brain tumor or an untreated endocrinological disorder (such as hyperthyroidism), or is currently abusing substances, a diagnosis of schizophrenia cannot be made until the physical condition has been treated or controlled.

To ensure that different hospitals and clinics use the same criteria to diagnose schizophrenia, specific diagnostic guidelines have been established (discussed further in Chapter 2). What is important to understand here is that the purpose of the interview is to determine whether the person has experienced any of the symptoms listed in the guidelines. Common symptoms of schizophrenia include hallucinations, delusions, and reduced emotional expressiveness. Other common problems include impairments in thinking and problems in functioning. Every person has a unique set of symptoms. To be diagnosed with schizophrenia, a person need not have every symptom or have them all the time. But all people with schizophrenia experience some problems in social functioning and ability to work, attend school, parent, or take care of themselves.

The symptoms and course of schizophrenia overlap considerably with those of several closely related disorders: schizoaffective disorder, schizophreniform disorder, and schizotypal personality disorder. Because of their similarities and the fact that the same treatments are effective for all, these illnesses are referred to as *schizophrenia-spectrum* disorders. Chapter 2 goes into more detail on the differences; for the sake of simplicity we use the term *schizophrenia* throughout this book. If your relative has any of the disorders in the spectrum, you'll find the information and suggestions in this book helpful.

What Is the Experience of Schizophrenia Like?

Having a better sense of the experience of the illness can help you offer appropriate guidance and support over the years. Schizophrenia has been described as "dreaming when you're wide awake." When we dream, we usually believe that the bizarre things we're experiencing are really happening. Your relative may feel that way when awake, having difficulty distinguishing between reality and the internal illusions taking place.

Practically every person with schizophrenia also has problems with attention. One person told us, "It's hard for me to concentrate on anything because I'm so easily distracted—like right now I'm listening to the cars on the highway outside the hospital." This difficulty can interfere with your relative's ability to work, attend school, parent, or participate in other activities that require sustained attention, such as reading a book. One reason people with schizophrenia have such trouble focusing their attention is that they are often exquisitely sensitive to, and easily overwhelmed by, sounds, sights, odors, and other stimuli. Imagine, as one person described it, playing tennis with many balls coming over the net at the same time.

Problems with motivation and enjoyment are also common. Another person with schizophrenia said, "We used to be a beach family, and I loved going to the beach. Now the beach is just a few blocks away, but I can't get the motivation to go there. Or if I do go, it's not fun." This problem can result in your relative's having fewer leisure activities and getting less enjoyment from social relationships than before the onset of schizophrenia.

Even with this understanding, the experience of schizophrenia is difficult to comprehend fully. If your relative is willing to talk about it, you may be able to understand more by discussing the experience. *Many people with schizophrenia lack insight into their illness, however, and are unable to talk about a problem they don't believe exists.* Reading books and watching videos of first-person accounts of schizophrenia can be illuminating (see the Resources section at the end of Chapter 2).

Prevalence

Approximately 1 in 100 people (1%) develops schizophrenia at some point during her lifetime. In the United States, 2–3 million persons have the illness. Schizophrenia occurs in men and women of all races, social classes, religions, and cultures. Some research has indicated that schizophrenia is more common in some cultures than others, but most researchers have found the rate fairly similar across cultures. Schizophrenia is, however, more likely to develop in those living in poverty, among ethnic/racial minorities (rates are slightly higher in African Americans, Afro-Caribbeans in Great Britain, and Dutch Antillean and Surinamese immigrants in Holland), and in urban areas. In all these cases, the higher incidence may occur because of interactions between biological factors responsible for the illness and environmental stress.

The cost of treating schizophrenia, to both families and society, is very high. More hospital beds are occupied by persons with schizophrenia than any other psychiatric illness. Most of the people in state psychiatric hospitals have this diagnosis. Approximately one-fifth of all chronic disability (including both physical and mental illnesses) is due to schizophrenia. The majority of people with schizophrenia are unable to live independently and live either with relatives or in supervised community residences. About 10% of all homeless individuals have schizophrenia.

How Schizophrenia Develops

Schizophrenia usually develops sometime during late adolescence or early adulthood, most often between the ages of 16 and 30, with women developing the illness at a slightly later age than men. Schizophrenia rarely develops after the age of 35. Childhood schizophrenia (onset before puberty) is rare and considered a different disorder. This book is intended for families with a relative who developed schizophrenia in adolescence or adulthood.

The onset of schizophrenia usually follows a gradual decline in functioning, including the ability to socialize and enjoy life. The earliest signs of schizophrenia often include depression, lack of pleasure in daily activities, and social withdrawal. Problems in cognition (thinking) are also common, such as not being able to focus when reading, finding math more difficult, forgetting things more easily, and not making logical connections as easily—all problems that can interfere with school, work, and friendships. Usually some time after these problems have developed the person begins to experience psychotic symptoms, such as hallucinations and delusions, which often lead to treatment and possibly hospitalization. The development of schizophrenia may take place over months or even years.

At first you may not have recognized these changes, or you may have attributed them to a "stage" that your relative was going through or to normal adolescent behavior. When families *do* recognize that something is wrong and seek professional advice, they may be told that their relative's behavior is normal and they need not worry. Many professionals who don't work with people who are seriously mentally ill are not trained to recognize the symptoms of schizophrenia. However, even professionals who are trained to detect schizophrenia often find it difficult to diagnose this illness during its earliest stages.

The question of whether people who develop schizophrenia differ from others in childhood or adolescence, before they become ill, has intrigued researchers for decades. The answer is both yes and no. Many people who develop schizophrenia were well adjusted before they became ill. Among those we personally know with schizophrenia are a high school class valedictorian, a virtuoso cellist who soloed with a major city orchestra, and a writer and illustrator who published his work in high school.

However, some individuals who develop schizophrenia *are* less well adjusted before they become ill, and these people's difficulties often date back to childhood. Two patterns of maladjustment have been described. Some people are unusually withdrawn before developing schizophrenia, have few friends growing up, and have few or no intimate relationships with others, such as a steady boy-friend or girlfriend. These social problems that started early in life often persist at a more severe level after the onset of schizophrenia. The second pattern of maladjustment involves disruptive behavior problems that first appear in child-hood—typically hyperactivity, attention problems, conduct disorder, and impul-sivity. These problems interfere with academic and social functioning and may also persist into adulthood.

It's important to know that most children and adolescents who experience these two types of problems never develop schizophrenia—which means we still can't accurately predict who will develop schizophrenia.

The Course of the Illness

Schizophrenia is an episodic illness with symptoms that vary in intensity over time. When episodes of the illness occur, persistent symptoms worsen and symp-toms that have been in remission reappear, at times requiring treatment in the hospital. Inpatient treatment is usually relatively brief (a few days) but may extend to several months. Even with substantial impairment, however, many peo-ple can be treated successfully in the community.

The course of schizophrenia is different for each person. Some people have a few episodes of the illness and return to normal functioning with treatment and illness management. Some experience more frequent episodes and only partly regain their former level of functioning between episodes. These individu-als may require more frequent hospitalizations at first and need to learn much more to manage their illness successfully, pursue personal goals, and achieve a degree of independence. A small proportion of people become extremely ill and require long-term inpatient treatment because they cannot care for themselves or are unsafe in the community.

Despite the serious impact of schizophrenia, there are good reasons to be optimistic about the long-term prospects. People with schizophrenia tend to improve gradually over time, not only from learning how to manage the illness but also due to a natural reduction in symptoms. A significant number of those with schizophrenia become free of symptoms later in life. We return to the issue of improvement and recovery from schizophrenia in Chapter 3.

Many people want to know whether the course and outcome of schizophre-nia can be predicted. In general, the answer is no. However, we do know that people who had social problems *before* they became ill tend to have a more severe course of their illness, including more intense symptoms or more frequent relapses. Early recognition and treatment of schizophrenia has also been found to be beneficial; the more rapidly someone is treated after developing the illness, the more quickly and more effectively the symptoms can be controlled. Women also tend to have a less severe course of the illness than men, including better functioning in the community and fewer hospitalizations. What is most critical in improving the course of schizophrenia is learning how to manage the illness and to take steps toward pursuing personal goals. People with better insight into their illness tend to have a better course. For some, this insight may develop gradually over time as they come to grips with the disorder and how to control it.

John developed schizophrenia at the age of 16. The next 15 years were rocky because he followed his medication regimen inconsistently, resulting in frequent relapses and rehospitalizations. Then, in his mid-30s, with the help of a family educational program, John began to develop a better understanding and awareness of his illness and started to follow his treatment recommendations, including taking his medication regularly. Gradually his symptoms improved, and he became interested in making social connections and getting back to work. Over the next 15 years John married, had two children, and went back to work part-time, despite continuing to experience mild symptoms of schizophrenia. John sees his psychiatrist and nurse every month to have his symptoms monitored, and he has not been in the hospital for treatment of a relapse in 20 years.

The Causes of Schizophrenia

Over the past 100 years scientists have proposed many theories to explain schizophrenia. Most scientists believe the illness has a biological cause involving some type of disturbance in the brain, but they still don't know exactly which biological factors are responsible. The task of researchers is complicated by the fact that no consistent biological differences have been found between people with the illness and others. One possible explanation for this lack of consistent differences is that schizophrenia is not one disease but several different or overlapping diseases. Extensive research continues to be conducted on possible biological causes of schizophrenia.

The Biology of Schizophrenia

Many theories of schizophrenia propose complex interactions between different parts of the brain (referred to as *neural networks*). For example, many recent theories stress the importance of the *prefrontal cortex*, a region of the brain required for planning, abstract thinking, and problem solving, and the *hippocampus*, a brain structure critical to memory.

The most prominent theory of the illness, the *dopamine hypothesis*, is based on the idea that schizophrenia is caused by an imbalance in chemicals in the brain. These chemicals play a vital role in all aspects of functioning, including the ability to think, feel, perceive, and act in a planned, goal-directed fashion.

Billions of nerve cells, called *neurons*, are densely packed and distributed throughout the brain. All neurons contain chemicals, or *neurotransmitters*, which communicate information from one part of the brain to another. The neurotransmitters are stored inside small sacs (*vesicles*) in the neuron. When a neurotransmitter is released from a vesicle, it leaves the neuron itself (the *presynaptic neuron*) and enters a small space (the *synaptic cleft*) before being absorbed by another neuron (the *postsynaptic neuron*). Some of the neurotransmitter is absorbed by the postsynaptic neuron, some of it is broken down by other chemicals and excreted through bodily fluids (such as sweat and urine), and some of it is reabsorbed into the vesicle (called *reuptake*) of the presynaptic neuron. The entire process of neurotransmitter release and absorption is referred to as *neurotransmission*.

NEUROTRANSMITTERS AND SCHIZOPHRENIA

Scientists have identified over 50 different kinds of neurotransmitters. An imbalance in the neurotransmitter *dopamine* is believed to exist in schizophrenia. Dopamine is an important neurotransmitter that regulates thoughts and feelings, both of which are disturbed in schizophrenia.

Animal studies of the effects of antipsychotic medications (the most effective medications for schizophrenia) on neurotransmitters have consistently found that these medications block dopamine neurotransmission in the brain. This finding has led scientists to hypothesize that people with schizophrenia have an excess of dopamine in certain regions of the brain. Research has not yet directly shown that people with schizophrenia have an imbalance in brain dopamine, because this is a difficult matter to demonstrate, given the technology currently available to scientists. Nevertheless, the dopamine hypothesis of schizophrenia is the most widely accepted biological theory of the illness, and it continues to stimulate much research into the causes of schizophrenia.

Genetic and Environmental Factors

How do some people end up with a chemical imbalance that results in schizophrenia? Research has shown that having a close relative with schizophrenia increases a person's chance of developing the illness. This familial connection indicates that vulnerability to schizophrenia may be caused partially by genetic factors. The same connection has been found for many other diseases, such as hypertension, diabetes, depression, and coronary artery disease.

As mentioned earlier, about 1% of people in the general population develop schizophrenia. If a person has a first-degree relative with schizophrenia, such as a parent or sibling, the chances are higher, about 1 in 10 (10%). If someone has more than one ill family member, the chances may be even higher. The table on page 12 summarizes the chances that a person will develop schizophrenia, based on whether a relative has the illness.

The significant role of genetic factors is supported by the fact that a person with an identical twin (a twin with the same genes) with schizophrenia has a greater chance of developing it than a person with a nonidentical twin who is ill.

Risk of Developing Schizophrenia	
Relative with schizophrenia	Chance of developing schizophrenia
No relative	1 in 100 (1%)
Ill aunt or uncle	2–3 in 100 (2–3%)
Ill parent or sibling	5–10 in 100 (5–10%)
Both parents ill	15–20 in 100 (15–20%)
Nonidentical (dizygotic) twin	5–10 in 100 (5–10%)
Identical (monozygotic) twin	50–70 in 100 (50–70%)

But a specific pattern of inheritance has not yet been identified, nor has a responsible gene (or combination of genes).

Another interesting question is why many families have only one person with this illness. If your family has few or no other relatives with mental illness, how did your relative develop schizophrenia? One possibility is that there are other individuals in your family who carry the genes that predispose them to schizophrenia, but these critical genes remain "unexpressed" (or only partially expressed)—meaning that the carriers do not develop schizophrenia but can still transmit the genes to another relative, who may very well develop the illness.

Another possibility is that some cases of schizophrenia may occur for reasons other than genetic vulnerability or because of interactions between very subtle genetic factors and the environment. The risk table shows that not every identical twin of a person with schizophrenia develops the illness—only 50–70% do—which suggests that genetic factors alone cannot explain who becomes ill. Some early environmental factors during pregnancy may increase the risk of developing schizophrenia later, such as the mother being exposed to the influenza virus, smoking cigarettes, or having poor nutrition, as well as obstetric complications during delivery, such as forceps delivery or fetal distress. In addition, the older the father at the conception of the child, the greater the risk of the child's later developing schizophrenia. Scientists don't understand how these environmental factors act, whether in concert with genetic factors or alone. Some have suggested that exposure to these types of environmental "insult" may cause small amounts of brain damage. This damage may become apparent only later in the person's development, when certain critical parts of the brain fail to mature in a normal fashion, such as during adolescence and early adulthood, eventually resulting in schizophrenia.

The Stress–Vulnerability Model of Schizophrenia

Everything that researchers and clinicians have learned about the causes of schizophrenia—its initial development and its course over time—indicates that four different factors are at work: biological vulnerability, stress, coping skills, and social support. Together they add up to what is called the *stress–vulnerability model.*

Biological vulnerability encompasses genetic factors, exposure to early biological risks (e.g., prenatal exposure to the influenza virus), or both, as just discussed. Among individuals with schizophrenia, the greater the biological vulnerability, the more severe the symptoms and course of illness. There is currently no direct measure of biological vulnerability.

Stress, as most of us are well aware, refers to negative aspects of the environment in which we live. Several types of stress can have a negative effect on those with schizophrenia. Significant life events, such as the death of someone close, loss of a job, or change in residence, can be stressful and lead to relapses. Living in an environment with a great deal of conflict or criticism can be stressful and cause relapses, as can living in a setting that places heavy demands on the person or lacks meaningful structure.

Coping skills allow an individual to handle stress and reduce its negative effects. Examples of coping skills are social skills and the ability to relax. Effective social skills enable people to establish rewarding relationships and to resolve conflicts. The ability to relax can help people cope with stress in any context, such as increased demands at work.

Social support is the help, acceptance, and caring received from family, friends, and others. High levels of support play a positive role in buffering the negative effects of stress on people with schizophrenia. Social support can effectively manage stress in several ways. First, support may prevent stress from occurring by addressing potential problem situations before they erupt, such as helping a person manage money to avoid rent defaults that might result in eviction. Second, social support can help a person with schizophrenia resolve a conflict with another person. Third, supportive others can prompt the person with schizophrenia to use coping skills in appropriate situations.

The stress–vulnerability model is illustrated on page 14. In addition to providing a framework for understanding the course of schizophrenia, this model is helpful in guiding treatment.

Treatment

The treatment of schizophrenia is guided by four general principles that follow directly from the stress–vulnerability model.

Reduce Biological Vulnerability

There is no cure for the biological vulnerability that causes schizophrenia. However, antipsychotic medications can reduce symptoms and the risk of relapse. These medications are the most powerful tools in treating schizophrenia, although they are by no means perfect. Adherence to the medication regimen is

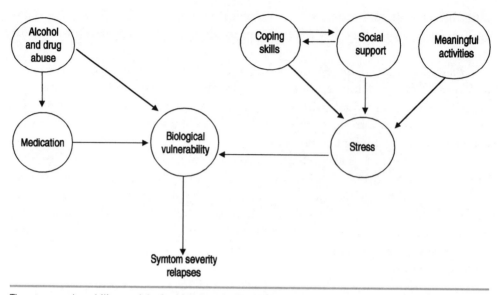

The stress–vulnerability model of schizophrenia. This model suggests that the course of schizophrenia can be improved by taking medications, avoiding alcohol and drug use, reducing stress, improving coping skills, and increasing social support.

important, as is monitoring of symptoms so that medication can be adjusted if symptoms change.

Treating substance use will also reduce biological vulnerability and improve the course of the illness. Alcohol use can interfere with the beneficial effects of antipsychotic medications. Drugs such as cocaine, amphetamines, and marijuana can worsen biological vulnerability, leading to more severe symptoms and relapses. Furthermore, biological vulnerability makes people with schizophrenia more sensitive to the effects of alcohol and drugs, so that even small amounts of substances can interfere with functioning and trigger relapses (see Chapter 22).

Reduce Environmental Stress

Stress can be reduced in a number of ways, as discussed in Chapter 11. Stress resulting from tense family relationships can be lowered by developing specific and realistic expectations for your relative's behavior and improving your skills at communicating (Chapter 14) and resolving problems (Chapter 15) with him. Chapter 16 provides additional information on strategies for creating a harmonious living environment. If your relative has little meaningful structure in her life, part-time work or school (Chapter 26) can add structure without creating excessive demands and expectations for rapid change. Striking a balance between understimulation and overstimulation in your relative's environment is vital to minimizing stress at home, work, school, and treatment program.

Improve Coping Skills

Much of this book is focused on the many different types of coping skills people can learn. Broadly speaking, coping skills can be divided into strategies that improve a person's ability to . . .

1. Solve problems and achieve goals (e.g., through social skills that resolve interpersonal conflict and improve relationships with others).
2. Deal with the negative experience of stress (e.g., through stress reduction techniques).
3. Cope more effectively with persistent symptoms and mood problems (e.g., hallucinations, delusions, anxiety, and depression).

Strengthen Social Support

Improving social support goes hand in hand with reducing stress and improving coping skills, and much of this book is aimed at helping families accomplish this increased support. Becoming knowledgeable about schizophrenia, developing realistic expectations, and supporting your loved one in following treatment recommendations and pursuing personal goals can maximize social support. People with schizophrenia often change gradually, and the road toward better living and recovery may be a rocky one, with setbacks along the way. Recognizing the small steps that your relative takes toward greater coping and self-sufficiency, and frequently encouraging him along the way, lets him know you appreciate his efforts and can see progress. Finally, letting your relative know you love her and conveying a sense of hope for the future are powerful influences that will help your loved one maintain the courage necessary to grow beyond the illness and pursue a fulfilling life.

Person–First Language

In the past, people with schizophrenia were often referred to by the diagnostic term, such as "they're schizophrenics" or "he's a schizophrenic." Although some people with schizophrenia feel comfortable using the term in this way—similar to saying "I am a diabetic"—many others prefer language that does not equate the person with the illness. Several alternative terms avoid implying that people with schizophrenia (or another mental illness) *are* that illness. For example, some individuals like the term *consumer of mental health services* (*consumer* for short), whereas others prefer the terms *client* or *patient*. There is also a growing emphasis on using language that puts the person, rather than the illness, first (e.g., "a person with schizophrenia" rather than "a schizophrenic person"). In this book, we have strived to use such person-first language to avoid suggesting that a person with schizophrenia *is* or *becomes* their illness. We encourage you to consider your use of language about your relative, and to remember that your loved one is a person first, with talents, strengths, and abilities, who also happens to have schizophrenia.

Hope for Those with Schizophrenia

You and your family may be just starting to learn how to manage schizophrenia, or you may have years of experience under your belt. Either way, you now know that schizophrenia is no one's fault and that you can do a lot to help your relative achieve a meaningful and rewarding life. Understanding schizophrenia prepares you to work collaboratively with your relative and her treatment providers.

Although schizophrenia is a serious illness, tremendous advances have been made in its treatment in recent years. New medications, rehabilitation programs, and coping strategies can now help people with schizophrenia manage their symptoms more effectively, enjoy relationships with others, become involved in meaningful activities such as work or school, and live as independently as possible. The prospect of learning how to cope with schizophrenia may seem frightening or overwhelming to you. However, with love and hope, up-to-date information, and realistic optimism based on scientific progress, you *can* help your relative move forward and develop a rewarding life.

Resources

Andreasen, N. C. (2001). *Brave new brain: Conquering mental illness in the era of the genome*. New York: Oxford University Press. A leading neuroscientist explains the current state of knowledge about the human brain, human genome, and mental illness in accessible terms, covering schizophrenia and three other major disorders.

Green, M. F. (2001). *Schizophrenia revealed*. New York: Norton. A highly readable, authoritative account of schizophrenia by a neuropsychologist and researcher.

Torrey, E. F. (2001). *Surviving schizophrenia: A manual for families, consumers and providers* (4th ed.). New York: HarperTrade. Detailed information from a leading researcher who has a sister with schizophrenia.

CHAPTER 2

Diagnosis and Symptoms

*D*iagnosis is a medical term that refers to the classification of an illness. A diagnosis must be based on a *pattern* of symptoms or signs of an illness, never on a single symptom. In fact, many of the symptoms of schizophrenia can be present in people with other psychiatric disorders. It's the unique combination of symptoms that distinguishes schizophrenia from other disorders.

Understanding how a diagnosis is made and the nature of the symptoms of schizophrenia-spectrum disorders will help you understand your relative's behavior and monitor his symptoms in the future.

Diagnostic Systems

A *diagnostic system* is a set of specific, objectively defined criteria for making a medical diagnosis. By carefully evaluating a person in relation to each criterion, a practitioner can make a reliable diagnosis of a psychiatric disorder. Two diagnostic systems are widely used throughout the world. The system used most commonly in the United States is the *Diagnostic and Statistical Manual of Mental Disorders*, developed by the American Psychiatric Association, now in its 4th edition (DSM-IV). Throughout the rest of the world, the system used most often is the *International Classification of Diseases*, developed by the World Health Organization, now in its 10th edition (ICD-10). The specific criteria for diagnosing schizophrenia in DSM-IV and ICD-10 are very similar.

How Diagnoses Are Made

As mentioned in Chapter 1, a diagnosis of schizophrenia must be based on interviews with the person and often with relatives or others who know the person well. These interviews focus on identifying specific symptoms, how long the symptoms have been present, problems in functioning, and the possible role of drug or alcohol abuse. Medical tests are often conducted to rule out physical causes of symptoms similar to those found in schizophrenia. The information obtained from the interviews and any medical tests is then used to arrive at a diagnosis based on the DSM or ICD criteria.

A number of different mental health professionals may be qualified to make the diagnosis of schizophrenia in your relative. All psychiatrists are qualified to make the diagnosis, because it is an essential part of their training. Many psychologists are also qualified to diagnose schizophrenia, as are some psychiatric social workers and nurses.

However, psychiatrists usually have the most experience in the area of schizophrenia, so finding a psychiatrist would be the most reliable route to go. Similar to the process of finding other medical specialists, you may start your search for a psychiatrist by asking others for their recommendations. You might be able to get good references for a psychiatrist from your local chapter of the National Alliance on Mental Illness (NAMI), your family doctor, or acquaintances who are mental health professionals or who have received mental health services.

If your relative has private insurance, start by finding out about the policy's mental health coverage. Does the company have a contract with a specific "network" of providers, meaning the level of reimbursement may depend on whether the psychiatrist consulted belongs to that network? Whatever coverage is provided, the American Psychiatric Association (APA) and the American Medical Association (AMA) maintain lists of member doctors, though these lists do not represent recommendations or indicate specialization in schizophrenia. Call the APA's "Answer Center" (888-357-7924 or 703-907-7300) to find out how to contact your state's Psychiatric Society, which will likely have a list of members who have given permission for their names to be given out to the public. The AMA's website (*www.ama-assn.org*) gives directions for requesting a list of local MDs with a psychiatric specialty. You can also find a psychiatrist by checking the yellow pages of your local telephone directory.

The alternative to finding someone privately is to contact your local community mental health center (see Chapter 5). All community mental health centers have professionals (including psychiatrists) who are experienced in diagnosing schizophrenia and similar disorders. At a community mental health center you will be charged on a sliding-fee scale, based on your ability to pay.

Although the criteria for diagnosing schizophrenia are clear, the evaluation process may differ from practitioner to practitioner. One person, for example, may conduct a half-hour interview with the person, whereas another may take more time with the individual and also meet with family members. As a rule, the more time spent and the more information obtained, the more accurate the diagnosis is likely to be.

How Reliable Is a Psychiatric Diagnosis?

If your relative has received several different psychiatric diagnoses since becoming ill, you may have wondered "Why can't they just make up their minds?!"

There are several reasons different psychiatric diagnoses may be given to the same person over time. One is that the symptoms themselves change, resulting in different diagnoses depending on which symptoms are currently most prominent. For example, most people with schizophrenia experience some problems with depression during their illness. A person who is evaluated during a period of severe depression may be diagnosed with major depression instead of schizophrenia. Similarly, someone who is evaluated during a period of extreme excitement may be diagnosed with bipolar disorder. Misdiagnosis of schizophrenia appears to be most common during the early stages of the illness, when the diagnostician has less patient history to go on.

During the first few episodes, some people are diagnosed with a less severe disorder, such as major depression or bipolar disorder, which is switched to schizophrenia when the symptoms and problems persist. This apparent misdiagnosis can happen when the diagnostician does not recognize the disorder, but it can also reflect the diagnostician's attempt to avoid alarming family members by giving such a serious diagnosis to a young person. When the symptoms of schizophrenia first appear during adolescence, professionals sometimes try to reassure concerned family members by saying that the teenager is "just going through a stage." The trouble is, delaying action sometimes means that people with schizophrenia and their families wait years before receiving an accurate diagnosis—or effective treatment.

Joe, 18, had been a good student and an avid weightlifter, but his academic performance had slipped dramatically in the last 6 months and his interest in lifting had waned. He had also become more distant from his parents and siblings, had begun to keep different hours than the rest of the family, and expressed odd beliefs, such as the thought that he was getting special messages from God. Joe was admitted to the psychiatric hospital when he threatened a neighbor whom he believed was putting thoughts into his head and interfering with his thinking. Joe's symptoms were consistent with a diagnosis of schizophrenia, but his psychiatrist felt such a diagnosis was premature and would be a hard blow to the family. He also thought it was possible Joe had bipolar disorder instead. Joe was discharged from the hospital in the doctor's care and treated for bipolar disorder. Over the next year Joe had three severe relapses and rehospitalizations before his psychiatrist changed his diagnosis to schizophrenia, and he finally began to receive the treatment he needed.

Schizophrenia–Spectrum Disorders

The schizophrenia-spectrum disorders have many similarities, including the treatments that effectively reduce their symptoms.

Schizophrenia

Schizophrenia is the most common of the schizophrenia-spectrum disorders. A diagnosis of schizophrenia requires certain symptoms that have lasted at least 1 month and that cause the person significant impairment in some aspect of social functioning, work, or self-care. Overall, the problems must have persisted for at least 6 months. The person must not have prominent symptoms of a mood disturbance (such as severe depressive or manic symptoms), or, if such symptoms are present, they must be relatively brief in relation to how long the person has been ill.

Schizophreniform Disorder

The diagnostic criteria for schizophreniform disorder are identical to those for schizophrenia, except that the symptoms must last for at least 1 month and then completely subside before 6 months. If later episodes last for less than 6 months, the diagnosis will remain schizophreniform disorder. Many with this disorder go on to develop schizophrenia.

Schizoaffective Disorder

The primary feature of schizoaffective disorder that distinguishes it from schizophrenia is mood episodes—significant symptoms of depression or mania for a substantial portion (but not all) of the time the person has been ill. Common symptoms of depression include feelings of sadness, thoughts of hopelessness or worthlessness, loss of appetite or increased appetite, sleep disturbance, loss of energy, thoughts of hurting oneself, and loss of pleasure. Common symptoms of mania include decreased need for sleep, irritability, grandiosity, and increased goal-directed behavior (e.g., the relentless pursuit of a business deal or romantic conquest). To be diagnosed with schizoaffective disorder a person must have experienced these mood symptoms for at least several weeks while having some of the symptoms of schizophrenia at times when mood symptoms are not present.

Schizophrenia and schizoaffective disorder are often difficult to distinguish from each other for two reasons. First, mood symptoms overlap with schizophrenia symptoms. For example, grandiose delusions (e.g., believing that one is the king of England) can be present in either mania or schizophrenia. Second, it can be difficult to determine how long significant mood symptoms have been present and whether this time period should be considered "substantial" compared to the overall duration of the illness. Fortunately, because the disorders respond to the same treatments and have a similar course, the distinction is not critical.

Schizotypal Personality Disorder

Schizotypal personality disorder is a little different from the other three spectrum disorders in that the symptoms tend to be milder—although impairment may not be. People with a schizotypal personality disorder are usually hospitalized less often, and many people with this disorder are never hospitalized. Despite the less prominent symptoms, many people with this disorder function only marginally better than people with schizophrenia; they often have few friends, have difficulty working, and get little satisfaction out of life. A significant number of people who develop schizotypal personality disorder at a younger age later develop schizophrenia, schizoaffective disorder, or schizophreniform disorder.

Subtypes of Schizophrenia

Since schizophrenia was first described over 100 years ago, many different subtypes (i.e., categories of most prominent symptoms) of the illness have been proposed. The subtypes of schizophrenia that are included in the DSM-IV are *paranoid, catatonic, disorganized, undifferentiated,* and *residual.* Many other subtypes have also been proposed. However, no consistent research shows that subtypes of schizophrenia respond differently to treatments or have a substantially different course of the illness.

The Symptoms of Schizophrenia

The symptoms of schizophrenia can be divided into five categories: psychotic symptoms, negative symptoms, cognitive impairment, mood problems, and behavioral disturbances. With the exception of behavioral disturbances, almost all people with schizophrenia have some symptoms in each category, though no one has *all* of the symptoms within each. No two people with schizophrenia have exactly the same symptoms; each person is unique. You'll hear many of the following terms throughout your relative's diagnosis and treatment. Familiarity with them and their meaning will help make you an informed participant in your loved one's ongoing care.

Psychotic Symptoms

Psychotic symptoms include perceptions or beliefs that reflect a break from reality and are not shared by people without mental illness. These symptoms are also called the *positive symptoms of schizophrenia* because they are defined by the presence of patently absurd or false thoughts, behaviors, or feelings. Two types of psychotic symptoms are most common in schizophrenia: hallucinations and delusions. For many people these symptoms fluctuate over time. They may be intense at certain times, requiring the person to be monitored closely or hospitalized. At other times psychotic symptoms may be mild or absent. Between 25% and 50% of people with schizophrenia experience some persistent psychotic symptoms. Chapter 17 focuses on strategies for coping with psychotic symptoms.

Hallucinations

Hallucinations are false perceptions—sensations that the person experiences but other people do not. These perceptions include hearing, seeing, feeling, tasting, and smelling things that are not present in the environment. About 70% of people with schizophrenia experience auditory hallucinations, 25% have visual hallucinations, and 10% have other types of hallucinations.

Auditory hallucinations are usually experienced as voices heard through the ears, but they may also be described as voices heard inside the head. The voices can seem quite real, as though they are coming from the next room or the street. Sometimes people think the hallucinations are real (e.g., a person who believes the voice is from God); other times people know the voices are not real. Examples of auditory hallucinations include:

- Two voices talking about the person and commenting on her actions.
- A voice saying she is a bad person and calling her names.
- The unclear murmuring of many people.

Auditory hallucinations are very distressing and distracting to most people. Some people readily admit to having hallucinations, whereas others do not. One indication of hallucinatory experiences is if your relative talks or laughs when no one is around. When this happens, the person is often responding to the hallucinations.

Delusions

A *delusion* is a false belief or a belief not shared by others in the person's culture or religion. Delusions appear quite real to the person but seem impossible or untrue to others. Many different types of delusions exist. These are some of the most common types that occur in schizophrenia.

PERSECUTORY (PARANOID) DELUSIONS

The person believes he is being persecuted unfairly or that people want to harm him for no good reason. Examples:

- Family members are secretly trying to poison his food.
- The Mafia, the CIA, and the FBI are conspiring to kill him.
- Family members are working together to drive him crazy.

DELUSIONS OF REFERENCE

This type of delusion involves the mistaken belief that something or someone is sending a message or referring (hence, *reference*) to the person with schizophrenia. The person may believe that the TV, radio, or newspaper has a special message for her or is referring specifically to her. Things in her immediate environment (e.g., the arrangement of objects, letters, or numbers) may be interpreted as conveying a symbolic message intended especially for her. Examples:

- The TV newscast referred to her last night on the news.
- The police are investigating her for a murder she did not commit.
- She sees the number 666 on the license plate on the car in front of her and believes it is a message from the devil that she is condemned to go to hell.
- People on the subway are talking about her.

DELUSIONS OF CONTROL

This type of delusion involves the belief that another person or force can control the person's thoughts or actions. Examples:

- A transmitter has been implanted in his stomach that controls his thoughts.
- Other people can put thoughts into his head (called *thought insertion*) and take thoughts away (called *thought withdrawal*).

GRANDIOSE DELUSIONS

The person erroneously believes that she is special, has unique talents, or is rich. Examples:

- She invented the Boeing 747.
- She is an unrecognized artistic genius.

Ricardo's behavior became stranger and stranger, and his parents just didn't know what to do about it. At first he began talking about how important he was and how he could control things at the snap of his fingers. He became more reclusive, refused to respond to his name, and began writing chapters for the Bible. Finally he decided he didn't need to eat because he could be "sustained from within" and began to lose weight. His parents took him to the psychiatric hospital. Even in the hospital he initially refused to respond to his name. While at first he was withdrawn with his psychiatrist, after they had developed a rapport Ricardo indicated to him that he was "the king of kings, the lord of lords, the master and creator of the universe." This grandiose delusion gradually faded away over several weeks as the antipsychotic medications were prescribed.

OTHER DELUSIONS

Delusions of persecution, reference, control, and grandiosity are the most common types of delusions in schizophrenia. Other types of delusions are also possible. Examples:

- Other people can hear his thoughts (*thought broadcasting*).
- His brain is rotting away (a *somatic delusion*).
- He has committed a terrible crime (a *delusion of guilt*).

Negative Symptoms

In contrast with psychotic (positive) symptoms, the *negative symptoms* of schizophrenia are characterized by the *absence* of normal thoughts, behaviors, or feelings. They can thus be harder to identify as signs of illness, but once you become familiar with your relative's specific negative symptoms, you will probably realize how prominent they can be. Negative symptoms also tend to be fairly stable over time, whereas psychotic symptoms may fluctuate more. Chapter 18 addresses coping strategies for dealing with negative symptoms.

Blunted Affect

Affect is the term that mental health professionals use to refer to the noticeable expression of emotion. People with schizophrenia often exhibit decreased facial and vocal expressiveness. For example, your relative may talk about something humorous or sad without showing any amusement or sadness in his facial expression or tone of voice. Sometimes professionals refer to lack of emotional expressiveness as *flat affect*. It's important to understand that not expressing emotion doesn't necessarily mean your relative isn't experiencing it. People with schizophrenia may feel the emotion but be unable to show it.

Alogia

Alogia is a psychological term for saying very little (also called *poverty of speech*) or not conveying much through speech (*poverty of speech content*). Poverty of speech is much more common in schizophrenia than poverty of speech content. You may have observed alogia in your relative when you tried to engage her in conversation and found it difficult to keep the conversation going for very long. It's not that your relative doesn't want to talk with you (although this is possible), but rather that she doesn't have that much to say.

Apathy

Your relative may not feel motivated to work toward personal goals or function more independently. This lack of motivation can interfere with even the most basic tasks, such as daily hygiene, and may be manifested in sleeping excessively or avoiding others. For some people, apathy reflects discouragement and hopelessness about the future, whereas for others it is just a genuine state of not caring. Having little energy and becoming fatigued easily are also related to apathy.

Anhedonia

Anhedonia is the decreased ability to feel pleasure or enjoyment. Activities such as reading, watching a movie, playing a game, or talking with other people may no longer make your relative feel good. Some people with schizophrenia are painfully aware of this change. One person said, "I used to love to watch the sunset, but now I just don't get anything out of it." You may find it difficult to get your relative with anhedonia involved in activities because he believes they won't be enjoyable.

Cognitive Impairment

Problems in cognition (thought processes) are one of the fundamental disturbances of schizophrenia. Undoubtedly you've noticed some of these problems in your relative, which can interfere with such basic activities as having conversations with others, going to work or school, and self-care. Lack of awareness of the illness may also have made it difficult to convince your relative to get help and follow treatment recommendations. Chapter 19 describes strategies for helping your relative cope with cognitive difficulties and Chapter 24 addresses problems related to lack of insight.

Basic Cognitive Functions

A variety of different problems in processing information are common in schizophrenia:

- Your relative has almost certainly experienced some *difficulties with attention and concentration*. People easily become distracted by their own thoughts or their environment. For example, a person may be distracted during a conversation by another person crossing her legs or the sound of a bus driving by.
- Decreased *psychomotor speed* is also very common, meaning that the person takes longer to process information and respond accordingly. For example, your relative may take longer to respond to your comments, making conversations feel strained and awkward.
- *Memory problems* are also quite common. Perhaps you've asked your relative to pick up something for you at the store, but he forgets.
- People with schizophrenia also have *trouble with executive functioning*, which is the ability to perform complex tasks that may require abstract reasoning, planning, and problem solving. As a result they frequently have difficulty managing their money because they are unable to budget it based on their future needs. They may find themselves unable to deal with conflict,

for example, at work; instead of trying to solve a problem with a coworker, a person with schizophrenia may walk off the job and get fired.

Social Perception

Social perception is the ability to recognize and understand important signals that occur during interactions with others. Recognizing another person's feelings through facial expressions and tone of voice and understanding what someone is upset about are examples of social perception. You may have seen problems in social perception in your relative when she has had trouble "getting the point" during a conversation with you. Problems in social perception make it difficult to understand another person's perspective and limit or eliminate the capacity for empathy.

Language Problems

Difficulties with thinking are immediately evident when a person uses language in an odd way that is hard to understand. Your relative may jump from one topic to another, remotely related topic (*loose associations*) or to an unrelated topic (*derailment*), making the conversation difficult to follow. He may stop talking in the middle of a sentence, having forgotten what he was going to say (*thought blocking*). He may make up new words (*neologisms*) or give an existing word a meaning that is confusing to others. For example, one person coined the word *ingrowability* to describe the ability to grow inward, as toenails can, or to have inner development or inner strength. Sometimes a person may speak incoherently, either because she does not speak clearly or because the syntax is mixed up (*word salad*).

Poor Insight

Many people with schizophrenia lack insight into the fact that they have a psychiatric illness. Your relative may believe there is nothing wrong with him, even if he has no friends, does not work or go to school, and is unable to fulfill even his most basic needs. The term *anosognosia*, most often used in neurology to describe a lack of insight into handicap displayed by many people following a brain injury, is sometimes used to describe the profound unawareness of illness and related disability in people with schizophrenia. Such lack of insight is not under your relative's direct control, although it may change over time.

Mood Problems

Mood problems, both long-standing and temporary, are common in schizophrenia. These may include depression and suicidality; anxiety; anger, hostility, and suspiciousness; labile mood; and inappropriate or incongruous affect.

Depression and Suicidality

You may have perceived some of the following signs of depression in your relative: feeling "blue"; feelings of hopelessness, helplessness, and worthlessness; a sad facial expression. Some people with schizophrenia have an awareness of their disorder, the limits it imposes, and the social stigma associated with it, and this awareness can contribute to their depression. Others experience depression without being aware of their illness and its social consequences.

Your relative may have talked about or tried to hurt himself. About 5% of people with schizophrenia die from suicide, with the risk being greater in the early years of the illness. Suicidal thinking occurs most often with depression. Some people also have chronic psychotic symptoms, which can be very distressful. For example, some people may experience persistent hallucinations of voices that insult them and instruct them to kill themselves. Advice for addressing depression and suicidal thinking is included in Chapters 12, 13, 17, and 21.

Anxiety

Many people with schizophrenia experience problems with anxiety that is often related to psychotic symptoms. Delusions, such as the belief that others want to hurt them, and hallucinations, such as hearing voices that put them down, can lead to anxious feelings and, in turn, to avoidance of certain situations. For example, a person who believes others talk about her on the bus and subway may be afraid of, and avoid, public transportation. On rare occasions people with intense fears (such as paranoid delusions) become aggressive when they feel threatened and have no escape. Anxiety is also common in social situations. People with schizophrenia often have limited skills for interacting with others, and this limitation may make them less comfortable in social situations. Chapter 20 provides suggestions for helping your relative cope with, and even overcome, anxiety.

Anger, Hostility, and Suspiciousness

When people with schizophrenia are angry and hostile, they have a strong effect on everyone around them. Sometimes people with schizophrenia have a "short fuse"—they're easily angered but then get over it quickly. Others may be more consistently hostile or suspicious, making them difficult to get along with. Angry or suspicious feelings often reflect psychotic symptoms, even when people deny such symptoms. For example, delusions, such as thinking that others are plotting against you or reading your mind, can lead to feelings of resentment and suspiciousness. Anger and hostility can also stem from the frustration of dealing with obstacles to working, establishing close relationships, and maintaining a decent standard of living. Chapter 23 focuses on strategies for helping your relative deal with these feelings.

Labile Mood

Your relative's mood may fluctuate rapidly from happy to sad or angry, for no apparent reason. When this happens (called *labile* mood), it can be confusing for people to understand what the person is feeling. Labile mood is usually accompanied by other severe symptoms, such as hallucinations or delusions.

Inappropriate or Incongruous Affect

Smiling or laughing when talking about a serious topic, such as the death of a friend, and other incongruous emotional responses, although relatively uncommon, can be very disturbing to family members and make it difficult to understand what your relative is feeling.

Behavioral Disturbances

Compared to some of the other types of symptoms, behavioral disturbances are rare in schizophrenia. *Catatonia* is a state in which the person maintains the same body posture for many hours or days. The person may be in a stupor, dazed, and unable to engage in any purposeful behavior. Sometimes people with schizophrenia engage in *catatonic excitement*, which is excited, purposeless motor activity not brought about by external stimuli. *Mutism*, refusing to talk, is another type of behavioral disturbance.

Understanding Your Relative's Symptoms

You've probably recognized many of these symptoms in your relative. Other symptoms may be more difficult to recognize if you haven't talked with your relative about them. Some people with schizophrenia are reluctant to talk about their symptoms, whereas others are willing. If you decide to talk with your relative, try to remember that he is the expert, because he knows what these symptoms are like. We've found that many people are willing to talk about their symptoms with family members once they've been assured they are the *real* experts.

The purpose of talking with your relative about symptoms is to understand what the experience is like and how the symptoms affect her life. If your relative prefers not to talk about this area, respect her desire for privacy. If your relative does talk, avoid challenging her. If she denies having the symptoms you've observed, or insists that certain delusions are true, show your interest in listening and try to understand her perspective.

To summarize the symptoms that your relative has experienced, complete Worksheet 2.1 at the end of the chapter. Appreciating the symptoms your relative has will help you understand how the illness has affected his life. Psychotic symptoms such as delusions and hallucinations make the world an unpredictable, frightening place. Negative symptoms, such as the loss of pleasure and apathy, lead people to withdraw and give up. Cognitive difficulties make it difficult for people to engage in rewarding interpersonal relationships, as well as to pursue goals such as work or school.

Understanding the Effects of Your Relative's Symptoms on You

Your relative's symptoms clearly have had a profound impact on her life. These symptoms have probably also had a major effect on your life and that of other close relatives. It hurts to see a family member unable to realize his full potential, and it's frustrating for an adult to be so dependent on you for basic living needs. In addition to these feelings, you may have also felt irritated at times, such as when your relative ignores something you say, forgets to do things, or won't "listen to reason." These reactions to your relative are quite natural, but they can have negative effects if you begin to blame your relative for having symptoms or if your feelings lead to arguments. The symptoms of schizophrenia are not your relative's fault, even though it may seem that she could try harder. You can help your relative function better and manage symptoms more effectively by working together as a team and by avoiding blame. Part III of this book offers help in these areas.

Is It Schizophrenia or a Mood Disorder?

After becoming familiar with your relative's symptoms, you may have questions about whether the diagnosis is correct. In particular, you may wonder whether your relative has a mood disorder rather than schizophrenia. The symptoms of schizophrenia do overlap with those of mood disorders such as bipolar disorder and major depression. As mentioned earlier, your relative has probably suffered from depression or mania at some point. Be aware, however, that there are significant differences between schizophrenia and mood disorders:

1. *The timing of the schizophrenia symptoms.* People with schizophrenia experience at least some periods of time during which they have psychotic symptoms but not significant mood symptoms. (If your relative has psychotic symptoms only while also having mood symptoms, the correct diagnosis may, in fact, be a mood disorder.)
2. *The age at onset.* People with schizophrenia tend to become ill at a younger age and to have symptoms that persist throughout life. Bipolar disorder and major depression tend to appear later and be more episodic.
3. *The level of functioning.* Many people with mood disorders have no symptoms and function quite well between episodes, whereas those with schizophrenia tend to have somewhat lower levels of functioning.

Understanding Your Relative's Illness

Schizophrenia is a complex illness that involves psychotic symptoms, negative symptoms, cognitive problems, and difficulties in functioning. People with schizophrenia also often have many other symptoms, such as depression and anxiety, which can complicate the diagnostic process. In the final analysis, a diagnosis is a judgment call that is not always easy to make. Regardless of the diagnosis, though, if your relative has many of the symptoms described here and does not function optimally, the recommendations we provide will be helpful.

Resources

First-Person Accounts and Biographies of People with Schizophrenia

Burke, R. D. (1995). *When the music's over: My journey into schizophrenia* New York: Basic Books. This sad but well-written book (the author committed suicide at age 32) provides an intimate description of the experience of schizophrenia compounded by substance abuse problems.

Chadwick, P. K. (1997). *Schizophrenia: The positive perspective*. London: Routledge.

Deveson, A. (1991). *Tell me I'm here: One family's experience of schizophrenia*. New York: Penguin Books. A mother's poignant description of schizophrenia in her son.

Kaplan, B. (Ed.). (1964). *The inner world of mental illness*. New York: Harper & Row. First-person accounts of the experience of mental illness.

Kytle, E. (1987). *The voices of Robby Wilde*. Washington, DC: Seven Locks Press. An excellent account of Wilde's struggle to work despite persistent hallucinations and delusions.

Miller, R., & Mason, S. (2002). *Diagnosis: Schizophrenia*. New York: Columbia University Press. Diagnosis, symptoms, medications, stigma, and coping skills described by two experienced clinicians and vividly illustrated by firsthand accounts.

Nasar, S. (1998). *A beautiful mind: The life of mathematical genius and Nobel laureate John Nash*. New York: Simon & Schuster. Biography about Nash's struggle with schizophrenia.

Schiller, L., & Bennett, A. (1994). *The quiet room: A journey out of the torment of madness* New York: Warner Books. First-person account of the author's journey from her early symptoms, diagnosis, and hospitalization to getting her life back.

Movies and Videos

A Beautiful Mind (2002). Universal Studios. Movie adaptation of the book by Sylvia Nasar based on the life of Nobel Prize laureate John Nash provides a good idea of the confusion of experiencing schizophrenia and the difficulty distinguishing between what is real and what is not. It is available in videotape or DVD format.

I'm Still Here (1996). Wheeler Communications Productions. Available from Direct Cinema Limited (*www.directcinema.com* or 310-636-8200). A poignant collection of the stories of several individuals and their families living with schizophrenia, with some functioning very well and others experiencing significant challenges.

Symptom Checklist

Instructions: Place a checkmark next to each symptom that your relative has experienced in the past (more than 1 month ago) or has experienced more recently. If you are unsure, leave the spaces for that symptom blank.

Symptom	Past	Present
Psychotic Symptoms		
Hallucinations		
Delusions		
Negative Symptoms		
Blunted affect		
Alogia		
Apathy		
Anhedonia		
Mood Problems		
Depression		
Suicidality		
Anxiety		
Anger, hostility, or suspiciousness		
Labile mood		
Inappropriate or incongruous affect		
Disturbances in Thinking		
Attention or concentration problems		
Memory problems		
Abstract reasoning impairment		
Social perception problems		
Peculiar logic		
Language problems		
Lack of insight		
Behavioral Disturbances		
Catatonia		
Mutism		
Disorganized or agitated behavior		

CHAPTER 3

Creating a Vision
of Recovery

C an people with schizophrenia get better? Can they recover? How often does improvement or recovery occur? These questions have been the topic of much debate since Kraepelin first described the illness over 100 years ago. Although Kraepelin believed that the illness had a downward course, research, doctors' observations, and personal experience now show that many people with schizophrenia recover either partially or fully from the disease. Furthermore, there are important steps family members, professionals, and people with schizophrenia can take to facilitate the recovery process. This chapter is devoted to helping you understand the nature of recovery and foster in your relative a vision of recovery imbued with hope, personal responsibility, and a sense of purpose.

Recovery from Schizophrenia

The term *recovery* means different things to different people. Some people view it as an *outcome* or a goal, similar to recovery from a medical illnesses, with permanent elimination of symptoms. In recent years, however, recovery has started to be viewed as a *process* that occurs independent of specific symptoms and impairments.

Recovery as a Medical Outcome

In conventional medical terms, *recovery* means no longer having the symptoms or related problems of the illness and being no more vulnerable to experiencing the illness in the future than anyone else—such as when someone recovers from pneumonia. In relation to schizophrenia, this would mean no longer hearing voices, having delusions, or experiencing negative symptoms, no longer having trouble holding down a job, and not being vulnerable to relapses or rehospitalizations. As one person with schizophrenia said, "Not having symptoms anymore is my definition of recovery."

Extensive research has provided compelling evidence that medical recovery from schizophrenia occurs in significant numbers of people and that many others improve substantially over time. The bar graph below shows that 42–68% of people with schizophrenia experience a full recovery or substantially improve over their lives.

Not surprisingly, scientists have also tried to understand why some people achieve such improvements. Robert P. Liberman, MD, and his colleagues at UCLA compared a group of people who currently experienced the symptoms and impairments of schizophrenia with a group of people who had recovered. Recovery was defined medically as not having any significant symptoms for the past 2 years; being employed at least half-time for the past 2 years; living independently and being able to manage money, shopping, food preparation, and personal hygiene; and having regular interactions with a friend, acquaintance (not family), or spouse. As shown in the table on page 34, 10 different factors were found to be related to recovery. This does not mean that every person who recovered from schizophrenia had every one of those factors working for him;

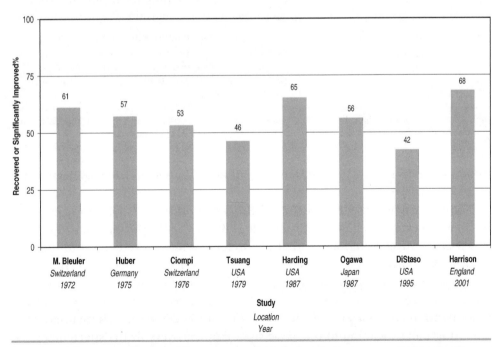

Long-term follow-up studies (over 20 or more years) of the longitudinal course of schizophrenia.

Factors Related to Medical Recovery from Schizophrenia	
Factor	Relationship to recovery
Family relationships	Low stress and high support facilitated recovery
Substance abuse	Recovery associated with little or no current/recent use of alcohol or drugs
Duration of untreated psychosis	People who recovered had received more rapid treatment for their psychosis after it developed
Initial response to medication	Recovered people experienced more benefit from their first trial on antipsychotic medication
Adherence to treatment	People who took medication and adhered to treatment recommendations were more likely to recover
Supportive therapy	Recovery was related to having positive and supportive relationships with psychiatrists, psychologists, social workers, or other mental health professionals
Cognitive abilities	People who recovered had good cognitive functioning, such as attention, concentration, memory, and ability to solve problems
Social skills	Recovered people had better interpersonal skills
Premorbid functioning	People who recovered functioned better before they developed schizophrenia in areas such as social relationships, educational level, and work
Access to care	Recovery was associated with better access to continuous care, including medication, psychotherapy, social skills training, family psychoeducation, vocational rehabilitation, and self-help groups

Note. Adapted from Liberman, Kopelowicz, Ventura, and Gutkind (2003). Copyright 2003 by Taylor and Francis. Adapted by permission.

rather, it means that the greater numbers of factors a person had, the more likely he was to recover.

To the extent that you can control the factors that contribute to it, medical recovery is certainly a goal worth pursuing. But many people with schizophrenia and their relatives would argue that it's preferable and more helpful to think of recovery as a *process* than as a single *outcome.* That's because medical recovery can span decades, even a lifetime. It's difficult for many families to keep going with their eyes on such a distant, often elusive, goal. Recovery as a process, on the other hand, keeps your eyes trained on shorter-term achievements that may actually bring more meaning to everyone's life than recovery in the strictly medical sense.

Recovery as a Process

Viewing recovery as a process rather than an outcome is a major shift in thinking that has provided many people with a renewed sense of hope and optimism, largely because it involves focusing on goals and aspirations instead of symptoms and limitations. When you focus all your efforts on overcoming a major illness, you make yourself responsible for an outcome over which you don't have total control—a demoralizing and depersonalizing prospect. The process view of recovery, on the other hand, allows you to focus on making whatever difference you can in your daily experience of mental illness, its consequences, and related hardships.

Patricia Deegan, who has written extensively about recovery based on her personal experiences and those of others, wrote:

> Recovery is a process, a way of life, an attitude and a way of approaching the day's challenges. It is not a perfectly linear process. At times our course is erratic and we falter, slide back, regroup, and start again. . . . The need is to meet the challenge of the disability and to re-establish a new and valued sense of integrity and purpose within and beyond the limits of the disability; the aspiration is to live, work, and love in a community in which one makes a significant contribution. (1988)

One of the most widely cited definitions of recovery was provided by William Anthony, the influential founder and director of the Boston Center for Psychiatric Rehabilitation, who described it as

> a deeply personal, unique process of changing one's attitudes, values, feelings, goals, skills, and/or roles. It is a way of living a satisfying, hopeful, and contributing life even with limitations caused by the illness. Recovery involves the development of new meaning and purpose in one's life as one grows beyond the catastrophic effects of mental illness.

Paul Carling, quoted below, helped to establish a vision of recovery that is oriented toward the values of community care for individuals with psychiatric disorders:

> Recovery involves a shift in consciousness of giving up the "sick" label, of seeing oneself, at core, as neither patient, nor even psychiatrically disabled, but as a unique individual with aspirations, strengths, and challenges, in short, a person in recovery.

Themes of Recovery

Common across all conceptions of recovery is the recognition that the person with the mental illness, and no one else, has the right to define recovery. Although definitions of recovery vary, a number of themes emerge:

Hope

Above all, hope is widely agreed to be the most fundamental ingredient of recovery, for without hope there can be no effort to rise above one's disability and to tackle the many challenges life offers. The importance of hope is underscored by the fact that people with mental illnesses have been often told that there is no cure for the illness, it is chronic, medication must be taken for life, and therefore there is no hope for recovery, for normalcy, or for a quality life. Such messages can deal a devastating blow to the individual, leading to resignation and moral defeat. No one, including mental health professionals, relatives, or "experts," can accurately predict the future of someone with schizophrenia (although many have tried!). The reason the future cannot be predicted is that it has not been written, and it is up to the person, with the help of family, to decide what her future will be.

Esso Leete, who has written eloquently about her experience of coping with schizophrenia, put it simply: "Having some hope is crucial to recovery; none of us would strive if we believed it a futile effort."

Empowerment and Responsibility

The concepts of recovery and empowerment have been intertwined since the earliest writings on the topic. *Empowerment* involves taking control of one's life, including the treatment of one's mental illness, and moving away from traditional hierarchical relationships with mental health professionals to collaborative ones based on shared decision making. Many people with mental illness have bitter memories of losing control over their lives when others have stepped in; they lost their voice, their freedom, and respect. Experiences with coercive interventions, such as involuntary hospitalization and pressure to take medication, lead to a mixture of feelings such as fury and resignation. The sociologist Althea McLean describes how such experiences with mental health treatment led to the emergence of the empowerment movement:

> Empowerment was evoked as a means to correct those violations and the pervasive debilitating consequences of their encounters with the mental health system. Thus, empowerment came to mean self-determination and control over their entire lives, not only their treatment.

Empowerment does not come without responsibility, however, and accepting responsibility for personal self-care is a critical part of recovery. Taking responsibility for oneself involves the development of better skills for self-managed care.

Dr. Daniel Fisher, the Director of the National Empowerment Center, has written, "Self-managed care draws on the power of each individual to direct their own healing."

The truly empowered person has the right to make choices and to bear the consequences of those choices, even when others may disapprove or disagree, be they professionals, friends, or families. Truly respecting that people with mental illness are independent people means allowing them to have the dignity of risk, including the possibility of failure, without always trying to protect them from the consequences of their decisions. Clay writes:

> The person most likely to get well—to become empowered—is the person who feels free to question, to accept or reject treatment, and to communicate with and care for the people who are caring for him. . . . Ultimately, patient empowerment is a matter of self-determination; it occurs when a patient freely chooses his or her own path to recovery and well-being. (quoted in Ralph)

Meaning and Sense of Purpose

The hopes and dreams of people with schizophrenia and other mental illnesses have often been dashed by the "slings and arrows of outrageous fortune"—their mental illness—resulting in a demoralized, passive acceptance of their lives. Out of fear of more disappointment, people stop pursuing their dreams and visions and settle back, watching their lives go by. Recovery involves regaining a sense of purpose in one's life.

Meaning and purpose are naturally defined by each person. For some people, they are found in being good parents, spouses, students, or employees. Meaning is multifaceted, and people can have many different activities in their lives that contribute to their sense of purpose. Advocating for social change, working at a peer support agency, becoming involved in the creative arts, being a mother, doing volunteer work, and caring for animals are just some examples of ways people create meaning and purpose in their own lives. One person with a mental illness stated about her job:

> I have to know that I am doing something that is meaningful for me, whether it is teaching kids or doing social change. If it is not personal at all, I couldn't do it. I always created my own job. (quoted in Provencher)

People need to be encouraged to define what is meaningful to them personally. Societal definitions of "adjustment" or "independence" should never take priority over people's own beliefs. Patricia Deegan warns of the hazards of rehabilitation programs that fail to help individuals develop their own meaning and sense of purpose in their lives and instead focus on traditional values defined by society:

> For some psychiatrically disabled people, especially those who relapse frequently, these traditional values of competition, individual achievement, independence, and self-sufficiency are oppressive. Programs that are tacitly built on these values are

invitations to failure for many recovering persons. For these persons, "independent living" amounts to the loneliness of four walls in the corner of some rooming house. For these persons, "individual vocational achievement" amounts to failing one vocational program after another until they come to believe they are worthless human beings with nothing to contribute. (1988)

Social Connection

Humans are naturally social creatures. Developing a mental illness can have a devastating effect on one's relationships with others and integration into the community. Close relationships are important in everyone's lives, and a common goal of people with mental illness is to establish closer relationships or to improve their quality. Shery Mead and Mary Ellen Copeland write of the importance of relationships with others and how people with psychiatric symptoms are able to connect with others:

> We are successfully establishing and maintaining intimate relationships. We are good parents. We have warm relationships with our partners, parents, siblings, friends and colleagues. We are climbing mountains, planting gardens, painting pictures, writing books, making quilts, and creating positive change in the world.

Dan Fisher notes that integration into society is a critical dimension of recovery, and he distinguishes this recovery approach from other approaches to working with people who have mental illness:

> Self-managed care is consumer-directed, multi-level, strength-building planning to genuinely assist a person to gain a meaningful role in society. This planning is contrasted to maintenance-based treatment planning which by its nature is professionally directed to correct pathology. (quoted in Ralph)

Many people with schizophrenia gain social connection, as well as a sense of purpose, through involvement in peer support groups (people with a mental illness meet and provide support to one another). Peer support, by its very nature, is nonhierarchical, and people report deriving great satisfaction from the process of helping others and from the help they receive in their equal relationships with others. Two people wrote of participating in peer support as follows:

> It brings companionship and a feeling of equality and respect. I am treated as an equal and as a competent person. That helps me to feel better about myself, and less depressed. (quoted in Provencher)

> I like working in a program like this because it makes me feel like I'm doing something not just for me but for other people, and to me that's important. Earning

money isn't so important in its own right. It helps me feel good about myself, and I know that I'm contributing to help other people. (quoted in Provencher)

Coping

People with schizophrenia and other mental illnesses often view recovery as the process of putting their lives back together through hope, meaningful activities, connections with others, and reintegration into their communities. However, the pursuit of these goals requires effective coping with symptoms and related problems. Coping is a "take charge" approach to problematic symptoms—it is the opposite of giving up. Coping efforts can be effective at changing the disturbing symptoms themselves, but more important, they are aimed at reducing the negative effects of symptoms on mood, behavior, self-confidence, enjoyment of life, and ability to pursue personally important goals. Esso Leete described the importance of coping with her schizophrenia in the following way:

> More than any other one thing, my life has been changed by schizophrenia. For the past 20 years I have lived with it and in spite of it—struggling to come to terms with it without giving in to it. Although I have fought a daily battle, it is only now that I have some sense of confidence that I will survive my ordeal. Taking responsibility for my life and developing coping mechanisms has been crucial to my recovery.

Coping is a broad concept. The inspiration and strategies for more effective coping can come from multiple sources, including the experiences of others with similar symptoms (as described in writings and peer support programs), family members, friends, religious or philosophical sources, or one's own creative mind. Directly addressing disturbing symptoms such as auditory hallucinations can be empowering in and of itself, as described by Patricia Deegan:

> The good news is that we no longer need to be alone and isolated with our voice-hearing experiences. We do not have to be passive victims of distressing voices. We can take a stand, find our own voice, and do something to help ourselves overcome distressing voices and reach our personal goals. (1996)

Personal lifestyle choices are another way of coping with the stress and symptoms of mental illness. These choices include a wide range of possible activities, such as exercise, meditation or prayer, involvement in the creative arts (writing, painting, acting), cooking, and socializing with friends and family. These activities are coping strategies because they help to bring much-needed balance into people's lives, provide opportunity for reflecting and processing personal experiences, and can reduce stress, energize, and strengthen feelings of well-being, inner peace, and optimism.

How Families Can Help

Recovery is a journey in which each person finds his own path. No one can take this journey for someone else, and the decision to begin it must come from within. At the same time, family members can do a lot to support and help a loved one pull his life together and work toward identifying and pursuing recovery goals.

Explore the Meaning of Recovery

Although it's important to respect the fact that your relative needs to develop her own understanding of recovery, you can help her begin the process by talking about it together, entertaining different options, and encouraging her to consider life's possibilities. Discussion about recovery best occurs in a low-stress, accepting environment in which each person feels free to talk openly without any commitment to change. It may be helpful to talk about what recovery means to different people to make it clear that there are many possibilities and no "right" definition of recovery.

Asking your relative directly about his ideas of recovery is one starting point. But you could also encourage your relative to use his imagination or even to fantasize about how things could be different. Questions like the following can help people think of their lives not as fixed and unchangeable but as fluid, malleable, and ripe with potential:

- "If you didn't have some of the difficulties you've been experiencing, what would you be doing that you're not doing now?"
- "If you didn't have schizophrenia [or a mental illness], how would your life be different?"
- "I remember that you were interested in [cite a specific interest] when you were growing up. How has that changed? Are you still interested in that?"

When talking about recovery and life changes, it's important not to push for goals too soon or to treat any goals that are identified as absolute commitments to which the person will be held. The last thing your relative needs is to be clobbered over the head with her own goals! At the same time, be careful not to discourage ambitions, for at least two reasons: First, no one, including you, knows whether an ambitious goal is attainable. Second, many positive changes occur in people's lives as they work toward achieving ambitious goals, even if the final goal is never attained. For many people, the process of striving toward a goal is more important and energizing than the actual attainment of that goal—or, as Robert Louis Stevenson wrote, "To travel hopefully is a better thing than to arrive." Once an ambitious goal has been identified, it can be broken down into smaller steps.

Materials about recovery also may be useful in stimulating dialogue. Sharing writings by people who have experienced recovery, watching videos, or surfing the Internet together are some possible strategies. Similarly, attending local lectures about recovery and exploring options for peer support are possible sources of inspiration. Examples of discussion questions include the following:

- "What does recovery mean to you?"
- "What changes in your life would make you feel you were on the road to recovery?"
- "Which of the following areas do you think are important to your personal recovery?"
  - Social relationships/feeling connected to your community
  - Work/school/parenting
  - Leisure time/spirituality/communing with nature/creative outlets
  - Health/exercise

Your relative may not see himself as having an illness to recover from, and he may be difficult to engage in a discussion about recovery. Lack of insight into having schizophrenia is quite common. In such circumstances it's best to focus on your relative's understanding of his difficulties and on helping him decide what can be done to make life better. You may not have a close relationship with your relative, or he may be very uncommunicative. In these situations, be selective in looking for the right time and place to initiate brief, positive talk about changes your relative may want in his life. Keeping your discussions short and simple may make it easier for your relative to warm up to you and realize that you're only trying to help.

Support Independent Decision Making

A critical part of recovery is becoming more independent and taking control over one's life. This involves learning how to make decisions and accepting responsibility for the consequences of those decisions. As a supportive family member, it's your job to encourage your relative to get involved and make decisions about her treatment and other aspects of her life.

Genuinely supporting your relative in running his own life requires you to accept his decisions, including any that may not seem like the best choices to you. Stepping in and taking control when you think the "wrong" decisions are being made can damage your relative's self-esteem, disempower him, and arrest the natural process of recovery. According to the "dignity of risk" concept alluded to in the "Empowerment and Responsibility" section earlier in this chapter, risk is an inherent part of life, and people learn from the decisions they make, including the bad ones.

It may be difficult to watch your relative make decisions you don't agree with. You might be concerned about decisions such as changing or discontinuing medication, moving, getting a job or going back to school, dropping out of a rehabilitation program, or resuming relationships with certain people. There are several strategies for minimizing the chance that your relative will make rash decisions while pursuing recovery goals. When goals involve the treatment of schizophrenia, your relative needs to understand how treatment for the illness works, such as the effects of medication on symptoms and relapses. In addition, although your relative has the right to choose the treatment she wants, she can be encouraged to talk over possible changes in treatment with members of the treatment team.

Of course, your relative's circumstances may not leave him in full control of all aspects of his life. He may be mandated to receive treatment, or you may have been assigned the responsibility for managing his money, and one of your duties is to make sure some of his funds are reserved for paying essentials such as bills and rent. Even with these limitations on your relative's free will, you can find ways to encourage self-determination. First, you can always empathize with your relative's lack of control in certain areas while continuing to support his autonomous decision making in other aspects of life. You can also ally with your relative in working toward the goal of his attaining greater control over important decisions in life, such as treatment and finances. To do this, you need to focus together on understanding why limits have been placed on your relative's decision-making authority and what might need to be done to remove them. For example, your relative may be motivated to learn how to budget his money with the goal of getting more control over his finances.

Being able to talk openly about your concerns while maintaining respect for your relative's right to make decisions is also important. As with discussing recovery in general, you can express your concerns directly or ask thought-provoking questions. Always take a collaborative planning and problem-solving approach. Chapter 15 describes effective techniques for weighing the potential advantages and drawbacks of a recovery goal your relative is considering. Once you've done that, it may be helpful to agree on some steps to take to minimize problems if the plan backfires.

If your relative's plan doesn't work or you disagreed with a decision from the outset, you (and others) can be available to process the experience and talk about where to go from there, while avoiding the tempting but counterproductive "I told you so." It's essential not to withdraw your love and support or act critically or judgmentally about your relative's choice. Above all, family members need to maintain positive and supportive relationships with a relative who is learning to take control over her life.

Check Out Local Peer Support Programs

Peer support programs are offered in a variety of settings, from freestanding clubhouses to drop-in centers. Because peer support can contribute to recovery in several ways, it's important for you to encourage your relative to seek out whatever programs are available locally.

Most obviously, peer support provides people with the chance to meet with others who have psychiatric disabilities on an equal footing, to share experiences, compare coping strategies, socialize, and experience the support of others facing similar challenges. Peer support centers provide a variety of helpful activities, including informal opportunities for socialization, support groups, advice on coping strategies, meals, recreational trips, jobs, and resources (e.g., library, video).

Possibly less evident but just as valuable, these programs allow participants to *give* support as well as to receive it. Helping someone else and receiving validation for his efforts can give your relative concrete evidence of his worth and ability to contribute to the lives of others. It can also help build the social skills needed to develop close and rewarding interpersonal relationships—an important goal for many people with schizophrenia. The positive effects of helping others are often greater than the benefits of the help that is received—a true instance where "it is better to give than to receive." Giving support to others shifts the focus of attention from oneself to someone else, which requires empathy, concern, and a desire to reach out and connect. By fostering these qualities, giving support often provides greater benefits than receiving it.

A final advantage of peer support is that it provides people with positive role models. At most peer support centers your relative will meet individuals who have learned to manage their illness effectively and who embrace the importance of recovery. More information about peer support programs and how to find one is provided in Chapter 5.

Help with Coping

The major symptoms of schizophrenia often lead to distress and difficulties in functioning. Helping your relative develop more effective coping strategies can both reduce stress and improve functioning. If your relative has established personal recovery goals, she will probably be highly motivated to learn coping strategies because they'll help her manage the symptoms that interfere with achieving those goals.

You can help your relative learn such strategies in a variety of ways. First, consider how motivated he is to cope better with his symptoms or day-to-day stress. If he experiences high levels of distress due to specific symptoms or is highly sensitive to the stress of everyday life, you may be able to tap into his desire to reduce that distress. You may also want to help your relative understand that the symptoms he is experiencing are not unusual and that many people have found relief from learning and practicing coping strategies.

If your relative doesn't seem motivated to alleviate her distress from symptoms or daily sources of stress, you might be better off focusing on the positive gains that can be made by improving functioning at work, in self-care, or in relationships. Then, when it becomes apparent that symptoms or stress are blocking your relative from achieving these goals, you can introduce the topic of coping strategies.

Either way, it's important to understand that motivation comes from *within*. Rather than explaining what *you* think and directly pointing out the problem, try asking your relative questions that will elicit his awareness of the factors that interfere with attaining his goals. Then you can share some of the suggestions for coping from this book and develop a plan for following up on those suggestions.

Keeping Hope Alive

The most important way you can help your relative develop a personal vision of recovery is to keep hope alive by always believing in her inherent ability to get better. Hope is the wellspring from which the energy to change one's life flows. Without hope and the belief that change is possible, recovery cannot take root.

Even if your relative has no hope—and many people lose hope in the despair and fog of mental illness—having hope for your relative and believing in him can have a profound impact. The fact that your relative has no hope does not mean that he cannot sense and feel *your* hope. Patricia Deegan describes the importance of never giving up hope for a loved one:

> Those of us who have given up are not to be abandoned as "hopeless cases." The truth is that at some point every single person who has been diagnosed with a mental illness passes through this time of anguish and apathy. . . . So it is not our job to pass judgment on who will and will not recover from mental illness and the spirit-breaking effects of poverty, stigma, dehumanization, degradation and learned helplessness. Rather, our job is to participate in a conspiracy of hope. It is our job to form a community of hope which surrounds people with psychiatric disabilities. (1996)

Sometimes family members get caught up in feelings of anger, sadness, and pity over the unfairness of schizophrenia striking their loved one. These feelings, although normal and understandable, can get in the way of instilling hope and belief in your relative's recovery. Focusing on the "unfairness" of mental illness sets your relative's experience apart from all others and implies that the challenges she faces are unique to her and others with psychiatric disorders. Although mental illness *is* unpredictable and can have devastating effects on people's lives, everyone experiences different challenges, setbacks, and traumas, and the experience of being in recovery is not unique to mental illness. Indeed, the experience of recovery is *universal*. By understanding your relative's mental illness as part of the human experience—and the will to recover as part of that experience—you may be better able to relate personally to your relative. You may also be able to maintain hope for the future, rather than dwelling on the past or feeling sorry for yourself or your loved one. Keeping hope alive is just as important for you as it is for your relative, for in hope lies the possibility for change and the belief in your relative's ability to recover.

Resources

Works on Recovery Cited in the Chapter

Anthony, W. A. (1993). Recovery from mental illness: The guiding vision of the mental health service system in the 1990s. *Psychosocial Rehabilitation Journal, 16*, 11–23.

Carling, P. J. (1997, September 5). *Recovery as the core of our work: The challenge to mental health systems and professionals.* Paper presented at the New Hampshire Partners for Change Conference on Recovery, Nashua, NH.

Deegan, P. E. (1988). Recovery: The lived experience of rehabilitation. *Psychosocial Rehabilitation Journal, 11*, 11–19.

Deegan, P. (1996). *Recovery and the conspiracy of hope.* Paper presented at the Sixth Annual Mental Health Conference of Australia and New Zealand, Brisbane, Australia.

Fisher, W. A., Penney, D. J., & Earle, K. (1996). Mental health services recipients: Their role in shaping organizational policy. *Administration and Policy in Mental Health, 23*, 547–553.

Leete, E. (1989). How I perceive and manage my illness. *Schizophrenia Bulletin, 15*, 197–200.

Liberman, R. P., Kopelowicz, A., Ventura, J., & Gutkind, D. (2003). Operational criteria and factors related to recovery from schizophrenia. *International Review of Psychiatry, 14*, 256–272. Available from *www.tandf.co.uk/journals*

Mead, S., & Copeland, M. E. (2000). What recovery means to us: Consumers' perspectives. *Community Mental Health Journal, 36*, 315–328.

McLean, A. (1995). Empowerment and the psychiatric consumer/ex-patient movement in the United States: Contradictions, crisis, and change. *Social Science and Medicine, 40*, 1053–1071.

Provencher, H. P., Gregg, R., Mead, S., & Mueser, K. T. (2002). The role of work in recovery of persons with psychiatric disabilities. *Psychiatric Rehabilitation Journal, 26*, 132–144.

Ralph, R. O. (2000). *Review of recovery literature: A synthesis of a sample of recovery literature 2000.* Portland, ME: Edmund S. Muskie Institute of Public Affairs, University of Southern Maine.

Books about Recovery

Carling, P. J. (1995). *Return to community: Building support systems for people with psychiatric disabilities.* New York: Guilford Press. This influential book describes how to create support networks in the community to facilitate integration and recovery for persons with major mental illness.

Chadwick, P. K. (1997). *Schizophrenia: The positive perspective*. London: Routledge. This is a remarkable book by an individual with schizophrenia who is also a psychologist and scientist and who has made significant contributions to the field.

Clay, S., Schell, B., Corrigan, P., & Ralph, R. (Eds.). (2005). *On our own, together: Peer programs for people with mental illness*. Nashville, TN: Vanderbilt University Press. Meeting other people with mental illness who are positive role models is one of the many advantages of participating in peer programs, especially if your relative experiences self-stigmatization. This is an excellent book that provides a history of peer support, describes different types of peer support programs (such as drop-in centers, and mentoring and educational programs), and provides information about finding a local peer support program.

Davidson, L. (2003). *Living outside mental illness: Qualitative studies of recovery in schizophrenia*. New York: New York University Press. Davidson studies the phenomenology of schizophrenia and the experience of recovery.

McLean, R. (2003). *Recovered, not cured: A journey through schizophrenia* Crows Nest, New Wales, Australia: Allen & Unwin. McLean describes his experience with schizophrenia, along with illustrations and photos. Available from *www.allenandunwin.com*.

Neugeboren, J. (1999). *Transforming madness: New lives for people living with mental illness*. New York: Morrow. This book describes the movement toward a recovery perspective for persons with psychiatric disabilities.

Ng, H. (2005). *Recovered grace: Schizophrenia*. Singapore: Harris Ng Yoke Meng. This interesting book is subtitled "A true, unusual and inspiring story; a heart wrenching journey through a dreadful mental disorder." It chronicles the recovery story of Harris Ng, who developed schizophrenia during the final years of studying for his degree in civil engineering. This personal account explains how he refused to take medications at first and suffered multiple relapses, but how with the support of his family he gradually came to an acceptance of the illness, learned how to manage it, obtained meaningful work, and fell in love and married. Available from *www.selectbooks.com.sg*

Ralph, R. O., & Corrigan, P. W. (Eds.). (2005). *Recovery in mental illness: Broadening our understanding of wellness*. Washington, DC: American Psychological Association. An excellent compilation of different perspectives on recovery.

Steele, K., & Berman, C. (2001). *The day the voices stopped: A memoir of madness and hope*. New York: Basic Books. Autobiography of a leading mental health advocate who developed symptoms at age 14.

Warner, R. (1994). *Recovery from schizophrenia: Psychiatry and political economy* (2nd ed.). London: Routledge. Warner brings to bear a wealth of evidence showing that recovery from schizophrenia is possible and, indeed, occurs often.

Wasow, M. (2001). Personal accounts: Strengths versus deficits, or musician versus schizophrenic. *Psychiatric Services, 52*, 1306–1307.

Websites about Recovery

www.chovil.com. Ian Chovil, who has schizophrenia, has developed an extensive website with information about the illness that he has collected in the course of reading, attending conferences, and giving presentations. He also tells his personal story.

www.fredfrese.com is a website hosted by Fred Frese, PhD, who is a clinical psychologist with schizophrenia. Dr. Frese is an eloquent spokesman on the experience of coping with schizophrenia and living a full, interesting, and professional life.

www.mentalhealthrecovery.com. Mary Ellen Copeland has developed a number of publications and programs for helping people in the recovery process, including the Wellness Recovery Action Plan (WRAP). Her website offers a free newsletter and articles and a list of workshops and publications that can be purchased.

www.nami.org. "In Our Own Voice" is an educational/recovery program developed through the National Alliance on Mental Illness (NAMI) to educate people about recovery from mental illness and reduce stigma associated with mental illness. Information can be obtained at the organization's website.

www.nsfoundation.org/sa. Schizophrenia Anonymous is a self-help organization whose website offers information about schizophrenia and stories of people who are in the process of recovering.

www.newyorkcityvoices.org. Mental health consumers, family members, and professionals offer mutual support for moving forward in their lives in this journal for mental health advocacy.

www.power2u.org. The National Empowerment Center provides information, programs, and materials on recovery from mental illness, including a newsletter and audiovisual materials; also refers people to local support groups and offers guidance for setting up new groups.

www.reintegration.com. The Center for Reintegration has a website that offers helpful information about schizophrenia, healthy lifestyles, and being involved in work and the community. It also publishes a free magazine, *Reintegration Today*, made possible by an unrestricted educational grant from Eli Lilly and Company, which produces medications. You can subscribe to the magazine on the Web or by calling 800-809-8202.

www.schizophrenia.com. This website includes several success stories that highlight people who have made progress in their own recovery.

Videotapes about Recovery

The Bonnie Tapes. (1997). Mental Illness Education Project (*miepvideos.org* or 800-343-5540). In a series of three videotapes (*Mental Illness in the Family*, *Recovery from Mental Illness*, and *My Sister Is Mentally Ill*), 27-year-old Bonnie and her family talk about schizophrenia and how it has affected them.

Living with Schizophrenia. (2002). New York: Guilford Press and Monkey See Productions (*www.guilford.com*). Four individuals with schizophrenia share their personal recovery journeys.

CHAPTER 4

Comprehensive Treatment of Schizophrenia

Chapters 1–3 should have left little doubt in your mind that the needs of people with schizophrenia are complex. A comprehensive treatment plan must provide medications to alleviate symptoms and prevent relapses, as well as meet needs in the areas of emotional well-being, social relationships, leisure activities, housing, self-care, and physical health. The mental health system, including your local community mental health center, is designed to implement such a plan. However, like any system, the mental health system is not perfect. To fill in the inevitable gaps, families often play a key role in helping their relatives get the treatment they need. Without your loving attention and care, many of your relative's most critical needs could go untreated. This chapter provides an overview of comprehensive treatment and helps you get a general idea of your relative's treatment needs so you're prepared to advocate effectively for him and to collaborate with professionals in ensuring that these needs are addressed.

General Treatment Needs:
The Stress–Vulnerability Model

As explained in Chapter 1, the stress–vulnerability model states that the severity and course of schizophrenia are affected by several factors, all of which need to be addressed through comprehensive treatment. *Biological vulnerability* is determined by genetic and other biological factors and contributes directly to the symptoms and impairments of schizophrenia. The effects of biological vulnerability can be minimized by *taking medication* and *avoiding alcohol and drugs*. In addition, *stress* can impinge on biological vulnerability and increase the risk of symptom relapses and decreased functioning. However, good *coping skills* and *social support* can protect people from the negative effects of stress on biological vulnerability. So, although the symptoms and impairments of schizophrenia are caused by a biologically based disorder, the course of the illness can be improved by taking concrete steps to minimize biological vulnerability and the effects of stress.

The implications of the stress–vulnerability model for treatment planning are clear. First, biological vulnerability can be reduced by taking medications and not using drugs and alcohol. Issues related to medication are addressed in Chapter 10, and strategies for reducing alcohol and drug abuse are covered in Chapter 22. Second, reducing stress can improve the course of the illness. Strategies such as relaxation techniques, exercise, leisure activities, improved communication, and effective problem-solving skills are covered in Chapters 11, 14, 15, and 28. Third, improving the ability to cope with persistent symptoms and other stressful experiences can improve resilience and reduce susceptibility to stress-induced relapses. Strategies for coping with common symptoms and other problems are covered in Part V of the book.

Fourth, improved social support can reduce the effects of stress on people with schizophrenia. For example, as family members improve their communication and problem-solving skills, they become better able to handle conflict successfully and reduce family stress. Research has shown that reduced levels of family stress result in decreased symptoms and relapse rates for people with schizophrenia. In addition, improved social support can facilitate the coping skills of people with schizophrenia. People who have positive, close, and loving relationships with family members and others in their lives often benefit from the suggestions of those people for how to handle stressful situations, thereby bolstering their coping skills and ability to handle stress effectively. (See Chapter 25 for more on improving social relationships.)

Specific Treatment Needs

The stress–vulnerability model provides a general framework for guiding treatment. To understand your relative's specific treatment needs, you need to consider her functioning and adjustment across a number of different life domains. The following 10 areas should be assessed in developing a comprehensive treatment plan for your relative.

1. Symptoms

The psychotic symptoms, negative symptoms, and cognitive problems at the core of schizophrenia can be distressing and interfere with enjoyment of life, interfere with functioning, and damage the quality and closeness of social relationships.

Therefore, interventions that address problematic symptoms focus on reducing distress and minimizing the interference that symptoms cause.

There are many different strategies for addressing persistent symptoms. Medications (see Chapter 10) have a powerful effect on symptoms, reducing many of the most flagrant symptoms of psychosis and exerting modest effects on negative and cognitive symptoms.

Coping strategies can also be very effective at reducing both the severity of symptoms and the interference they cause in functioning and relationships, as described in Part V. As Chapter 3 discussed, you can play a vital role in helping your relative identify and practice coping strategies.

2. Emotional Well-Being

The quality of your relative's life is greatly influenced by how he feels about himself and his experience of contentment, joy, and happiness. Emotional well-being is determined by the circumstances of one's life as well as the experience of positive and negative emotions. Housing and work are important contributors to emotional well-being. People experience lower life satisfaction when they are homeless or in jail, and higher life satisfaction when they have stable housing and receive sufficient support to live independently. Chapter 27 describes strategies for addressing housing issues. People also experience a greater sense of well-being when they are working or involved in some type of meaningful activity (such as school or parenting) that gives them a feeling of purpose. Strategies for helping your relative pursue employment goals or return to school are described in Chapter 26.

People with schizophrenia often experience fewer positive emotions, either because of *anhedonia* (loss of pleasure), addressed in Chapter 18, or due to lack of rewarding relationships or activities, discussed in Chapters 25 and 28.

Depression, Anxiety, and Anger

Depression can have a devastating effect on people with schizophrenia, making it difficult to do things, to take care of themselves, enjoy time with others, and go to work or school. In fact, depression can be so severe that it makes them feel like life is not worth living—a state that may lead to suicidal thoughts and attempts. Many different ways of addressing depression in schizophrenia are described in Chapter 21.

Anxiety can be debilitating when it causes people to avoid situations and activities that would otherwise bring them happiness, a sense of accomplishment, or greater self-sufficiency. Anxiety is a particular problem in people with schizophrenia because of the psychotic symptoms they often experience—threatening voices and persecutory delusions—and because of the awkwardness they feel in social situations. People with schizophrenia may also experience anxiety related to the upsetting experience of developing a severe mental illness, the stigma associated with it, and unpleasant treatment experiences, such as involuntary hospitalizations. Finally, people may have anxiety because they have experienced traumatic events, such as being physically or sexually assaulted, being in a natural disaster or accident, or witnessing something terrible happen to someone else. Chapter 20 provides guidelines for addressing anxiety problems.

[Problems with anger in schizophrenia may be related to paranoid delusions or general suspiciousness.] Also, many people get angry because they feel trapped by their illness. Substance use can cause angry behavior, either by leading to conflict with others in the pursuit of alcohol or the drugs on which the person has become dependent or by lowering inhibitions and allowing freer expression of anger. Finally, anger can be a product of the many frustrations experienced by people with schizophrenia: from the absence of satisfying relationships and interesting activities to the meager economic resources, poor living conditions, and enduring social stigma. Chapter 23 describes strategies for addressing problems related to anger and violence.

3. Role Functioning

The term *role functioning* refers to the ability to fulfill socially defined roles, such as at work, at school, as a parent, or as a spouse/partner. Impaired role functioning is one of the defining problem areas in schizophrenia. Evaluating which areas of role functioning your relative has difficulty in and which areas she most wishes to change is critical to helping her develop meaning, a sense of purpose, and greater fulfillment in life.

Work

Employment is a common goal of people with schizophrenia, yet rates of competitive work are low. Most people with schizophrenia want regular jobs in the community that pay competitive wages and provide ongoing contact with nondisabled workers. Chapter 26 describes strategies for helping your relative get work, including those of "supported employment," a rehabilitation approach that helps people find jobs.

School

[Schizophrenia often causes people to drop out of school, which can lead to feelings of low self-esteem and inferiority and also limit the potential to find interesting and rewarding work.] For many people, therefore, reaching educational goals takes priority over finding work and may be an important part of their treatment. Many mental health programs and colleges have special programs for helping people with mental illness increase their educational level. In addition, the principles of supported employment (outlined in Chapter 26) can be adapted to help your relative get back to school.

Parenting

Many people with schizophrenia, especially women, have children, yet schizophrenia can interfere with their ability to parent effectively. In many cases, family members are drawn into helping a relative with schizophrenia care for her children, and sometimes they assume primary parenting responsibility, including legal guardianship over the child. Regardless of the extent of responsibility the person with schizophrenia has for caring for her children, a common goal is to improve the quality of her relationships with her children, including better parenting skills. Chapter 9 offers strategies people can use to improve their parenting skills and their relationships with their children. Special classes for people with a mental illness may be available in your local community.

Spousal/Partner Relationships

A significant number of people with schizophrenia marry, particularly women, but divorce rates are much higher than in the general population. The symptoms of schizophrenia and associated challenges can place a burden on a marriage. Also, people with schizophrenia often have trouble doing their share of household tasks and parenting and meeting other typical expectations of an intimate partnership (such as emotional availability).

Chapter 8 describes strategies for improving spousal and partner relationships. The role of medications in contributing to lethargy and low energy may need to be evaluated (see Chapter 10). Couples may benefit from reviewing and practicing more effective communication and problem-solving skills, as described in Chapters 14 and 15. Couples counseling may help partners address relationship issues and develop a fair division of shared responsibility between them. Skills training may be useful to teach basic homemaking skills such as cooking, cleaning, and laundry (Chapter 27).

4. Social Relationships

One of the most common problem areas for people with schizophrenia is their social relationships. High levels of conflict in close relationships are typical, as is the absence of, or only few, close relationships. Fortunately, there are many options for helping people improve their social relationships. Social skills training is one effective approach for improving the quality of social interaction and involvement in leisure activities. Skills training programs are available at most mental health centers, and the steps of skills training are described in Chapter 25. Peer support programs, such as psychosocial clubhouses, provide another opportunity for people to expand their social networks and socialize with others in a comfortable environment (see Chapter 3). Exploring local organizations can provide still other avenues for making connections with people, such as a local nature or outing club, the Rotary Club, the YMCA, the local amateur astronomy association, a reading group, or a bowling league (see Chapter 28). Chapters 14 and 15 describe strategies for improving communication and problem-solving skills, which can enhance the quality of social relationships. Negative symptoms, including reduced social drive and difficulties experiencing pleasure, can interfere with having good relationships with others; Chapter 18 describes strategies for dealing with these types of problems.

5. Leisure and Recreational Activities

Your relative may have no hobbies, sports, or other interesting activities, instead spending inordinate amounts of time sleeping, eating, watching TV, and using drugs and alcohol. This lack of recreational activities is partly due to the fact that schizophrenia typically appears during late adolescence or early adulthood, when people are in the process of developing their interests. A common goal for people with schizophrenia is to improve how they spend their leisure time. Leisure activities are often social in nature, so many of the strategies described above for improving social relationships are also effective for increasing the number and enjoyment of recreational activities (see Chapters 25 and 28).

6. Self-Care and Living Skills

Living independently is a common goal of many people with schizophrenia. The quality of a person's self-care skills has an important bearing on functioning in many areas, including the maintenance of health and the enjoyment of daily life. Grooming, hygiene, money management, use of transportation, shopping, care of clothing, safety, and mental and physical illness self-care are all aspects of independent living that need consideration.

Many mental health programs have classes designed to teach living and self-care skills. Supported living services are also available at many mental health centers. These services can help people meet their basic living needs, while maintaining their independence, through the assistance of training provided in their natural living environment. In many mental health centers, these services are provided by assertive community treatment (ACT) teams. ACT teams, which are described in Chapter 5, provide intensive outreach services to people living in the community and teach them basic living skills so that they can get their practical needs met. In cases where such assistance is not available, family members, friends, or other members of the community (e.g., clergy) may be involved in helping people with schizophrenia meet their basic daily living needs.

7. Physical Health

People with schizophrenia often have medical problems that are inadequately detected, monitored, and treated. Two of the difficulties in recognizing their medical conditions are that (1) they are less likely to report physical symptoms, and (2) professionals may take their complaints less seriously. The result is that untreated illnesses take a heavy toll, contributing to increased disability and premature death. Helping your relative identify any medical conditions that require treatment is an important part of a comprehensive treatment plan.

People with schizophrenia often have medical needs due to smoking, infectious diseases (such as hepatitis C and HIV), diabetes, cardiovascular problems, and poor dental hygiene. Smoking is a major problem for people with schizophrenia; approximately 80% of individuals smoke cigarettes (see Chapter 22). The high rate of infectious disease in people with schizophrenia is related primarily to the high level of drug abuse. Anyone who has had a drug abuse problem should be evaluated for possible infectious diseases. Other diseases, including diabetes, cardiovascular problems, and dental problems, are common in people with schizophrenia because of their poor dietary habits, sedentary lifestyle, and lack of self-care skills. If your relative has not received appropriate dental care in the past year and has not been medically evaluated for these illnesses, you should arrange for these evaluations to be conducted.

Some severely ill individuals with schizophrenia consume extremely high quantities of liquids (such as drinking several gallons a day), including coffee and caffeinated sodas, but also water and noncaffeinated beverages. Drinking such large amounts of liquids can be hazardous to the person's health and even fatal if preventive action is not taken. If you are concerned that your relative may have this condition (referred to as *polydipsia*), contact his doctor to evaluate this possibility; careful monitoring and restriction of your relative's drinking may be necessary.

8. Alcohol and Drug Use

Problems related to substance use are common in people with schizophrenia. Substance abuse in schizophrenia is associated with a more severe course of psychiatric illness, as well as health, legal, economic, and social problems. Thus, addressing substance abuse is an important priority in persons with schizophrenia. Chapter 22 provides guidance for addressing substance use problems in a relative.

9. Spiritual Needs

People with schizophrenia, like others, have spiritual needs. However, because of concerns about confusing spiritual needs with the religious themes of many delusions, these needs are often overlooked. Many people with schizophrenia endorse the importance of their belief in God, or some other transcendent connection such as nature, through yoga or meditation. The comfort of getting spiritual needs met can become a satisfying source of support and coping. Furthermore, involvement in spiritual pursuits can help people make deep and meaningful connections with others, which can be both rewarding and helpful.

10. Recovery

Never lose sight of the importance of recovery as the overarching goal of all treatment. As discussed in Chapter 3, recovery means different things to different people, and each person with mental illness can develop his own understanding of what recovery means. Talking about recovery with your relative leads quite naturally to personal recovery goals. These goals should always be at the forefront of treatment planning. Indeed, engagement and active participation in treatment are most effectively accomplished when the person sees how treating his mental illness will improve his ability to achieve personal goals.

Assessing and Prioritizing Your Relative's Treatment Needs

We encourage you to use Worksheet 4.1 at the end of this chapter for "Identifying Treatment Needs" in collaboration with your relative and her mental health professionals. Further information on many treatment components is provided in this book. Information about community resources that may be helpful in the treatment of your relative is addressed in the next chapter.

Of course, some treatment needs take priority over others. There are three basic levels of priority, as follows:

1. Resolving Crises

Of utmost priority is any situation in which your relative is in imminent danger of harming herself or someone else—a crisis that must be attended to immediately. For example, Antoine, who had not yet received a diagnostic evaluation, became convinced that his family members were not real, but robot replacements, and made serious threats to "destroy" them. His family responded to this crisis by seeking an emergency psychiatric evaluation and began the process of getting a diagnosis and appropriate medication for their son. Chapter 13 provides more information on responding to crises related to schizophrenia.

2. Managing Symptoms

If your relative experiences troubling symptoms, even if he is not in crisis, it is still vital to get a diagnosis and appropriate medications. If he has received a diagnosis and is already taking medications, the priority is to work with a psychi-atrist (or other prescriber) to optimize his relief from symptoms.

Since receiving a diagnosis of schizophrenia, Tatiana had been regularly taking the medication prescribed by the doctor. However, she continued to hear voices that told her she was an evil person who should stay away from others so as not to "contaminate" them. She expressed distress at hearing these voices and spent much of her time alone in her room. With her family's encouragement, she talked to her psychiatrist about the unpleas-ant auditory hallucinations, and he tried changing the dose of the medication. That led to sedation but no lessening of symptoms, so after a reasonable trial period he tried a dif-ferent medication. The doctor was able to prescribe a dose of this medication that was more effective in controlling the voices and did not have a sedating effect. When Tatiana experienced fewer distressing symptoms, she was able to focus on other treatment needs, such as locating a supported employment program to help her find and maintain a job.

3. Addressing Problems in Functioning and Quality of Life

When everything has been done to manage your relative's symptoms as well as possible, it's important to move on to discussing other treatment needs related to improving her functioning and quality of life, such as increasing her social rela-tionships, getting a job doing volunteer work, living independently, pursuing hobbies, etc. Some people with schizophrenia may continue to experience persis-tent symptoms (such as hearing voices) after every effort has been made. Never-theless, it is vital not to delay other treatment needs indefinitely. For those indi-viduals, learning strategies for coping with persistent symptoms (as described in Chapters 17, 18, and 19) is an important component of treatment that can help them pursue goals in other areas.

Leo experienced his first episode of schizophrenia when he was 20. After receiving a diagnosis, he worked with his doctor for almost a year to identify the most effective medica-tion and dosage. He shared an apartment with a roommate and visited his parents at least once a week, but had no other relationships and was not involved in activities that were meaningful to him. When his parents brought up the idea of exploring what he would like to be doing with his time, he was receptive. Using the Identifying Treatment Needs worksheet, he realized he would like to go back to school to take classes in comput-ers, but he hesitated to do this because he was having trouble concentrating. This realiza-tion led to the identification of two main treatment needs: getting some help with cogni-tive symptoms and finding a computer course in the community.

WORKSHEET 4.1 Identifying Treatment Needs (p. 1 of 2)

Treatment needs	Going well or not a problem	Problematic, could use improvement	Specific improvement desired
Managing Symptoms			
Psychotic symptoms			
Negative symptoms			
Cognitive symptoms			
Emotional Well-Being			
Meaningful activities			
Managing depression, anxiety, anger			
Role Functioning			
Work or school			
Parenting			
Spouse/partner			
Homemaking			
Social Relationships			
Friends/roommates			
Family/spouse			
Coworkers			
Boyfriend or girlfriend			
Leisure Activities			
Hobbies			
Sports			
Playing music or creating artwork			
Listening to music or looking at artwork			
Creative writing			
Reading for pleasure			

(cont.)

Treatment needs	Going well or not a problem	Problematic, could use improvement	Specific improvement desired
Self-Care and Other Living Skills			
Grooming/hygiene			
Money management			
Use of transportation			
Shopping/food prep			
Laundry			
Safety			
Eating nutritiously			
Stable housing			
Physical Health			
Medical checkups			
Regular dental care			
Avoiding risky sexual behavior			
Smoking cessation			
Avoiding risky drug-taking behavior			
Chronic disease management (e.g., diabetes)			
Alcohol and Drug Use			
Addressing problems related to drug and alcohol use			
Integrated treatment			
Spiritual Needs			
Involvement in religious activities			
Experiencing nature			
Meditation/yoga			
Recovery			
Developing a personal definition of recovery			
Setting and working toward personal goals			

CHAPTER 5

Community Resources

Once you've helped your relative identify his needs, as you did in Chapter 4, the next step is to work together to identify how to get those needs met. Determining which services your relative is most likely to benefit from requires a team effort involving you, your relative, and mental health professionals. To be an effective team member and a successful advocate for your relative, you need to be informed. This chapter describes different services, resources, and benefits available in most communities. To help you sort it all out, we also describe *evidence-based practices*, which are specific treatment methods shown in carefully controlled scientific research to be effective in improving the lives of people with schizophrenia. Through collaborative work with mental health professionals and your relative, you can help your loved one get his treatment and personal needs met and thereby make progress toward recovery goals.

Naturally, you may have to do some detective work to discover which resources are actually offered in your own community. How do you start if you don't yet have a treatment team in place? If your relative has already been diagnosed, the professional who made the diagnosis should be able to refer you to appropriate service providers to initiate treatment. If your relative has not yet been diagnosed, see Chapter 2 to find a practitioner who is qualified to conduct a professional evaluation.

Where to Find Mental Health Services

Mental health services can be found in a variety of places or contexts in your community:

Community Mental Health Centers (CMHCs)

Currently over 800 community mental health centers (CMHCs) are funded in the United States to serve as the major focal point in the community for providing outpatient mental health services. CMHCs are funded directly by each state but receive reimbursement from many different federal programs (such as Medicaid and Medicare). They are widely available across the country, in rural areas as well as cities. Each center provides services to a local region, referred to as a *catchment area*. Many centers have multiple satellites throughout their catchment area to reduce transportation costs. In addition, most do some outreach by going to the homes of families.

CMHCs provide services for a wide range of disorders, but their most critical mission is to provide treatment for disorders that are severe and persistent (often called *severe mental illnesses*, or *SMIs*) and result in significant functional impairment. Because schizophrenia is the most debilitating mental illness and the costs of treating it can be staggering, many people get treatment for it at CMHCs. And because this practice is so common, the treatment available at CMHCs is actually better, in many cases, than in the private sector.

The CMHC in your catchment area is required to provide services to you and your family member. Fees are determined based on insurance coverage, eligibility for medical assistance, and your ability to pay.

CMHCs provide a wide range of services, including evaluations, case management, medication services, psychoeducation, individual therapy, group therapy, day treatment/partial hospitalization programs, emergency services, vocational rehabilitation, family therapy, family psychoeducation, residential services, and referrals to other services, such as peer support programs. These services are described later in this chapter. Many centers are also affiliated with community residences, transportation, and vocational and educational programs.

A comprehensive treatment plan for schizophrenia usually includes services that are available at the CMHC. If your relative has a private psychiatrist, she may make a referral to the local CMHC and arrange for an interview, or you or your relative can call to arrange an interview. Phone numbers can usually be found in the government listings pages of the phone book under "Mental Health."

During the first appointment, sometimes referred to as the *intake interview*, your relative's needs will be evaluated and appropriate services determined. Your relative should be prepared to answer questions about current medications, symptoms, hospitalizations, living situation, sources of social support, finances, and personal goals. Certain types of information—insurance cards, medical assistance cards, a list of current medications, and Social Security information—will be helpful to have at the intake interview. The intake interview is an excellent opportunity for your relative to learn which services are available at the CMHC, because no CMHC will provide everything an individual needs. Some examples of questions to ask include:

- "Who will my doctor be?"
- "Will I have an individual therapist or counselor?"
- "What kind of treatment programs are offered?"
- "Is transportation provided?"

- "Are vocational rehabilitation/educational services available?"
- "Can I call you in case of an emergency? If not, whom should I call?"
- "May I have a tour of the facility?"

Private Service Providers

Private-sector alternatives to CMHCs are also available, such as private mental health agencies, local hospitals, private therapists, rehabilitation programs, private psychiatrists, and even family doctors or general practitioners. Your relative's insurance and your financial resources will be the major determinants of eligibility. Ask directly about costs and payment procedures when you inquire about services from a private agency. Don't assume private treatment will not be affordable; many agencies accept insurance and don't charge extra for their services.

Peer-Based Programs for Those with Mental Illness

Some self-help and advocacy groups operate volunteer programs for people with mental illness to gain work experience that may lead to employment. Others provide support groups and social opportunities helpful in recovery. Each state has different organizations available; see the Resources section at the end of the chapter.

National Alliance on Mental Illness

The National Alliance on Mental Illness (NAMI) is an important resource for advocacy, education, and support for individuals, family members, professionals, and anyone else interested in improving the outcome of mental illness. Every state has a NAMI chapter, and many communities have their own chapters. They often offer educational and support groups for family members or individuals with mental illness or both. Other national organizations include the National Mental Health Consumers' Association and the National Mental Health Association. The Resources section at the end of the chapter lists these organizations.

Types of Services and Benefits

Once you've identified the sources of mental health services that you might be able to tap, you'll need to know what types of services are typically offered so you can help determine which might be helpful to your relative.

Professional-Based Outpatient Services

The largest category of services for individuals with mental illness are those provided by professionals in an outpatient setting. You and your relative can use

Worksheet 5.1 at the end of this chapter to check off the services he is already receiving and those he is interested in trying.

Mental Health Evaluations

Your relative's diagnosis and treatment will be based largely on a mental health evaluation conducted by a psychiatrist, psychologist, social worker, or nurse. During the evaluation, your loved one will be asked questions about psychiatric symptoms, what makes her symptoms better or worse, use of alcohol or drugs, what is and is not going well in her life, what kind of social support she has, and what her goals are. The diagnostic process is described in Chapter 2. You may be able to get a diagnostic evaluation at a CMHC or from a private provider; Chapter 2 also tells you how to find a qualified diagnostician in your community.

Medication (Pharmacological Treatment)

Medication is the mainstay of treatment for schizophrenia. Psychiatrists (medical doctors with special training in psychiatric disorders) can prescribe medications, as can general practitioners (such as a family practice doctor). Some clinical nurse specialists can also prescribe medications, as can nurse practitioners and physician assistants. Psychologists generally *cannot* prescribe medications except in certain settings (e.g., in Louisiana specially credentialed psychologists can prescribe medication). When medication is prescribed, the practitioner sees the individual regularly, usually once every month or two, and more often if necessary, to evaluate how well the medication is working and to monitor side effects. Chapter 10 provides more information about medications.

Case Management

Case management is offered as a routine service at most CMHCs, as described later in this chapter. Case managers work with individuals to establish specific treatment goals, address social and financial needs, and coordinate and monitor overall treatment, as well as with members of the treatment team, such as the psychiatrist and therapist or counselor. They make referrals to treatment services and assist people in applying for financial benefits such as Social Security Disability Insurance (SSDI). Case managers often need to coordinate referrals and applications for services with the person, family, psychiatrist, and other mental health treatment providers.

The case manager is usually the first person your relative should contact if she is not getting the services needed. With your relative's permission, you can assist by initiating phone calls or by helping her practice what to say to the case manager. Once your relative has established a relationship with her case manager, she and the case manager will meet on a regular basis to monitor progress toward goals. If your relative agrees, you can also stay in contact with the case manager. Ongoing contact is important to ensure that information is shared among your relative, family members, and the treatment team. Your relative may be asked to sign a *release of information* form so that staff at the mental health center can share information with family members.

Intensive Case Management

Intensive case management services can be helpful to people whose mental illness is severe and results in repeated or prolonged hospitalizations, homelessness, or problems with the law. Intensive case management involves *outreach*—which means that workers provide most needed services to people in their natural living settings, such as their home, rather than at the local CMHC. A comprehensive array of services may be available, such as transportation to appointments, medication monitoring, shopping assistance, training in daily living skills, assistance with accessing financial benefits, and emergency interventions. The overall goal is to strengthen people's skills for coping with their mental illness and living independently in the community. The most widely used intensive case management program is *assertive community treatment (ACT)*, which is described later, in the section on *evidence-based practices*.

Mental Illness Management Programs

These programs focus on providing information and teaching skills for managing mental illness and pursuing personal recovery goals. Programs commonly include information about mental illness and relapse prevention, strategies for taking medication as prescribed and coping with persistent symptoms, and help in pursuing personal goals. More information about these programs is provided in the section on *evidence-based practices*.

Individual Therapy and Counseling

Many people with schizophrenia find it helpful to have a therapist or counselor to talk things over with. The approaches to therapy most helpful to people with schizophrenia are those that provide support, education, practical problem-solving skills, and strategies for coping with symptoms. Cognitive-behavioral therapy is one approach that has widely been studied and shown to improve outcomes in people with schizophrenia. Therapy that focuses primarily on developing insight and exploring the person's past, such as psychodynamic approaches, has not been found to be beneficial for most people with schizophrenia.

Group Therapy and Skills Training

Therapy can also take place in a group format. This format provides participants with social support, feedback, ideas, and role models from others who have had similar experiences. Groups vary in their goals, content, and procedures. Depending on the group's purpose, the sessions may focus on providing emotional support, increasing knowledge, encouraging personal growth, or building coping skills. A wide variety of topics can be addressed, as indicated by the following examples of group names: Coping with Mental Illness, Building Self-Esteem, Anger Management, Communication Skills, Friendship and Dating, Current Events, Problem Solving, Healthy Lifestyle, Stress Management, Relapse Prevention Skills, Men's Issues, Women's Issues, Trauma Empowerment, and Support Group. Groups may be time-limited (such as meeting for 12 sessions) or open-ended (no set number of sessions). Social skills training is one type of group treatment that is an evidence-based practice, which is described in more detail later in this chapter.

Family Education (or Psychoeducation) and Family Therapy

These programs aim at educating families about schizophrenia and reducing tension in the family. Family programs can be provided to individual families or a group, where several families share their experiences and offer each other support and suggestions for solving common problems. Family psychoeducation programs are often offered by local CMHCs and usually involve the whole family, including the person with schizophrenia.

Family psychoeducational services are also available from nonprofessional organizations. NAMI, introduced earlier, is composed primarily of family members, people with mental illness, and concerned professionals. Many NAMI affiliates provide "Family-to-Family," a 12-week program led by family members who have a relative with mental illness and who have been trained to teach families about mental illness, treatment principles, and coping methods. Individuals with schizophrenia are not included.

Substance Abuse Treatment

Many people with schizophrenia and other major mental illnesses also have problems with alcohol or drugs (called *dual disorders*). Programs that simultaneously treat mental illness and substance abuse in a cohesive, integrated fashion are most effective. Sometimes people with dual disorders need inpatient treatment to detoxify from the effects of substances, as described later in this chapter. Chapter 22 provides more detail about the nature and treatment of alcohol and drug problems in people with schizophrenia.

Partial Hospital/Day Treatment Programs

Partial hospital programs (also called *day treatment* or *continuing day treatment programs*) are designed to provide a structured therapeutic environment on an outpatient basis. These programs are usually open daily for about 6 hours, but some people attend for fewer hours a day. Partial hospital programs have a daily routine that usually includes group therapy, skills training, educational groups, and activities such as creative expression, relaxation training, and cooking. They also provide important opportunities for regular socializing.

Vocational Rehabilitation and Educational Programs

Vocational rehabilitation programs help people enter or reenter the work force. A wide range of vocational programs for people with mental illnesses is available, including supported employment programs, an evidence-based practice for helping people find and keep competitive jobs in the community. Some vocational programs exist within CMHCs; others are freestanding agencies. See Chapter 26 for details.

In additional to vocational programs, a growing number of programs help people with mental illnesses pursue educational goals. Some mental health centers have supported educational programs, similar to supported employment programs, designed to help people resume their education. Also, many school districts, trade schools, and colleges have special programs aimed at helping people with psychiatric disabilities get the education they need. Chapter 26 provides more information on helping your relative achieve his educational goals.

Medical and Dental Care

People with schizophrenia have the same medical and dental needs as everyone else, but these needs are often not met. If your relative has not been medically evaluated for illnesses such as diabetes and cardiovascular disease or has not received dental care in the past year, you should arrange for these evaluations to be conducted by the appropriate health care professional. It's important for individuals with schizophrenia to have yearly physicals and biannual dental checkups and to receive prompt treatment for any medical or dental problems that emerge between checkups.

Inpatient Services

Sometimes individuals with mental illnesses need more structure and intensive treatment than can be provided in an outpatient program. Psychiatric hospitalization and detoxification are the primary types of inpatient services.

Psychiatric Hospitalization

Significant increases in symptoms sometimes require hospitalization to protect the person from herself or to protect others. Common services provided by inpatient facilities include medication evaluation, group and individual therapy, classes on managing mental illness, occupational therapy, recreational therapy, and discharge planning. Most hospitalizations are short, ranging from a few days to a few weeks. However, some people with severe symptoms who pose a grave threat to themselves or others require longer inpatient treatment. Sometimes people recognize that they need hospitalization and voluntarily seek admission, but at other times their symptoms may hamper their judgment and they may refuse hospitalization, even when it would ensure their own or others' safety. Guidelines for involuntary admission to a hospital are included in Chapter 13.

Detoxification

People who become addicted to drugs or alcohol may require *detoxification* to withdraw from those substances. Detoxification involves closely monitoring a physically dependent person who has stopped using substances and providing support (and sometimes medication) to manage the withdrawal symptoms. Outpatient detoxification is often successful, but inpatient detoxification may be needed to address significant medical concerns or ensure abstinence.

Peer-Based Services

People who have experienced the symptoms of psychiatric disorders often find it helpful to share information, support, and encouragement with those who have had similar experiences—called *peers*, *consumers*, or *psychiatric survivors*. Peer-based services are available in a variety of forms.

Consumer-Led Programs and Peer Support

Consumer-led programs offer support groups, education, wellness strategies, drop-in centers, and recreational opportunities, among other services. Some consumer-led programs are provided by independent organizations, such as the Wellness Recovery Action Plan (WRAP) developed by Mary Ellen Copeland of Brattleboro, Vermont, which has helped thousands of people across the country.

Self-Help Groups

Self-help organizations have been important to individuals with many different life challenges, particularly addictive disorders, with the largest and oldest such organization being Alcoholics Anonymous (AA). Variations of AA have been developed for persons who also have a major mental illness; Dual Recovery Anonymous (see Chapter 22) is one example. See the Resources section at the end of the chapter for help in finding self-help groups, or try a computer search, newspaper announcements, or your local phone directory.

Advocacy Organizations

In addition to *Family-to-Family* (described on p. 64), NAMI sponsors a variety of programs, including *In Our Own Voice* (educational presentations in which consumers talk to community audiences about their experiences with mental illness and recovery), *Peer-to-Peer* (a consumer-led educational program for other consumers about coping with mental illness and moving forward in recovery), *NAMI Care* (consumer-led support group), and *Hearts and Minds* (a health program focused on providing information about diabetes, diet, exercise, and smoking). Some NAMI affiliates also have lending libraries that make available books, videos, and other resources for coping with mental illness. Other advocacy organizations can be found in the Resources section at the end of this chapter.

Residential Programs and Housing Services

Housing and residential services are generally aimed at helping people with a mental illness live as independently as possible while providing support that allows them to meet their basic living needs. The housing options available to your relative depend on the level of assistance or support needed, financial resources, and what types of housing are available in your community. Keep in mind that you can help your relative improve skills for living independently and caring for himself, as described in Chapter 27.

Residential Programs

A variety of different residential programs may be available, depending on your state and area. The names of these programs vary across regions and include *board and care homes, domiciliary care, personal care group homes,* and *community residential rehabilitation centers*. Residential programs typically provide a range of services to help the people live in the community, such as supervision (24 hours or less for more independent individuals), meals, rehabilitation, and training in independent living skills such as cooking, grooming, and money management. Some housing programs limit how long a resident can stay. Although levels of structure and supervision vary, most residential programs have a formal admission process and specific rules, and some require residents to be involved in a treatment program or activity during the day.

Supported Housing

Through this service people receive support from professional staff to live in their own apartments. Housing support staff may check in to make sure your relative's needs are met, but your relative will be responsible for meal preparation, laundry, and other aspects of independent living. Supported housing allows people to live in their own place but may make them feel more socially isolated than those living in residential programs. Strategies for addressing this isolation are described in Chapter 25.

Rental Assistance Programs

Section 8 is a tenant-based rental assistance program available through the U.S. Department of Housing and Urban Development (HUD). Under this program, a person pays either 30% of her adjusted income, 10% of gross income, or the welfare assistance amount designated for housing. A certificate or voucher pays the remainder of the rent to the landlord. Section 8 assistance is in great demand, and there may be a waiting list.

HUD's Chapter 9 Housing Program offers landlords an incentive to provide housing for people with disabilities, but the demand for this housing is also high.

Respite Care

Some communities have special respite residences or crisis centers where your loved one can spend a few days under close supervision while a crisis abates, thereby avoiding hospitalization. Respite residences may be staffed by professionals, consumers, or a combination.

Financial and Health Insurance Benefits

A variety of benefits programs help people with insufficient resources meet their basic needs. If you or your family member with schizophrenia feel embarrassed about needing assistance, remember that your family is part of a larger community in which everyone deserves this support.

Financial Benefits

Your relative's case manager, social worker, or benefits counselor can assist you and your loved one in understanding the benefits available and how to apply for them. Application procedures can be confusing and time-consuming, so your relative may appreciate your help, too.

Organization and good will go a long way toward securing the benefits your relative is entitled to. Keep all of your relative's documents in one place and record dates and the names of people you talk to during the application process. This will prove especially critical if you have to apply for a benefit more than once.

Social Security Disability Insurance and Supplemental Security Income

Most major benefits are provided by the federal, state, or county government, though anyone who has served in the military may be eligible for benefits from the Veterans Administration. Social Security Disability Insurance (SSDI) and Supplemental Security Income (SSI) are given to individuals whose psychiatric (or physical) disability prevents them from working enough to support themselves, as documented by a qualified mental health professional.

To be eligible for SSDI, your loved one (1) must have worked a significant amount in the past and contributed money to Social Security, (2) must be currently unable to work, and (3) will not be able to work for at least the next year because of the psychiatric illness. SSDI is provided to people regardless of whether they have other (non-work-related) sources of income.

SSI is given to people who are currently unable to work because of their psychiatric disorder and have not worked in the past or worked for only a short time. To be eligible, your relative's income and assets must not exceed a certain amount (not including any financial support you may be providing).

Public Assistance

Financial benefits provided by different states or local communities are often referred to as *public assistance, temporary assistance for needy families* (TANF), or *welfare.* To be eligible for public assistance, your relative must have insufficient income from other sources (including SSDI or SSI) and, in some cases, show that he is unable to work because of illness. Eligibility requirements vary by location. Payments from public assistance are usually quite modest. Your relative can apply for public assistance at the Office of Public Assistance (welfare office).

Food Credits

Low-income individuals may also be eligible for stamps or an electronic benefits transfer card that can be used to buy food (but not non-food items such as cigarettes or alcohol). Your loved one can apply for food credits at the Office of Public Assistance.

Transportation Benefits

Ask your relative's case manager or check the government listings of the telephone directory to find out about transportation benefits. Some mental health and vocational agencies provide transportation to their programs, and your city, state, or county may provide transportation for people who receive medical assistance or have a disability. Advance registration for these programs is required.

Some bus and subway companies offer reduced fares for those with mental illness, but possibly only to people who are receiving other mental health benefits, such as Medicaid, SSI, or SSDI. Consult regional transportation companies or your relative's caseworker.

The table on page 71 summarizes the major financial benefits available to people with mental illnesses. The specific eligibility criteria and the amount of the financial award may vary from year to year. Call the appropriate federal office (look under "Social Security Administration" in the phone book) or state office (look under "Public Assistance" or "Public Welfare") to get current application information or ask your relative's case manager.

Health Insurance Benefits

Health insurance benefits for people with mental illness are provided by local (state or county) and federal governments, as well as by the VA for those who have served in the military.

State health care insurance is usually called *medical assistance* or *Medicaid*, and is available to those with insufficient income from personal resources and, in some cases, to those who can prove they are disabled by illness. Covered expenses—inpatient bills, outpatient bills, prescriptions, etc.—vary by state and depend on the severity of the illness.

Federal health insurance is part of the Medicare program. Your loved one will be eligible for Medicare if he has been disabled by a psychiatric illness, cannot work full-time, and has been receiving SSDI for more than 2 years. Like SSDI, Medicare is provided whether or not your relative has other (non-work-related) sources of income. If she receives SSI and is not eligible for SSDI, her medical assistance/medicaid will probably cover most routine medical expenses incurred by the illness.

The table on page 72 summarizes available health insurance benefits.

Appealing Decisions

The Social Security Administration and local state programs have procedures for appealing eligibility decisions. If you feel a decision was not made correctly, you have the right to file an appeal, so inquire about the appeal process when you apply.

Community-Based Resources Not Related to Mental Illness

As part of pursuing recovery, expanding their social relationships, and becoming more active in their own community, many people with schizophrenia enjoy participating in activities available to everyone, such as religious services, classes, clubs, volunteer opportunities, and the arts. In thinking about what would be

Benefit	Who is eligible?	Based on disability?	Based on financial need?	Health care insurance provided?	Where to apply?
Social Security Disability Insurance (SSDI)	Persons who are now disabled but worked in the past and contributed to Social Security (or in some cases, whose parents contributed)	Yes	No	After 2 years of receiving SSDI, people are eligible for Medicare	Social Security Administration office
Supplemental Security Income (SSI)	Persons who are disabled and do not qualify for SSDI (or qualify for only small amounts of SSDI) and have limited income and assets	Yes	Yes	Medicaid	Social Security Administration office
Public assistance or welfare	Low-income adults who have serious mental health problems and meet state criteria	Yes, but criteria are not as stringent as Social Security Administration programs	Yes	Usually Medicaid is provided	Office of Public Assistance or welfare office
Food stamps	Low-income adults who meet state criteria	No	Yes	No	Office of Public Assistance or welfare office
Transportation	Varies by state	Varies by state	Varies by state	No	Office of Public Assistance, local mass transit companies, community mental health centers

Financial Benefits for Individuals with Mental Illness

| Health Insurance Benefits for Individuals with Mental Illness | | | | |
Benefit	Who is eligible?	Based on disability?	Based on financial need?	What is usually covered?	Where to apply?
Medicare	Disabled persons who have been entitled to SSDI for more than 2 years	Yes	No	Inpatient and outpatient bills, subject to deductibles, copayments, and "ceilings" for certain services	Social Security Administration office
Medicaid, also known as medical assistance	Low-income persons who meet state or county criteria	Yes	Yes	Inpatient and outpatient bills, subject to small copayments and restrictions on reimbursements	Office of Public Assistance
Private insurance	Varies by policy	Varies by policy	No	Varies by policy	Check with your insurance provider

helpful to your relative, it's important to include community-based resources that are open to everyone.

Clergy

Members of the clergy can be very helpful in addressing your relative's spiritual needs, and many also have some training in counseling and are especially understanding of people who have mental illnesses. Although interest in religion varies from person to person, many individuals with schizophrenia find that religious services are comforting and make them feel part of a larger community.

Classes

Community educational opportunities can help your relative pursue personal interests while meeting people. General equivalency diploma (GED) courses and classes at local colleges or music schools can allow your loved one to further his education. Your relative might also enjoy hands-on lessons in art, cooking, or computer skills. Many communities have evening adult education classes for exploring subjects such as history, travel, foreign languages, and yoga.

Volunteer Opportunities

Volunteer opportunities are available in most communities, such as delivering meals to senior citizens ("Meals on Wheels"), assisting in an animal shelter or zoo, shelving library books, working in a soup kitchen, and participating in home-building/repair programs such as Habitat for Humanity.

Lectures

The events/weekend section of the local newspaper often lists lectures that are open to the public. These lectures may be sponsored by bookstores, libraries, museums, churches, colleges, high schools, or clubs. Sometimes they include free screenings of films.

Musical Performances

Free or low-cost concerts are often sponsored by music schools, churches, museums, universities, and municipalities. In the summer free outdoor concerts in parks or city squares may also be offered.

Museums

Your relative may be interested in exploring a museum's collection, whether it's a museum of art, history, science, paleontology, anthropology, or natural history. Most museums have free or reduced-admission days, and larger art museums sometimes offer weekly or monthly concerts or films that are included in the price of admission. Some museums also offer low-cost classes related to their collections.

Special-Interest Organizations and Clubs

Your relative may have an interest that he could pursue by participating in an organization or club devoted to nature, conservation, folk music, folk dancing, hiking, history, sports, travel, or any of various hobbies. Attending the meetings of such organizations also allows your relative to meet others with similar interests.

Family-Based Resources

You and your family are probably an important resource for your loved one with schizophrenia. Part V of this book describes the role families can play in helping a loved one cope with common symptoms in schizophrenia. Part VI focuses on how families can work with a relative toward achieving common recovery goals, including social relationships, work (or completing school), leisure and recreational activities, and self-care skills and independent living.

Evidence-Based Practices

As described in the first part of this chapter, many professional-based services and resources address the needs of people with mental illnesses. Some of these services have been evaluated rigorously in carefully controlled scientific studies and have been shown to improve functioning in people with schizophrenia. These services are called *evidence-based practices*. A variety of different researchers and groups have been involved in defining evidence-based practices, and although they generally agree on the criteria, there is some disagreement regarding the exact practices themselves. Evidence-based practices BPs are usually defined as interventions that . . .

- Are standardized.
- Have been studied in multiple rigorous (controlled) scientific studies.
- Have been studied by different investigator teams.
- Have been shown to improve important outcomes in well-defined groups.

Researchers from the Substance Abuse and Mental Health Services Administration (SAMHSA) and Robert Wood Johnson Foundation have identified a set of five psychosocial evidence-based practices (plus one focused on medication) available in the form of implementation toolkits that can be downloaded from the Web (*mentalhealth.samhsa.gov*). Other groups have proposed their own lists. Our list includes all the SAMHSA psychosocial practices, plus three others that have good evidence supporting them. Exclusion from this list does not mean that other interventions are not also effective; they simply may not have been carefully evaluated yet in scientific studies or research is underway.

The table on pages 75–77 summarizes the evidence supporting these practices. The pages that follow describe current evidence-based practices for schizophrenia so that you can help determine which services are most important to access for your relative.

Medication

Antipsychotic medications are crucial to the treatment of schizophrenia, with hundreds of studies documenting their effectiveness. A standardized approach to prescribing medication and evaluating its effects is called *medication management approaches in psychiatry* (MedMAP). MedMAP is a systematic method of help-

Psychosocial Interventions for Schizophrenia That Are Supported by Research

Psychosocial treatment	Goals	Treatment description	Research evidence[a]
Assertive community treatment (ACT)	• Engage people in treatment who do not regularly attend outpatient clinics • Improve coordinated delivery of services to people who are prone to frequent relapses, rehospitalizations, and long-term institutionalization	• More intensive services provided because staff members are responsible for treating fewer people than in traditional services (e.g., staff:client ratios = 1:10 in ACT vs. 1:30 or more in traditional services) • Most services provided in person's natural environment (e.g., home, street) • Most services provided directly by ACT teams rather than by other treatment providers • 24-hour responsibility for individuals • Clinicians on ACT team share responsibility for a group of individuals, rather than each clinician being solely responsible for a set number of people	• Reduced symptoms and rehospitalizations • Improved housing stability and quality of life • High satisfaction with services • Less costly for people who need the most services
Family psychoeducation	• Establish a collaborative relationship between person, family, and treatment team • Improve monitoring of psychiatric illness and response to early signs of relapse • Reduce burden of care on family • Increase family support for person with schizophrenia	• Long-term (>6 months) • Single-family or multiple-family formats • Future oriented, not past oriented • Focus on psychoeducation, improved communication, and problem-solving skills • Focus on helping *all* family members pursue shared and personal goals	• Reduced relapses and rehospitalizations • Decreased family stress and care load

(cont.)

Psychosocial Interventions for Schizophrenia That Are Supported by Research (*cont.*)

Psychosocial treatment	Goals	Treatment description	Research evidence[a]
Supported employment	• Help find and keep regular jobs in the community	• Focus on competitive jobs • Attention to person's preferences in job type and employment support • Rapid job search rather than extensive assessment and training process • Integration of vocational and clinical services • Provision of follow-along support	• Improved rates of competitive employment, hours worked, wages earned
Social skills training	• Increase social skills in making friends, having conversations, resolving conflict, expressing feelings, assertiveness, dealing with problems on the job, and developing leisure and recreational activities	• Group skills training occurs over at least several months • Trips provided to the community (or other natural settings) to practice skills	• Improved social and leisure functioning
Training in illness management skills	• Improve understanding of schizophrenia and its management • Increase medication adherence • Prevent relapses and rehospitalizations • Enhance coping with distressful symptoms	• Education about illness • Development of strategies for taking medication regularly • Development of relapse prevention plans	• Increased knowledge about schizophrenia • Increased medication adherence • Fewer relapses and rehospitalizations • Reduced distress due to symptoms

Intervention	Goal	Methods	Outcomes
Cognitive-behavioral therapy for psychosis	• Reduce severity of persistent psychotic symptoms	• Exploration of events and circumstances in person's life when psychotic symptoms develop • Consideration of different explanations for delusional beliefs or hallucinations • "Behavioral tests" to examine beliefs related to psychotic symptoms	• Reduced severity of psychotic symptoms • Reduced severity of negative symptoms
Integrated treatment for mental illness and substance abuse	• Decrease substance abuse	• Treatment of schizophrenia and substance abuse provided by the same team of clinicians • Outreach used to engage reluctant individuals • Motivation-based interventions geared to keep people interested in treatment • Reducing harmful consequences of substance abuse is a major focus	• Decreased substance abuse

[a]Research evidence supporting psychosocial interventions for schizophrenia:

Assertive community treatment (ACT): Bond, G. R., Drake, R. E., Mueser, K. T., & Latimer, E. (2001). Assertive community treatment for people with severe mental illness: Critical ingredients and impact on clients. *Disease Management and Health Outcomes, 9,* 141–159.

Family psychoeducation: Pitschel-Walz, G., Leucht, S., Bäuml, J., Kissling, W., & Engel, R. R. (2001). The effect of family interventions on relapse and rehospitalization in schizophrenia: A meta-analysis. *Schizophrenia Bulletin, 27,* 73–92.

Supported employment: Bond, G. R., Becker, D. R., Drake, R. E., Rapp, C. A., Meisler, N., Lehman, A. F., et al. (2001). Implementing supported employment as an evidence-based practice. *Psychiatric Services, 52,* 313–322.

Social skills training: Bellack, A. S. (2004). Skills training for people with severe mental illness. *Psychiatric Rehabilitation Journal, 27,* 375–391.

Training in illness management skills: Mueser, K. T., Corrigan, P. W., Hilton, D., Tanzman, B., Schaub, A., Gingerich, S., et al. (2002). Illness management and recovery for severe mental illness: A review of the research. *Psychiatric Services, 53,* 1272–1284.

Cognitive-behavioral therapy for psychosis: Pilling, S., Bebbington, P., Kuipers, E., Garety, P., Geddes, J. R., Orbach, G., et al. (2002). Psychological treatments in schizophrenia: I. Meta-analysis of family intervention and cognitive behaviour therapy. *Psychological Medicine, 32,* 763–782.

Integrated treatment for mental illness and substance abuse: Drake, R. E., Mueser, K. T., Brunette, M. F., & McHugo, G. J. (2004). A review of treatments for clients with severe mental illness and co-occurring substance use disorder. *Psychiatric Rehabilitation Journal, 27,* 360–374.

ing prescribers and individuals work together to find medications that work best for them. When a new medication is being started, the individual meets with the prescriber on a frequent basis to discuss symptoms. Symptom severity, side effects, and functioning are evaluated at each visit. With the permission of the individual, family members can offer helpful input about symptoms and side effects.

Family Psychoeducation

Several different approaches to teaching families about mental illness and how to cope with it have been shown to be effective. Some involve teaching specific communication and problem-solving skills to help family members get along better and deal with common problems. Some involve working with individual families, in the home or clinic, whereas others involve multiple-family groups. Unlike the family-led programs offered by organizations like NAMI, family psychoeducation is provided by mental health professionals.

Illness Management and Recovery

Illness management and recovery (IMR) is a step-by-step program that helps people set meaningful goals, learn to manage their psychiatric illness, and make progress toward their recovery. The program, provided weekly in either individual or small-group sessions, helps people put strategies into action in their everyday lives. The structured curriculum consists of the following 10 modules:

- Recovery strategies
- Practical facts about mental illness
- The stress–vulnerability model
- Building social support
- Using medication effectively
- Substance use
- Reducing relapses
- Coping with stress
- Coping with problems and symptoms
- Getting your needs met in the mental health system

Supported Employment

Supported employment programs help people find and keep competitive jobs in the community. These programs are staffed by employment specialists who are often members of the treatment team and who meet regularly with other team members to integrate employment goals with mental health treatment. These specialists help people look for jobs in their areas of interest soon after entering the program and provide support as long as it's needed.⏋

Integrated Mental Health and Substance Abuse (Dual Disorders) Treatment

This approach offers mental health and substance abuse services in one setting, at the same time. The same clinician or team develops a personalized treatment plan with the individual that addresses both disorders. A variety of services are offered, such as basic education about the disorders, case management, specialized counseling to enhance motivation, cognitive-behavioral counseling, and help with housing, money management, and relationships. Clinicians take a long-term perspective, and services are not time-limited.

Assertive Community Treatment

Assertive community treatment or ACT is an intensive team approach that helps people with very severe symptoms avoid hospitalization, incarceration, and homelessness and enables them to function as well as possible in the community. ACT services are provided by practitioners who work closely together and provide most services in the community (e.g., in the home or at a local coffee shop) rather than at the local clinic. A wide range of different services is provided by ACT teams, such as assistance in meeting daily needs, skills training, and teaching people how to manage their mental illness. Services are provided for as long as they are needed.

Cognitive–Behavioral Therapy for Psychosis

Cognitive-behavioral therapy reduces the severity of, and interference caused by, persistent psychotic symptoms such as hallucinations and delusions. The therapist develops a collaborative relationship with the person, and then explores the development of psychotic symptoms, considering various coping strategies, and creating alternative explanations for those experiences. Cognitive-behavioral therapy is usually provided on an individual basis but may also take place in a group format.

Social Skills Training

Social skills training is a systematic approach to teaching people more effective interpersonal skills that foster closer, more comfortable relationships with others. The training is most often done in a group and involves breaking down complex interaction skills into more manageable steps and then practicing these steps in role plays and real-life situations. Groups may focus on a wide range of social skills, such as making friends, having conversations, resolving conflicts, self-assertion, developing leisure activities, and handling social situations at work.

Confidentiality

As mentioned earlier, to protect your relative's right to privacy, mental health agencies must have written permission from him (commonly called a *release of information*) to give out information, even to family members. Each agency has a printed release form, which usually specifies the type of information that can be released, the person (or agency) to whom it can be released, and the time period covered (such as six months).

Most people with schizophrenia see the value of keeping their family involved and informed about their illness and its treatment, but if your relative's illness makes him suspicious about signing forms or causes delusions about family members, he may refuse to sign the release. Some states, therefore, have special regulations that allow family members access to information that is crucial to the health and well-being of their relative (diagnosis, admission to or discharge from a treatment facility, the name and possible side effects of the medicine prescribed, treatment plans, behavioral management strategies) without consent. The person with the illness must be living with the family member, or the family member must be providing direct care.

Getting What You Need
from the Mental Health System

People sometimes have difficulty getting their needs met in the mental health system. This difficulty is compounded by the uncertainty of where to go to get questions answered. Common questions of family members include:

- "What can be done about medication side effects?"
- "What kind of educational programs are available to help me and my relative learn more about schizophrenia?"
- "What types of support are available to help my relative live independently in the community?"
- "How can my relative learn better social skills for making friends?"
- "Is there some therapy available to help my relative cope better with symptoms?"
- "How can my relative overcome his depression?"
- "Is there any help my relative can get for learning how to parent her young child?"

- "Are there any new medications that might be more effective for my relative?"
- "How can my relative get supported employment?"
- "What can be done to help my relative stay out of the hospital?"

One key to helping you get what you need from the mental health system is to develop a good relationship your relative's treatment team. Staff members usually appreciate hearing from caring family members. If possible, identify a staff member who might be helpful as an advocate or spokesperson for your concerns. It's reassuring to feel that someone understands your point of view and shares your desire to help your relative. When problems do come up, the following guidelines may help you address them.

1. *Keep a record of the details of the problem and what you've tried to do about it.* Write down the dates, who was involved, and whether you spoke to someone about your concern. Keep a copy of any applications you made or letters you wrote concerning the problem. Keep all the information in one folder.

2. *With your relative's permission, talk over the problems with the treatment provider most directly involved.* For example, if your relative needs a referral, speak to the case manager. If you have questions about the rules of a community residence, consult the residence director. If you're concerned about medication side effects or worsening symptoms, speak to the psychiatrist or nurse. Keep in mind that it is generally not helpful to complain to secretaries and other office staff members, because they are not involved with your relative's treatment.

3. *Communicate your concerns calmly and clearly.* Be as well informed and organized as possible in your interactions with mental health professionals. You may find it useful to make notes about your concerns before raising them. When speaking, be assertive but also listen to what the other person says. Stay focused on the problem and persist in seeking a solution.

4. *Take additional action if you're not satisfied after speaking with a staff person.* Sometimes you'll have to speak with more than one person to get your relative's needs met. If you don't get what you need from one staff member, try talking with another, who may be able to intercede on your behalf. In some cases you may have to talk with a supervisor.

5. *Follow through promptly on suggestions that require action from you.* You may choose not to take every suggestion, but act as quickly as possible on those that seem reasonable so you'll know the results. When one doesn't work, the person may be able to make another suggestion. It also helps to check back with others to see if they have followed up on what they agreed to do. Persistence often leads to a solution, even when the problem initially seems overwhelming.

6. *Let people know you appreciate their efforts.* Expressing your appreciation makes others more likely to continue helping you and your relative, and it creates a positive atmosphere.

7. *If your attempts to find a solution fail, contact the "designated problem solver" at the agency.* Most CMHCs and inpatient facilities have at least one staff member (often called the *consumer advocate* or *consumer liaison*) assigned to help people solve problems with receiving services. There may be a department designed to assist in this process, called something like the *Office of Consumer Affairs*. You can also call the director of the agency. In addition, organizations such as NAMI will help advocate for families.

8. *Keep trying, even in the face of obstacles.* You may not be able to get every need fully met. However, persisting in an assertive, diplomatic manner usually results in important improvements.

Many Hands Make Light Work

Determining your relative's needs and accessing necessary services and other community resources may seem like a formidable challenge. However, you don't need to shoulder this responsibility alone. Collaboration with others—mental health professionals, your relative, other family members, friends, and advocacy organizations such as NAMI—can lighten your burden and increase your success in helping your relative get her needs met. Your family and community contain a rich variety of resources that can be tapped through creative thinking, reaching out, and networking with others who have common concerns.

Putting It All Together

The goal of Part I of this book has been to guide you in working with your relative and mental health professionals to make sure he gets an accurate diagnosis, develops a vision of recovery, and receives the services that will meet his treatment needs. Josh's family (described below) has been through this critical process, with everyone focused on the priority of Josh's treatment needs. Like Josh, your relative's needs will vary over time.

For several weeks, Josh, a college student, had been easily distracted and found it difficult to concentrate on his schoolwork. At times he thought he heard a voice calling his name, even though no one was around. He felt very uneasy but didn't tell anyone. Although he had been an occasional drinker, he began to drink two or three beers daily in an effort to relax and take his mind off his worries. When he came home at spring break, his parents noticed several changes in his behavior, including sleeping a lot and avoiding interaction with family members. He made no effort to get together with friends and didn't return their phone calls. When his parents expressed concern, Josh said that he wasn't feeling like his usual self but didn't get more specific. He agreed to get a checkup from his regular physician, who found no physical problems.

When Josh returned to school, he continued to have problems with concentration, and the voice he had been hearing became louder and began telling him he was stupid and would never succeed at college. His grades declined dramatically, and he became paranoid that his roommate was the source of the critical voice he heard. He was drinking four or five beers every day. One day near the end of the semester, Josh became afraid and tearful and called his parents, asking them to pick him up because "I can't go on with all this pressure." They could get no more details from their son on the phone and were extremely concerned, so they drove to the university and brought him home.

When Josh finally told his parents about hearing voices, they realized his problems were more complex than they had originally thought and required going further than their regular doctor. While his father sat with Josh, his mother called as many people as possible to get references for a psychiatrist, including their physician, a friend who worked as a social worker at a psychiatric clinic, and a neighbor who had been receiving treatment for depression. Two of their contacts recommended the same psychiatrist, and Josh's mother called her immediately. Because Josh was becoming more anxious and fearful, one parent stayed with him at all times while they waited for the appointment with the psychiatrist the next day.

To diagnose Josh's symptoms, the psychiatrist talked to both him and his parents. After carefully interviewing everyone, she told Josh and his parents that he was experiencing the symptoms of schizophrenia and explained the basic facts about the disorder and how medication can help relieve the symptoms. At first Josh refused to take medications, saying he was just under stress at school and now that he was home he would be fine. After the doctor explored his concerns further and discussed the advantages and disadvantages of taking medications, he agreed to "give them a try." The psychiatrist gave Josh and his parents handouts about schizophrenia, referred them to books about the subject, and suggested contacting NAMI.

For the next 6 months, the treatment priority was to get Josh's symptoms under control. During this time Josh's parents read about the illness and attended two NAMI meetings. The first medication helped reduce the voices, but he still heard them and was distracted by them. An increase in the dosage decreased the voices further, but Josh said he felt "foggy and sleepy all the time." The second medication the psychiatrist tried was more successful in controlling the hallucinations without sleepiness, and for a few weeks Josh said, "I feel like my old self." However, he then decided that he was "cured" and no longer needed to take medications.

Without telling anyone, Josh went to the medicine cabinet each day as if he were going to take his pills–but instead threw them in the trash. When his symptoms returned and his parents noticed he was more irritable, talking to himself, and drinking more beer, they became concerned. Although he insisted nothing was wrong, he agreed to see his psychiatrist "just to get you guys off my back." After much discussion, Josh admitted to his psychiatrist that he had stopped taking his pills. He also acknowledged that he had heard fewer voices and felt less fearful while taking the medications, and reluctantly agreed to resume taking them. This time his parents asked him to use a weekly pill box and to take his medication at mealtimes so they could monitor it.

When Josh had been taking his medication consistently for several months, his symp-

toms were under better control. However, he was spending all his time at home, without any outside activities, and was continuing to drink three or four beers a day. Josh's parents suggested meeting with the psychiatrist so they could work together to figure out the next steps in Josh's treatment. At the appointment, the doctor said the first priorities of treatment (receiving an accurate diagnosis and getting symptoms under the best control possible) had been accomplished; it was time to look at other treatment needs so Josh could move on with his life.

The psychiatrist reviewed a list of possible treatment areas, and Josh said he was most interested in treatment that would help him get back to school. He said he still felt "shaky" about interacting with other people, however, and wanted to "build up to returning to college." His parents said they were also concerned about his drinking because it was interfering with his concentration and motivation. Josh disagreed, saying he did not have a drinking problem and did not want to pursue treatment in that area. The psychiatrist recommended that Josh contact the local CMHC, which offered classes in social skills, to help him build up his confidence about talking with others. She also proposed a supported education program, which, she explained, helped people with mental illness return to school. Lastly, the psychiatrist recommended an integrated treatment program at the CMHC for people who have mental illness and use drugs or alcohol.

Josh benefited from the social skills program and supported education program. His parents completed the NAMI Family-to-Family program and learned more strategies for coping with their son's illness. After receiving a ticket and large fine for driving while intoxicated, Josh finally agreed to take part in the integrated treatment program for mental illness and substance use. About 2 years after receiving a diagnosis, with the ongoing support of his parents and his continued participation in treatment, Josh felt ready to resume his college classes.

Resources

Information, Self-Help, and Advocacy Organizations

Center for Mental Health Services (CMHS)
800-540-0320 (contact person for anti-stigma resources center)
www.mentalhealth.samhsa.gov/cmhs/

— Provides information on a variety of services and programs for people with a mental illness, including information about the illness, housing assistance, and anti-stigma campaigns.

Consumer Organization and Networking Technical Assistance Center (CONTAC)
800-598-8847
www.contac.org

— Provides technical assistance to adults with psychiatric disability throughout the United States.

GROW
Illinois Branch Center
2403 West Springfield
Champaign, IL 61821
217-352-6989 or 618-632-7366
— A self-help organization that encourages people to share their experiences and strengthen each other through support and encouragement.

Mental Health Recovery
802-254-2092
www.mentalhealthrecovery.com
— This program, developed by Mary Ellen Copeland, has books and programs for helping people in the recovery process, including the Wellness Recovery Action Plan (WRAP). The website offers a free newsletter and articles and a list of publications and workshops that can be purchased.

Mental Illness Education Project (MIEP)
800-343-5540
miepvideos.org
— Seeks to improve understanding of mental illness through the production of videotapes for people with psychiatric disorders, their families, mental health practitioners, administrators, educators, and the general public.

National Alliance on Mental Illness (NAMI)
800-950-NAMI (helpline)
www.nami.org
— A support and advocacy organization of people with mental illness, their families and friends. It provides educational and support groups for families and consumers, supports increased funding for research, and advocates for adequate health insurance, housing, rehabilitation, and employment for people with psychiatric disabilities. Each state has a chapter, and many communities have their own chapters.

National Empowerment Center (NEC)
www.power2u.org
— An award-winning provider of mental health information, programs, and materials with a focus on recovery. It can refer you to a local support group or help you set up a new group. Newsletter and audiovisual materials are also available.

National Institute of Mental Health (NIMH)
www.nimh.nih.gov
— A government-funded organization engaged in research on the causes and treatment of mental disorders. Its website provides educational materials and an excellent list of free publications on psychiatric disorders, including a comprehensive listing of resources.

National Mental Health Association (NMHA)
www.nmha.org
— Provides information and referral services for people in the process of recovery.

National Mental Health Consumers' Self-Help Clearinghouse
www.mhselfhep.org
— Provides information about psychiatric disorders, technical support for existing or newly starting self-help groups, and a free quarterly newsletter for people with mental illness. They sponsor an annual conference. Spanish language services are available.

National Mental Health Information Center
800-789-2647
www.mentalhealth.samhsa.gov
— Part of the Substance Abuse and Mental Health Services Administration (SAMHSA), this clearinghouse formerly known as the Knowledge Exchange Network (KEN) offers free information about mental health, including publications, references, and referrals to local and national resources and organizations. Click on "Publications" and select "Online Publications" for helpful handouts, booklets, and information.

Recovery, Inc.
www.recovery-inc.com
— Encourages a program of attending weekly meetings and reading books by Abraham Low, MD.

United States Psychiatric Rehabilitation Association (USPRA)
601 North Hammonds Ferry Road, Suite A
Linthicum, MD 21090
410-789-7654; fax, 410-789-7675
www.uspra.org
— USPRA, formerly known as the International Association of Psychosocial Rehabilitation Services, is a nonprofit organization committed to promoting, supporting, and strengthening community-based psychosocial rehabilitation services and resources. It also publishes a journal, newsletters, and a resource catalog.

WRAP
See "Mental Health Recovery" listing.

Note: Many states and local communities have self-help and advocacy organizations, such as **the Pennsylvania Mental Health Consumers' Association** (717-564-4930 or *www. pmhca.org*) and Advocacy Unlimited (860-667-0460 or *www.mindlink.org*) in Connecticut.

Books

Clay, S., Schell, B., Corrigan, P., & Ralph, R. (Eds.). (2005). *On our own, together: Peer programs for people with mental illness*. Nashville, TN: Vanderbilt University Press. Meeting other people with mental illness who are positive role models is one of the many advantages of participating in peer programs, especially if your relative experiences self-stigmatization. This is an excellent book that provides a history of peer support, describes different types of peer support programs (such as drop-in centers, peer support and mentoring, and educational programs), and provides information about finding a local peer support program.

Smith, G., Kennedy, C., Knipper, S., & O'Brien, J. (2005). *Using Medicaid to support working age adults with serious mental illnesses in the community: A handbook.* Rockville, MD: U.S. Department of Health and Human Services, Office of the Assistant Secretary for Planning and Evaluation. Medicaid is an important source of funding for mental health and related services for people with schizophrenia and other severe mental illnesses. This handbook explains how Medicaid options and services are used by states to finance a range of community supports and services for people with severe mental illnesses and describes what aspects of those services are funded by Medicaid. Can be downloaded from: *http://aspe.hhs.gov/daltcp/reports/handbook.pdf.*

Winerip, M. (1994). *9 Highland Road: Sane living for the mentally ill.* New York: Pantheon. This book provides an excellent account of the lives of persons with a mental illness living in a community group home, and their relationships with each other, professional staff, and family members.

Evidence-Based Practices Noted in This Chapter

SAMHSA Implementation Resource Kits

The Substance Abuse and Mental Health Services Agency (SAMHSA) is a cosponsor of a project that identified six evidence-based practices to be developed into implementation resource kits. These practices include supported employment, integrated dual disorder treatment, family psychoeducation, and assertive community treatment. These practices are described in this chapter and on their website: *www.samhsa.gov.*

Social Skills Training

UCLA Social Skills Training Modules, Psychiatric Rehabilitation Consultants
805-484-5663
www.psychrehab.com

Bellack, A. S., Mueser, K. T., Gingerich, S., & Agresta, J. (2004). *Social skills training for schizophrenia: A step-by-step guide* (2nd ed.). New York: Guilford Press.

Cognitive-Behavioral Therapy for Psychosis

Fowler, D., Garety, P., & Kuipers, E. (1995). *Cognitive behaviour therapy for psychosis: Theory and practice.* Chichester, West Sussex, UK: Wiley.

Kingdon, D. G., & Turkington, D. (2004). *Treatment manual for cognitive therapy of schizophrenia.* New York: Guilford Press.

Morrison, A. P., Renton, J. C., Dunn, H., Williams, S., & Bentall, R. P. (2004). *Cognitive therapy for psychosis: A formulation-based approach.* New York: Brunner-Routledge.

Outpatient and Residential Services

Instructions: Review this worksheet with your relative and check off the services that he or she is receiving and those that he or she would like to try. Help your relative make a plan for accessing the services that he or she is interested in.

Type of service	Already receiving	Interested in receiving
Professional-Based Services		
Mental health evaluation		
Medication services		
Case management		
Intensive case management/assertive community treatment		
Illness management programs		
Individual therapy		
Group therapy		
Social skills training		
Family education and family therapy programs		
Treatment for substance abuse		
Partial hospital/day treatment programs		
Vocational rehabilitation programs		
Educational programs		
Medical care		
Dental care		
Peer-Based Services		
Consumer-led programs		
Peer support programs		
Self-help groups		
Advocacy organizations		
Residential Programs and Housing Services		
Residential programs with onsite supervision		
Supported housing		
Rental assistance		
Respite programs		

Special Issues
for Family Members

CHAPTER 6

Parents

A family member's schizophrenia affects everyone. Depending on the particular relationship and role in the family, each person has to make adjustments in response to the symptoms of the illness. Probably no one is affected as much as parents, however, who often bear many of the responsibilities for caring for their son or daughter.

For this reason, we begin Part II with help for parents struggling with the issues raised by schizophrenia. This chapter is intended for anyone who acts as a parent, whether grandparent, aunt, uncle, or guardian. Chapters 7, 8, and 9 address the needs of other family members. Specific help for you can be found in the chapter that applies to your relationship to the person with schizophrenia, but you might find it helpful to read about how other family members are being affected as well.

In fulfilling the considerable responsibilities that schizophrenia imposes, it's critical to understand that your emotional reactions are normal and shared by many others in the same position. Your son or daughter's illness *does* have an impact on your life and relationships. This chapter helps you come to terms with that fact and also offers specific strategies for reducing stress to yourself and other family members.

Common Reactions of Parents

Schizophrenia is a difficult illness to understand and to deal with, for both family members and professionals. It's particularly troublesome for you, as parents, because you feel responsible for your children's welfare and want to help them. The situation is even more complicated when your child is an adult and has established (or partially established) independence from you. This can make it more difficult for your son or daughter to accept your help and support, even when needed. Other children in the family, regardless of their age, may struggle with the behavior change in their sibling and dealing with their own fears and reactions—which is yet another concern for you. The following examples describe a variety of reactions and feelings that parents commonly report.

Helplessness

When individuals begin to develop the symptoms of schizophrenia, their parents often report that they try their best, but nothing they do seems to help. As one mother said, "My husband and I had raised three other kids by the time our youngest son was 16, and I thought we were prepared for about anything that might come up. But when he came to me saying that he heard threatening voices coming from the walls of his bedroom, I felt totally out of my element. I had no idea how to answer him or what I could do to help." Especially in the early stages of the illness, you may be flooded with questions: "What is happening to my child?" "What can I do to help him?" "Is she safe?" "Are other family members in danger?" "Will he ever be normal again?" You have plenty of questions, but few solid answers.

Confusion and Frustration

It is upsetting to see your son or daughter behave in a way you don't understand. One father reported being totally confused when his son started wearing several layers of clothing in the summer, explaining that "the clothing will protect me from evil in the air." One mother said she had no idea how to respond when her daughter refused to eat meals with the family because she thought the food was "from another planet" and therefore not digestible by humans. Frustration can run very high, especially when your attempts to help are unsuccessful. One mother said she tried to convince her son that the refrigerator was not recording their conversation by unplugging it. She was taken aback when he told her that it didn't make any difference, because the taping could be done by auxiliary battery power. Parents are further frustrated when the mental health system is not responsive to their concerns or lacks adequate resources. Of particular urgency are situations in which the person is a danger to herself or others and yet cannot be admitted to a psychiatric hospital unless she agrees to a voluntary admission.

Guilty Feelings

When children experience problems, their parents often look to themselves for the reason. Although it is no one's fault when a family member develops schizophrenia, parents frequently worry that something they did (or failed to do) has brought on the condition. Their feelings of guilt may be worsened by the fact that many people still believe families cause mental illness, despite scientific evidence to the contrary. Sometimes parents worry that a single event may have caused the illness. One mother, for example, thought her daughter's schizophrenia was caused by her having fallen off a bike when she was 6 years old. She truly believed "If only I hadn't let her ride her bike that day, this would never have happened." Even though research shows that families do not cause schizophrenia, it can be difficult for parents to accept that they are blameless.

Sadness

It naturally makes you sad to see your child suffering, whether with physical or emotional pain. "My son had always been such a good student," said one mother, "it was hard to see him struggle to work out math problems that had been easy for him before his illness." Parents often feel a sense of loss when their child has difficulty following through with goals because of mental illness. "My daughter had to leave college and move back home," said one father. "I worry that she won't be able to return to school." Some parents also mourn the loss of the close relationship they had with their son or daughter before the illness, such as the father who said, "I hope there will come a time when my son and I can enjoy going to football games again. I miss that."

Embarrassment

Sometimes it's embarrassing for you when your son or daughter acts in ways that draw unwanted attention. One mother reported feeling embarrassed when she was shopping for groceries with her son, who sometimes took items off the shelves and put them in his pocket because he thought he owned everything in the store. It can ease some of the embarrassment to know the behavior is prompted by the symptoms of a mental illness and it is not the person's intention to embarrass someone. However, other people observing the behavior may not be so understanding and may make critical remarks, which can hurt. "If my son was in a wheelchair," one parent said, "people would understand his condition and empathize. But they look at Manuel, who is physically fine, and they have absolutely no idea of the mental pain and confusion he's experiencing."

At other times the source of discomfort is not public behavior but rather the implicit judgment of other people. One father felt uncomfortable at parties when other parents talked about their grown children and their many accomplishments. Even though he was proud of his daughter for her strength in dealing with schizophrenia, he was silent, fearing that other parents would not understand this as an accomplishment.

Anger

There are many reasons to feel angry when your son or daughter develops schizophrenia. It's natural to feel angry that he or she has to experience pain. It's also natural to experience anger over the upheaval the illness is causing in your family life. You may also feel angry when continually frustrated in your attempts to improve the situation. "Nothing I did turned out right," said one parent. "I started to feel furious that all my efforts were wasted." As many parents do, you may look around and wonder "Why me? Why my son? Why my daughter?" and feel resentful that schizophrenia happened to someone in your family and not in others. One parent said, "I hated myself for it, but it took me a long time to be able to visit my sister's family and not feel angry that things were going so well for her children."

Impact on Your Life and Relationships

Schizophrenia affects many aspects of a person's life, but it also has a strong impact on the lives of family members, including parents.

Disruption of Your Usual Routines

Parents often find that many of their routines at home and at work are disrupted when their son or daughter first develops the symptoms of schizophrenia. "I was spending so much time responding to my son's fears and delusions that I didn't have time for shopping and cooking," said one mother. "It seemed like we ate take-out almost every night the year before he was diagnosed correctly and started taking medication." Another mother reported that instead of enjoying a relaxing lunch break with coworkers, she spent all her lunch hours holed up in her office, talking on the phone to mental health care providers.

Neglect of Your Own Needs

Some parents devote so much time to their son or daughter with schizophrenia that there is no time left for their own needs. These parents may stop pursuing interests and hobbies that they found rewarding. "I used to attend church regularly and sing in the choir twice a month," said one single mother. "I stopped doing that because I was too worried when my daughter was home alone." A father said that he gave up jogging and participating in a softball league because it took too much time. Some parents even find it difficult to pursue hobbies at home, such as reading or sewing, because they are too tired at the end of a day. Many parents find it difficult to keep up friendships, both because of the time involved and because they feel that other people don't understand what they are going through. "My friends didn't have a clue about what schizophrenia was. It was hard to have conversations with them."

Relationship with Your Son or Daughter

Even though you are now spending significant amounts of time with your son or daughter, you may feel the relationship is not the same as it was before the symptoms developed. "We used to laugh and joke a lot before, and I miss that aspect of our relationship," said one mother. "But I do see some of my son's sense of humor coming back, which makes me hopeful." Because of the symptoms, some people with schizophrenia may become hostile or angry with their parents, which is difficult to accept. "My daughter thinks I'm working for the FBI and spying on her," said one father. "I wish she didn't think I was against her." On the other hand, you may find your relationship becoming closer in the process of coping with the illness. "My son says I was the only one who helped him when he was down and out," one parent reported. "Our relationship is better than it was when he was a teenager."

Separating from parents is a normal developmental process that occurs throughout adolescence and early adulthood. This process is often disrupted when the person develops a mental illness, and the disruption can lead to struggles between the parents and the child. It can be difficult to know when to be protective and when to encourage your son or daughter to make her own choices, even if those choices are not guaranteed to be successful. "My son told me to stop hovering over him," said one parent. "I was only trying to help, but he felt I was holding him back."

Relationships with Your Other Children

When you have other children, you may find your time and energy stretched very thin. It can be difficult to attend to the needs of your son or daughter with schizophrenia and still have time to spend with the other children. In some situations you may overlook your other children's accomplishments. One parent said, "I was so relieved that Elliott's brother was doing so well and didn't need much from us. I think at times I failed to pay as much attention as I should have to his being on the honor roll and playing on the soccer team." In an attempt to protect your other kids from upsetting information, you may resist talking openly to them about their brother or sister's mental illness. Unfortunately, this may make them feel left in the dark and even more confused and worried. They may also be angry with their sibling because they don't understand that the troublesome behavior is related to symptoms of schizophrenia, or they may resent the amount of attention the person with the illness gets from you.

Relationship with Your Spouse or Partner

Mental illness in a son or daughter can place strains on any marriage or partnership. Spouses or partners may disagree about the nature of the problem, the best course of action, or how involved to be. These disagreements can lead to arguments and tensions between them, which adds to their stress. "My husband and I both wanted desperately to help our daughter," said one mother, "but he thought we should use 'tough love,' and I thought we should be as gentle as possible. It was like we were on different planets."

Isolation

In spite of many advances in the understanding and treatment of schizophrenia, many people are woefully misinformed and subscribe to negative stereotypes about the illness. These stereotypes make it difficult for parents to share with others what they are going through. "People either make jokes about people with mental illness or talk about how they are all 'psycho killers.' They don't realize what it's like." You may be fortunate to find others who understand and empathize, or you may feel isolated and alone as you deal with the many challenges of helping your child.

Strategies for Helping Your Son or Daughter

In spite of the many challenges of having a son or daughter with schizophrenia, there are strategies you can use to help him or her cope more effectively.

- *Learn about the illness.* By reading this book, you are already taking an important step. The more you learn about the illness, the less overwhelmed you will feel and the more you will be able to assist in coping with symptoms, making treatment decisions, participating in treatment, and preventing relapses. As you develop a recovery vision, you will also feel more confident in encouraging your son or daughter to pursue personal goals and move forward.
- *Support participation in comprehensive treatment.* As described in Chapter 4, the course of schizophrenia can be improved through participation in a comprehensive treatment plan that includes taking medication as prescribed, avoiding the use of alcohol or drugs, minimizing stress, developing coping skills, and increasing social support. You can help by reinforcing the message that treatment is beneficial, by facilitating access to mental health services, and by noticing and praising the progress made in treatment.
- *Support medication adherence.* Medication is one of the most powerful tools available for reducing symptoms and preventing relapses. For the best results, medications must be taken regularly. You can assist by helping to set up a system that makes taking medication part of the daily routine. For example, some people like to take their medication at breakfast, so they place their bottle of pills next to the coffeepot. Other people like to use reminders or cues, such as notes on the calendar or pill organizers. In addition, your son or daughter may appreciate receiving assistance with transportation to the doctor's office or pharmacy. She may also appreciate the opportunity to talk about medication side effects and her concerns about using medication on a regular basis. Chapter 10 pro-

vides more information about medications and strategies for helping your relative use them effectively.

- *Communicate with the treatment team.* You are an important part of the treatment team and at many mental health agencies you will be invited to be a part of the treatment planning meeting. Also, with your son or daughter's permission, you can contact the treatment team when you have information that would contribute to treatment, from reports on progress to concerns you might have to advocating for services that would be beneficial. Chapter 5 contains suggestions for advocating effectively.

- *Recognize early warning signs of relapse.* Schizophrenia is subject to relapse. Small changes in thinking and behavior often occur days or weeks before a relapse or episode of illness. These changes are referred to as *early warning signs* of relapse. When you or other family members observe these signs, you can help your relative recognize them and take appropriate action. Taking action early can make a dramatic difference, because the earlier the intervention, the more likely a relapse can either be averted or reduced in severity. Although each person with schizophrenia has a unique pattern of early warning signs, some common examples include increased tension, agitation, eating problems, concentration problems, sleep disturbance, social withdrawal, and discontinuance of medication. Chapter 12 contains more information on recognizing early warning signs of relapse.

- *Develop a relapse prevention plan.* It's very important to have a plan of action in case your son or daughter begins to experience signs of an impending relapse. This plan is best made during a calm period, when there is no crisis at hand, and should include input from you, the person with the illness, other family members, and treatment team members. A comprehensive relapse plan includes (1) recognition of situations or events that were associated with previous relapses, (2) early warning signs experienced, (3) steps to take to help reduce symptoms or distress, and (4) people (or agencies) to be contacted for assistance. Chapter 12 provides further information about developing an effective plan.

- *Encourage independence.* Doing *everything* for your son or daughter may be helpful in the short run but harmful in the long run. The more independent the person is, the more options he will have in the future. There are many ways you can promote independence. For example, if your son or daughter lacks skills for living away from home, you can teach skills such as budgeting, shopping, cooking, laundry, and cleaning, and by setting reasonable expectations that specific chores will be done. You can also help by encouraging independent problem solving and decision making. Discussing the risks and benefits of specific decisions may be desirable, but it's important to respect your son or daughter's decisions. Chapter 3 contains suggestions for supporting this autonomous decision-making process.

- *Encourage the pursuit of personal goals.* Most people in the process of recovery from schizophrenia report that it has been essential to pursue their own goals, whether the goals are large or small. You can help your child identify personal goals by reviewing what's important to her as an individual, what she would like to accomplish, and what she would like her life to be like. Sometimes it's helpful to reminisce about what she used to enjoy doing or what she aspired to, and explore whether she is still interested in pursuing some aspect of that area of her life. Encourage your child to think of herself as being able to grow and change and accomplish things that are important to her.

• *Provide a low-stress environment.* Based on the stress–vulnerability model described in Chapter 1, we know that stress can contribute to relapses of schizophrenia. Two types of behavior—criticism and extreme self-sacrificing behavior—are usually stressful to the person even if done for his own good, as are repeated prompting, correcting, and suggestions for improvement. All these behaviors may lead to an increased risk of relapse. You can become more aware of how you communicate and try to reduce nagging and criticism. Disagreements are bound to occur, but it is important to keep communication as positive as possible. Chapters 14–16 provide suggestions for reducing stress in the home environment, such as expressing positive feelings, using a step-by-step method for solving problems, and taking a break when discussions get heated.

• *Encourage alternatives to alcohol and drug abuse.* Individuals with schizophrenia are highly sensitive to even small amounts of alcohol or drugs, which can make their symptoms worse. It's therefore important to encourage avoidance of alcohol or drugs and participation in other activities instead. A person who has developed a strong habit or addiction to using alcohol or drugs may need professional help. Your son or daughter may also benefit from brainstorming with you about other enjoyable activities or other people to spend time with who don't use alcohol or drugs. Chapter 22 provides more strategies for dealing with substance abuse.

• *Maintain a positive relationship.* It's important to have a relationship that extends beyond helping your son or daughter cope with the illness. Make time to talk about non-illness-related topics and to participate in enjoyable activities together. Let your child choose the activity, whether it's playing a game of cards, taking a walk, watching a television show, listening to music, playing catch, or discussing a news article. Take opportunities to offer praise and to demonstrate your confidence in the person with the illness. Encourage an atmosphere where everyone in the family can talk freely about hopes and dreams.

The positive communication skills described in Chapter 14 can help you avoid resentments and conflicts when problems arise, as can using the step-by-step problem-solving method described in Chapter 15. If, for example, your relative repeatedly leaves the front door unlocked at night, try making a positive, noncritical request: "I'd appreciate it if you locked the door when you get home after eleven—it would make me feel safer." If the door still ends up unlocked, explore why your relative forgets and brainstorm alternative solutions.

• *Maintain household routines.* People with schizophrenia report that having structure and routine in their lives helps to counteract the inner turmoil they experience as a result of symptoms such as hallucinations, delusions, and cognitive disorganization. One way to promote stability is to maintain as many of the basic elements of your family's household routine as possible. For example, if your family normally had dinner together every night, try to continue this practice. If your family usually went to religious services every week, keep going. Increased demands on your time may make it necessary to have pizza occasionally instead of home-cooked meals or to eat together 4 nights a week instead of 7. Continuing to celebrate birthdays and holidays together is also important. As one individual with schizophrenia said, "It made me feel better to see that life could still go on, that we could still be a regular family, even though I had this illness." You may need to simplify holiday events by scheduling shorter or smaller gatherings if your child tends to get overstimulated.

• *Establish household rules.* You have the right to live in a home in which you feel safe and comfortable, your privacy is respected, and all family members contribute something to the ongoing operation of the household. Many people find it helpful to establish a few basic household rules so that everyone knows what is expected of them. One mother told us, "Until we set up some rules, everything revolved around my son's sleeping all day and staying awake all night. The rest of us were constantly walking on eggshells, which would have a been a disaster in the long run." Chapter 16 provides suggestions for setting up rules that everyone can live with.

Helping Other Children in Your Family

Although your other children must decide for themselves how they will cope and what level of involvement they want with their sibling, you can help them with these decisions in many ways. For example:

• *Educate yourself about schizophrenia.* Educating yourself about schizophrenia will, of course, help *you* cope better as well as your other children, who may look to you as a model of how to behave and react. If you are well informed, your children can ask you questions about their sibling's illness and receive accurate answers.

• *Openly discuss the illness.* Although parents naturally want to protect their children from upsetting information, most siblings report that they don't want to be kept in the dark. As one sibling said, "For years I knew something was wrong with Daniel, but no one would tell me what it was." If you don't discuss the condition openly, your other children (even as adults) may develop misconceptions about it. "I was so surprised to hear that my kids thought Brad was a dangerous criminal," said one parent. "They didn't realize that he had a mental illness."

Keep your other children informed about what's happening. If their sister is displaying symptoms, explain how these behaviors are related to the illness. Your other children may also appreciate knowing about their sibling's treatment, including medication, counseling, and day programs. They will feel less confused and more in control when they are told more of the facts.

• *Make time to spend with your other children.* The needs of your son or daughter with schizophrenia are real and compelling. At times it is necessary to focus all your attention on averting a crisis or responding to a problem caused by the condition. However, it's important to balance the needs of the ill person with those of your other children. Try to make time to talk regularly with your other children, acknowledge their problems and achievements, and be available to support them in their lives.

Sometimes it can be helpful to divide responsibilities with your spouse or partner. For example, if your son or daughter has symptoms that make it difficult to be around other people, you might stay home while your partner goes to the sibling's birthday dinner. However, avoid having one spouse always take responsibility for the person with schizophrenia, which can be stressful and deny that spouse the experience of being involved with the other children. Sometimes friends or relatives can help free up some time for you to spend with your other children. One parent said, "My sister has been invaluable. Without her bringing over meals during the crises with Anna, I never could have spent any time with Maria and Victor."

• *Get to know how your other children feel.* Siblings experience a range of emotions when a brother or sister has schizophrenia. These emotions naturally include some negative ones, such as anger, fear, resentment, guilt, and embarrassment. Try to listen to your other children's feelings without judging them. These emotions are unavoidable, but if your children are allowed to talk about them, and they see that you understand their position, they will be better able to cope. It may also be helpful to suggest professional counseling or a support group to your children. Some National Alliance on Mental Illness (NAMI) affiliates offer sibling support groups that give siblings a place to share their thoughts and feelings with others who have similar experiences.

• *Avoid pressuring your other children.* Some siblings feel comfortable with their brother or sister with schizophrenia and want to help, but others don't. Siblings must determine, on their own, what is the right amount of contact and responsibility. Forcing siblings to be involved can foster resentment, which can be sensed by the sibling with schizophrenia and be detrimental to their relationship.

On the other hand, some siblings are more interested in being involved than you might think. "When Victor told me that he wanted Anna to come to dinner at his house once a week, I was surprised," said her mother. Allowing your children to determine their own level of involvement will avoid the negative repercussions of trying to force more closeness or responsibility than they can handle.

Helping Yourselves as Parents

If you allow yourself to get stressed out and run down, you won't have the inner resources or energy you need to take care of your loved ones. Other parents have told us that the following strategies are helpful.

- *Take care of your own needs.* As we noted, some parents devote so much time to their son or daughter with schizophrenia that they have no time left for their own needs. It's important to continue to pursue the interests and hobbies that you find rewarding. First, doing so will help you relieve your own stress. As one mother said, "When Alice was in the hospital, I was worrying about her all the time. If I hadn't been able to take a break and work on my knitting, I would have been totally stressed out." Or as one father said, "I needed to go to the gym two or three times a week to let off steam; otherwise I wouldn't have been able to stay calm for my son." Second, pursuing your own interests will help relieve the stress your child may feel about interfering with your life. As one daughter said, "I didn't want to be responsible for my mother not singing in the church choir any more; she enjoyed that and I didn't want her to stop because of me."

- *Maintain a positive relationship with your spouse/partner.* When a son or daughter develops a mental illness, spouses or partners may disagree about the nature of the problem, the best course of action, or how involved to be in their child's adolescent or adult life. It's important to communicate directly with your spouse or partner about what you're experiencing, including your feelings and opinions. When disagreements arise, try to listen to each other's point of view and resolve differences without one person forcing his opinion on the other. Seeking additional information may be helpful in resolving differences. One couple who disagreed about the inadvisability of their son's daily beer drinking were able to come to agreement after their doctor confirmed that three beers is approximately equivalent to three ounces of whiskey—both of which are contraindicated for people with schizophrenia.

Make time for enjoyable activities on a regular basis. Continue to do the hobbies and activities you previously enjoyed together, such as going to movies, eating out, watching videos, dancing, listening to music, etc. As one mother said, "My husband and I try to go out once a week, even if it's just for coffee, to stay close as a couple. We have a rule that we're not going to talk about problems while we're out." Express your affection and appreciation to your spouse or partner as often as possible and let her know that you notice the positive things that she does. Some of the suggestions about effective communication and problem solving found in Chapters 14 and 15 will be helpful in your relationship with your spouse as well as with your child.

- *Maintain your friendships.* Avoid isolating yourself by maintaining your friendships; try to continue to do things with friends, such as hobbies and activities you used to enjoy. With some friends, you may feel comfortable talking about your child's experience with mental illness, whereas with others you may be uncomfortable and want to focus only on having fun. "I kept up my weekly poker game with Antonio and a couple of friends," said one father. "Usually we would just talk about work and joke around while we played cards. But sometimes I would stay after the game and talk to Antonio about what was happening with my daughter. Our friendship got me through some rough times."

• *Stay healthy.* Sometimes parents become so concerned with the welfare of their children that they neglect their own health. It is important to make sure that you have regular physical checkups and to see a doctor whenever you have a health problem. Try to eat a healthy diet, exercise regularly, and avoid excessive smoking and drinking. The healthier and stronger you are, the more you can help your child—and enjoy your life.

• *Participate in family programs and support organizations.* Many families find it helpful to participate in family programs, such as family psychoeducation, behavioral family therapy, and Family-to-Family, which teach people about mental illness and strategies for coping with it. Organizations such as NAMI can be invaluable resources for families; not only can they learn more about mental illness, but they can also meet other families who have gone (or are going) through similar experiences. Chapter 5 describes family programs offered through NAMI. One mother said of NAMI, "The best part was finding out that I was not alone. Other parents knew exactly what I was talking about."

• *Get help for yourself when needed.* Professional counseling may help you cope with the experience of having a child with schizophrenia. A counselor or therapist can listen, understand, and empathize with your experience and give you practical suggestions for coping and getting on with your life. You can get a recommendation for a good therapist by contacting your local chapter of NAMI, asking other health professionals you trust (such as a member of your relative's treatment team), asking friends who have received counseling, or contacting your local community mental health center. You can also look up therapists and counselors in the Yellow Pages.

Putting Schizophrenia into Perspective

Raising a child is hard work, filled with unexpected challenges that force you to adapt and invent and discover strengths you may not have realized you possessed. Like all parents, you care deeply about your children's well-being and happiness, and it's hard to see your offspring suffer. Life can seem unfair when a son or a daughter develops a serious illness like schizophrenia, and it's easy to get trapped in sorrow over the person's "lost potential" and the hardships you have to endure. In such circumstances it's important to remind yourself that your family is not so unique and that *everyone* experiences unexpected challenges in their lives. In the words of Billy Lampert, an employee at the Fountainhouse Psychosocial Clubhouse in New York City, "life throws everybody curveballs."

Appreciating your child for who he *is*, rather than who you wish he could be, is the key to an accepting and rewarding relationship. Such a relationship is also critical to forming an alliance with your son or daughter aimed at coping more effectively with schizophrenia and achieving personal goals. By balancing your son or daughter's needs with those of your own and other family members, you can move forward individually and as a family, without allowing schizophrenia to dominate your lives.

Resources

Beard, J., & Gillespie, P. N. (2002). *Nothing to hide: Mental illness in the family*. New York: New Press. Contains first-person accounts and photographs of several families who have a member with mental illness.

Deveson, A. (1992). *Tell me I'm here: One family's experience of schizophrenia*. New York: Penguin.

Swados, E. (1991). *The four of us: A family memoir*. New York: Farrar, Straus, & Giroux. Describes how the mental illness of one member affected everyone in the family, as told from the perspective of the person, the mother, the father, and the sister.

Wyden, P. (1998). *Conquering schizophrenia: A father, his son, and a medical breakthrough*. New York: Knopf. Describes how a father helped his son find an antipsychotic medication that worked for him.

CHAPTER 7

Siblings

*I*f you have a sibling with schizophrenia, understanding the issues that arise can help you cope with the changes the illness brings while also strengthening the bonds between you and your brother or sister. If you're a parent, knowing what your other children may be going through will make it easier to help them cope in the ways suggested in Chapter 6 and also improve the overall resilience of the family.

Common Emotional Reactions to Having a Brother or Sister with Schizophrenia

One sibling's illness evokes emotions in the other siblings that must be reconciled with the usual feelings of affection and rivalry that occur in any family. When the illness causes bizarre and sometimes frightening behavior, children and adolescents may feel confused and overwhelmed. Even if you're an adult, you may be familiar with some of the following reactions to a sibling's developing schizophrenia.

Confusion and Frustration

It is very confusing to see your brother or sister do strange, unexplainable things, especially before the diagnosis has been determined. A loved one who is paranoid and accuses you of stealing and conspiring against him is frightening. It's also frustrating when your sibling doesn't respond to reason or behaves strangely in front of your friends. Such behavior is even harder to understand when you haven't been informed of your sibling's diagnosis.

Anxiety about Developing the Illness

Siblings often worry that whatever caused their brother's or sister's illness will also cause them to become ill. If you've heard something about the genetic aspects of schizophrenia, you may naturally be concerned. Even though the risk of developing schizophrenia is higher when a family member has the illness, the chances are still far against you or one of your children developing the illness (see Chapter 1). It can be helpful, however, to talk to a genetic counselor about any concerns you have for yourself and for your (planned or present) children. "After my sister was diagnosed with schizophrenia, it took a long time for me to relax and stop checking myself daily for symptoms," one sibling said.

Distress

It's upsetting to see your brother or sister suffering, especially if you've been close to your ill relative. You may even be able to empathize with your sibling. In many ways, siblings grieve for the loss of the brother or sister they knew. For example, Alice missed the closeness she once had with Dan and wished she still had the kind of older brother she could turn to for advice and protection.

Feeling Self-Conscious

Embarrassment is a common reaction to some of the behavior typical of schizophrenia. Before his first hospitalization, Mark would frequently get into arguments with salesclerks and waiters when he was out with his family. As a teenager, his sister Danielle found it especially mortifying to have people's attention drawn to her or her family. Adults are not immune to this reaction. Rosa felt embarrassed when the neighbors called to report that her brother, Xavier, unknown to the family, was standing on the front porch in his underwear smoking cigarettes. Remembering that such behavior is prompted by the symptoms of a mental illness can ease your embarrassment. But you might also plan outings to minimize the potential for embarrassing situations, such as eating at informal instead of formal restaurants.

Resentment and Anger

It's natural to feel angry about the disruptions that schizophrenia can cause. You may feel it has robbed you of your parents' attention and forced unwelcome changes on the whole family. Resentment is understandable and doesn't mean you don't still care deeply for your brother or sister.

"By the time I was 15," said one man, "my older brother was already beginning to develop schizophrenia, and that consumed most of the attention my parents had to give. No matter how hard I tried—making the honor role, acting in the school play, playing sports—my parents hardly seemed to notice. It was almost as though my accomplishments were taken for granted."

Survivor Guilt

Siblings often feel guilty when things are going well for them but not their brother or sister with schizophrenia. "It shouldn't have been Dan," Alice complained, "He was so talented and I was just average." If you feel this way, try to remind yourself that you didn't choose to have your sibling develop schizophrenia any more than he or she did.

How Schizophrenia May Affect Your Life and Relationships

Because schizophrenia can affect so many aspects of family life, the illness is bound to have an impact on siblings. Indeed, siblings often feel the strongest effects in the areas of relationships and level of involvement with their family.

Your Relationship with Your Parents

As mentioned earlier, you may feel that your parents focus (or focused) all their attention on the ill child, to the exclusion of you and your other siblings. Although intellectually you may understand that your brother or sister needs this attention, emotionally it may be difficult to accept. "I don't think my parents even knew I was president of my class my junior *and* senior years," said one sibling, "because they were going through such a bad time with my brother." Children who are used to seeing their parents handle difficult situations are often jolted by seeing them visibly "undone" and uncertain of how to respond to the disruptive or disorganized behavior of their ill child. "It was so scary watching Mom and Dad try to deal with Xavier," said his sister. "Even though they worried about his illness all the time, no one seemed to know what to do."

Your Relationship with Your Sibling

Depending on the age of the siblings and the severity of the illness, schizophrenia can disrupt even a strong sibling relationship. "I thought I would always be able to turn to my older brother," said one young man, "but now he won't even talk to me because he thinks I'm poisoning his food." If the bond is not strong or there is conflict between siblings, the emergence of schizophrenia in one can intensify the sense of disconnection. "I didn't have much in common with James before he got sick," said his sister, "but afterward it seemed impossible." In contrast to these experiences, some siblings actually become closer after schizophrenia develops, because of the brother or sister's strong empathy and willingness to help. "I always looked up to my oldest sister, who was very popular in school," said Kayla. "After she developed schizophrenia, she had some rough times and would talk to me about it. Sometimes she still says I understand her best."

Your Involvement with the Whole Family

When one member becomes ill, the family dynamics change. Your reactions to this change may range from withdrawal to intense involvement. "I was a teenager when Cassie got sick," said her brother. "I felt so shaken up by her talking to voices and thinking that there were hidden cameras in her bedroom that I ended up just staying away from the whole situation. I spent most of my time at friends' houses and hardly ever came home." Even as an adult you may withdraw when your sibling becomes ill—calling and visiting less often—out of confusion and distress, rather than lack of concern.

You may, however, find yourself intensely involved, acting more like a parent than a brother or a sister. You might take on the role of protector, even taking your sibling to the hospital and advocating for the best treatment possible. You could, in fact, focus so much on your brother or sister that you neglect your own interests and goals. "I never seemed to have time to find a boyfriend," said Andrea, "because I was so busy trying to keep Thomas out of the hospital."

Your Relationships with People Outside the Family

"I was so embarrassed when my buddy came over and Franco was dressed in strange clothes and was ranting about conspiracy theories," Carl said. "After that I always went to his house." Being afraid to bring a friend home is just one way having a sibling with schizophrenia can affect your other relationships. You might also find that you become more secretive with friends and acquaintances after your brother or sister develops symptoms of mental illness. One sibling reported, "I couldn't tell anyone what was happening at our house anymore or how I was feeling about it." Being cautious about disclosing your relative's schizophrenia is understandable, given the stigma of mental illness in our culture. Yet being excessively secretive can interfere with your ability to form close or intimate relationships, as discussed in Chapter 29.

Strategies for Coping with Your Sibling's Schizophrenia

In spite of the many challenges of having a brother or sister with schizophrenia, it's never too late to improve the situation. There are several strategies you can use to cope more effectively with the illness.

• *Learn about schizophrenia.* Knowing more about schizophrenia will help you understand your sibling better. Reading Chapters 1 and 2 of this book would be a good start, because what you learn about symptoms will help you understand some of the behavior you've seen in the past. You'll find informative publications at libraries and through NAMI, and several are in the Resources sections at the ends of Chapters 1 and 2.

Also try discussing the illness directly with your parents and your sibling. When you show that you care and are interested in the answers, they will probably try to be open with you. If your sibling is reluctant to discuss such matters, respect her decision and consult your parents, but keep in mind that your sibling might be more receptive to talking about her experience at a later time.

Reading Chapter 3 will help you develop a vision of recovery for schizophrenia, which will make you feel more confident in encouraging your sibling to pursue personal goals and move forward in his life. Having optimistic and supportive siblings can be extremely helpful to anyone with schizophrenia.

• *Encourage your sibling to participate in treatment.* As described in Chapter 4, the course of schizophrenia can be improved by comprehensive treatment. You can help your sibling by reinforcing the message that treatment is beneficial and by noticing and praising progress made in treatment.

• *Discourage your sibling from using alcohol and drugs.* People with schizophrenia are highly sensitive to even small amounts of drugs or alcohol, which can make symptoms worse. As a peer, you probably carry more weight than your parents and should both avoid using substances with your sibling and encourage her not to use alcohol and drugs.

• *Maintaining your relationship.* In spite of the changes your sibling has experienced since developing schizophrenia, the two of you can have a rewarding relationship. It may be different from the one you had before the illness—you may not be able to spend as much time together or converse about the same subjects—but with effort you can form a new relationship and develop new interests in common.

You can also focus on the aspects of your sibling's personality that you once enjoyed and that are still present in some form. For example, many siblings can still enjoy each other's sense of humor, taste in music, or love of certain foods. "Before the illness, Jack and I used to talk about sports nonstop," said one brother, "and we still enjoy watching a baseball game together on TV once in a while. We're both diehard Red Sox fans."

Don't wait for a crisis to become involved. You won't get a sense of your sibling's strengths and capabilities if you know him only in crisis.

• *Determine a comfortable level of involvement.* Siblings differ in their degree of involvement with the brother or sister with schizophrenia. A great deal depends on your relationship with your sibling and your other responsibilities. "At first I thought there was nothing I could do," said one sibling, "but when I visited my brother in the hospital I could see that it did him good just to talk to me. So now, that's what I try to do on a regular basis—be available when he wants to talk about what's on his mind." Some siblings are closely involved in day-to-day matters and may even have their brother or sister live with them. Others feel comfortable keeping more of a distance, staying in touch by phone once a month and being supportive to the principal caregivers. "My brother lives with Mom, and she does the lion's share of the work. But since neither of them drive, I give them rides to the grocery store and to appointments." Still another sibling said, "I try to stay in regular touch with my parents. We talk about a lot of things, including what's happening with my sister. There are very few people they can talk to about this. I still care about her, and they know that."

At a minimum, try to remain informed about how things are going for your sibling and how treatment is progressing so you'll hear about the positive things she's doing and assuage any fears you have about her welfare. Staying informed will also allow you to know when to help out, if only temporarily. When Ben's mother ended up hospitalized with pneumonia, he was glad he knew his brother had recently moved to his own apartment and temporarily needed help with shopping. While their mother was in the hospital, Ben drove his brother to visit her and also to the grocery store.

• *Pursue your own interests.* Avoid becoming so involved in your sibling's care that you neglect your own interests and ambitions. It's important to balance your own needs with those of your ill relative. Everyone needs to determine her own level of involvement, but it's usually not beneficial to devote yourself solely to your sibling. "My sister was traveling everywhere, ending up in emergency rooms in every state," said Juanita. "I used to take a bus or train to wherever she was and bring her home. Now, instead, I spend time on the phone talking to the staff at the hospital, telling them which medication she is on, which ones were tried in the past, how they might convince her to be admitted voluntarily, and so on. I think I'm still helping her, but now I have time for my own life too."

• *Get support.* Many siblings feel alone in having a brother or sister with mental illness. Finding someone to talk to can help, whether it's an understanding friend, a spouse, or a counselor. Many siblings benefit from being involved with support groups, such as the Sibling and Adult Children Network, a subgroup of the National Alliance on Mental Illness (NAMI). This group brings siblings together to talk about their experiences and to share strategies and information about resources. You're not required to speak when you attend such a group, and some people prefer to listen, especially at first. Whether they speak or not, most siblings leave these meetings feeling relieved that they are not alone, that others share their experience and care. Siblings are also encouraged to participate in family programs (in either the single-family or a multiple-family group format) such as the ones described in Chapter 5. The more you and your family are on the same page regarding information and strategies for helping your sibling, the better it will be for all concerned.

• *Remind yourself of the nature of the illness.* Sometimes siblings can lose touch with how much schizophrenia influences their relationship with their ill brother or sister. It helps to repeat the following reminders to yourself:

— "Despite having a mental illness, my brother is still capable of having relationships and experiencing enjoyment in life."
— "My sister's symptoms are the cause of her upsetting behaviors."
— "My efforts to help my sibling are important, no matter how big or how small."
— "My sibling may appreciate my involvement, even if it is difficult for him to show that appreciation."
— "Underneath the illness, this is still my sister."

Special Concerns about the Future

Surveys conducted with siblings in young adulthood indicate they have two main questions on their minds: "What is going to happen to my sibling?" and "What will be expected of me when my parents are no longer able to care for my sibling?" Although the answers to these questions are complicated and depend a great deal on the individual circumstances involved, we offer broad-based responses here.

Your Sibling's Prognosis

The course of schizophrenia is impossible to predict. Some people are able to live independently and hold a full-time job. Others are bothered by constant symptoms that interfere with their ability to work or take care of themselves. Most people with schizophrenia fall somewhere in between these two extremes, and many vary over time. This variability makes it especially difficult to know what the future may bring for your brother or sister. As described in Chapter 3, the research about the long-term course of schizophrenia is encouraging because it shows that many individuals recover either partly or fully. Ongoing advances in treatment offer additional reasons to be hopeful.

To understand your sibling's prognosis, talk with his treatment team. Because of their knowledge of your sibling and their extensive experience with others who have schizophrenia, they can discuss short- and long-term goals for your sibling. One sibling, after speaking to her brother's psychiatrist, told us, "I didn't realize that Martin would probably be living in the community residence for several months. I thought it was just for a few days or weeks, while he got back on his feet." After speaking to his sister's treatment team, another sibling told us, "I'm more optimistic now. I thought that Sylvie would never be better than she is now. The staff told me that treatment is helping her a lot and that she will most likely continue to increase her independence." Stay informed of your sibling's "clinical status" (how well the person is doing) and treatment on an ongoing basis, so that you will have a broad perspective of her capabilities.

What Might Be Expected of You

As parents become less able to care for a child with schizophrenia, siblings naturally wonder how much care and involvement might be expected of them. "I never had much contact with Kathy because it was too upsetting for me," said her sister Joanie, "but I was petrified that when Mom died I would suddenly find out I was supposed to take total responsibility." To avoid this scenario and ensure that there are no such surprises for either you or your sibling, openly discuss the situation, reviewing the needs of your sibling and considering all the options. Don't postpone this kind of discussion until the last minute. Be sure to involve as many family members as possible. It's crucial that you make an informed decision about the level of responsibility you're willing to take. This level depends on your relationship with your sibling, your past involvement with him, your other responsibilities, your capabilities, and what you truly want to do. As mentioned in Chapter 6, feeling pressured to be more involved than you want can have negative consequences.

There are other ways to be helpful besides assuming full responsibility for providing care. You could, for instance, participate in discussions, help to come up with possible solutions, and assist the primary caregiver with specific tasks, such as taking your brother or sister shopping on a regular basis or being available during emergencies.

Coming to Grips with Schizophrenia

Having a sibling with schizophrenia can be a bewildering experience that has a dramatic effect on every family member's life. Becoming knowledgeable about the nature of the illness and understanding its effects on your sibling and on your relationship with him is crucial in sorting out your own feelings and deciding how involved you want to be in his life. You are not alone in your experience, and it takes time and help to process it. By choosing to learn more, by reading this book, and by talking to others about your experiences and feelings, you are taking important steps to cope with the effects of schizophrenia on you and your family and to move forward in your individual and shared lives.

Resources

Readings and Videotapes

Hyland, B. (1986). *The girl with the crazy brother*. London: Franklin Watts Publishing Group. Written for adolescents by a member of NAMI, available through NAMI. It was released on videotape by Godhil Home Media, International, in 2000.

Marsh, D., & Dickens, R. (1997). *Troubled journey: Coming to terms with the mental illness of a sibling or parent*. New York: Tarcher/Putnam Books.

Moorman, M. (1992). *My sister's keeper*. New York: Norton. The author describes how she learned to cope with her sister's schizophrenia. A movie by the same title is available on videotape through the NAMI bookstore.

Neugeboren, J. (1998). *Imagining Robert: My brother, madness and survival.* New York: Henry Holt. The author describes the many stages of his relationship with his brother, who has had schizophrenia for over 30 years. A documentary videotape by the same title was produced by Florentine Films in 2002.

Secunda, V. (1998). *When madness comes home: Help and hope for children, siblings, and partners of the mentally ill.* New York: Hyperion.

Wagner, P. S., & Spiro, C. S. (2005). *Divided minds: Twin sisters and their journey through schizophrenia.* New York: St. Martin's. Told in the alternating voices of twin sisters, one of whom has schizophrenia, this book is an account of the illness and the complex effects it can have on sibling relationships.

Websites for Siblings

"Coping Tips for Siblings and Adult Children of Persons with Mental Illness" can be found at *www.nami.org/copingtipsforsiblings*.

"The Sibling Voice," which describes a variety of siblings' experiences, can be found at *www.newyorkcityvoices.org/siblings.html*.

CHAPTER 8

Spouses and Partners

*I*f your spouse or partner[1] has schizophrenia, we don't have to tell you how deeply the illness can affect your intimate relationship. From working toward shared goals and dividing up household responsibilities to making parenting decisions and enjoying intimacy and sex, schizophrenia can disrupt your life as a couple. This chapter helps you understand the feelings you may be experiencing and offers some suggestions for how you and your partner can cope effectively.

Experiences of Partners

Deciding to get married or make a permanent commitment to another person is one of the most significant and most complex decisions in life. When your intended partner or spouse develops an unanticipated illness such as schizophrenia, all your expectations may seem to be threatened, and many emotions are likely to arise. Even if you were already aware of your partner's schizophrenia, the illness may worsen or otherwise change in the future. In either situation, you may end up experiencing some of the following common reactions.

Confusion and Frustration

It's upsetting to see your partner behave in ways you don't understand, especially if it occurs in the early stages of the illness when a diagnosis has not been determined. One husband, for example, reported being baffled when his wife came home from the grocery store after several hours without purchasing a single item. When he asked her about this, she said, "I kept walking around the store,

---

[1]In this chapter we use the term *spouse* or *partner* to refer to individuals who are married or in a committed relationship, and *marriage* to mean the spousal relationship or the committed partnership, including gay couples.

but I kept forgetting what I was supposed to be buying. I finally left." One woman said she didn't know how to respond to her husband when he told her he, not John Lennon and Paul McCartney, had written all the Beatles' songs and planned to sue to get the royalties he deserved.

Partners can find it frustrating when their attempts to help are unsuccessful. For example, one woman said she ate a few bites from her partner's dinner plate to convince him his food was not poisoned. When he replied that the poison would affect only his body and not hers, she didn't know what to say or do next. People who are able to convince their partners to seek professional advice may be further frustrated when doctors are unable to diagnose the problem or when inadequate treatment is available. "I took my husband to the doctor," said Leila, "but the doctor just said he was having problems concentrating because he was under stress at work. I knew it was more than that."

Guilty Feelings

Although it's no one's fault when a person develops schizophrenia, people frequently worry that something they did caused the illness. For example, Jacob said he thought his working late several nights a week while his partner was home with their two toddlers had been so stressful that it caused her to develop schizophrenia. Spouses' feelings of guilt may be worsened when their partner's family mistakenly blames them, saying things like "He was okay until he met you." Although scientific research shows that families (biological or nonbiological) do not cause schizophrenia, it can be difficult for partners to accept that they did nothing to cause their loved one's schizophrenia.

Sadness and Loss

Partners experience sadness and distress when they see their loved one suffering from schizophrenia. "My husband had always been so proud of his work and ability to take on challenges," said one wife. "It was painful to see him having trouble solving even the most basic problems on his job." Depending on the severity of the illness, some people also grieve for the loss of the special relationship they had with their partner prior to the illness. One man said, "We used to be able to talk about everything, both the good and the bad things that happened. It's much harder to have intimate discussions like that now. I'm hoping it will improve in the future."

Embarrassment

People may feel embarrassed when their partner with schizophrenia acts in ways that attract attention. One woman felt embarrassed when a friend dropped by for a cup of coffee and her boyfriend warned the friend not to sit in the chair next to the window because it was reserved for the president when he visited.

One man was uncomfortable when he and his wife ran into a couple they knew at the mall and she looked down, unable to respond to their greeting or friendly questions. It can be especially difficult for partners because other people cannot see any outward signs that the person is experiencing difficulties. "She looks the same as ever," Haiping said of his wife. "It's not like she has a bandage wrapped around her head or anything. People just don't understand."

Anger

Partners have many reasons to feel angry when their loved one develops schizophrenia. For example, they may feel angry when the illness creates problems in their relationship or disrupts their household routine. Partners may also feel angry that they have been thrust into this situation. "I thought I knew what I was getting into when I married Ross," one woman said. "It may be unfair to think this way, but I feel like other people knew he'd been having problems and they didn't tell me before we got married." Spouses may look at their married friends and relatives and wonder "Why *me*? Why my husband or wife? What did I do to deserve *this*?" Feeling resentful that schizophrenia occurred in their relationship and not in others is not an uncommon response.

Concern about Finances

Many partnerships depend on the earning power of the person with schizophrenia, which can result in financial concerns for immediate needs and long-term security. For example, Anita reported that she had depended on Jerome's job as a foreman to pay their monthly mortgage payments. "I knew Joe had schizophrenia when we got married, but he had always been able to work full-time. Now he's had a relapse and needs to cut back on his hours, so he's under less stress. I've taken a part-time job, but we still have to budget carefully so we don't lose the house." One husband said, "We were saving for college for our two sons when my wife developed schizophrenia; we've had to dip into that account to cover some of our medical expenses."

Concern about the Future

Many couples find that their plans for the future are challenged when one of them develops schizophrenia. These plans may include further education for one or both partners, job advancements, children, traveling, or moving. "I wasn't sure how to proceed," explained one wife. "Our plans involved my husband working full-time while I stayed home with the children—and suddenly that had to be reevaluated."

All these concerns are normal and understandable, so don't give up hope! The pages that follow describe how couples can learn to adapt to schizophrenia, pursue their personal and shared goals, and grow beyond the illness and its effects on their lives.

Impact on Your Life and Relationships

Your partner's schizophrenia can affect your life and relationships in numerous ways.

Your Routines and Chores

People often find that routines at home are disrupted when their partner develops the symptoms of schizophrenia. "We have young children, and our household routine was to have an early dinner, give the kids their baths, then read each of them a story before they fell asleep," said one woman. "Then we would have a cup of tea or hot chocolate and talk about our day before we went to sleep ourselves. It became very hard to do this when Jim was hospitalized so often. I would take the kids to a fast-food restaurant, then to my mom's, then I'd visit Jim, then rush to my mother's to pick up the kids, then rush home to get them to bed. It was so hectic."

Sometimes it can be difficult to share the labor when your partner is experiencing symptoms of mental illness. "Sandy had schizophrenia when we first got together. She always insisted on dividing up the household chores evenly," said Nathan. "Sandy still wants to do her share, and I appreciate that. But I'm doing more of the chores because she's had more trouble with symptoms lately."

Your Needs

Some partners devote so much time to their loved one that there is no time left to pursue their own goals. They may stop participating in activities they used to find rewarding. "I wanted to go back to school," said one man. "When I married Sarah, her illness was stable and hardly ever presented a problem. But she recently has had some relapses, so I had to put school on hold to get her health taken care of." For many spouses it's difficult to find time for themselves. "I've been so busy looking after my husband," said one woman, "that I haven't been going to the gym to work out—which used to be very important to me. My own health is starting to slide."

Your Partner

Schizophrenia can place strains on any relationship. Partners often disagree about the nature of the problem, what course of action to take, and how to handle daily chores and financial responsibilities. "We used to work things out calmly," said one man, "but after Lucinda developed schizophrenia, we found ourselves yelling at each other in frustration." Some people find they go out less often as a couple and don't have as much fun as they did before schizophrenia developed.

Some couples report retaining the emotional and sexual intimacy they had shared before schizophrenia is challenging. As one woman said, "I miss being able to tell David about things that bothered me about the kids or my job. He used to help me see the humor in some of the situations. It's hard for him to do that now." Sexual relationships may also be affected. "I still love my husband," said one woman, "but we have sex less often now. It just seems like there's no time or that the mood is not right. Sometimes I feel more like a sister or a mother than a wife."

Although many couples experience difficulties in their relationships related to schizophrenia, some also say they feel closer as a result of going through hard times together. Partners often discover strengths in each other that they had not known. "Tony is the strongest person I know," said one woman. "Other people would have given up if they had had even one of the experiences he had with schizophrenia. Not my Tony." And as Tony said of his wife, "She stayed with me throughout this ordeal. She even went to bat for me at the hospital to get the doctors to change my medicine. She was so quiet before—I didn't know she could be so tough!"

Your Parents and In-Laws

When a partner develops schizophrenia, it not only affects their relationship with each other but also with both sets of parents. Sometimes parents and in-laws can be supportive and provide significant assistance. "My mother-in-law has been a great help to me with Alexander's schizophrenia," said Lina. "When he was having a rough time, she would come over every night with a meal for us and to take the kids out for a few hours. She was invaluable." At other times, parents and in-laws may not understand the nature of the illness and may be the source of added pressure and tension. "My parents meant well," said Len, "but they kept stirring things up by insisting that all Alicia needed was a better diet and fresh air. They didn't understand the situation at all."

Your Friends and Neighbors

Many people don't understand schizophrenia and have negative images of people with the illness. They may think all people with schizophrenia are violent, abuse drugs, or have "split personalities," stereotypes that make it difficult to share with others what they are going through with their partner. It may even be difficult to be open with people who were once close friends. Some friends may want to maintain the relationship but fear saying or doing something to upset the person with the illness. "We used to see the Goldmans every week for bridge," said one man. "We tried to keep that up, but they always acted like they were walking on eggshells. It was very uncomfortable, and we eventually stopped seeing them."

Your Children

As discussed in Chapter 1, those who have a first-degree relative with schizophrenia (such as a mother or father) have a higher risk of developing schizophrenia than people whose first-degree relatives do not have schizophrenia. This increased risk is often a concern to couples who are considering having children or who have them already. Some couples seek genetic counseling to help them decide whether to have children. Even with the help of counseling, however, it remains a very individual decision. A great deal depends on the severity of the illness and how both partners feel about becoming parents.

When there are already children in the family, parents may find their time and energy stretched very thin when one of them develops schizophrenia. Parenting can be stressful and demanding under the best of circumstances; it can be especially challenging when the father or mother is dealing with the symptoms of schizophrenia. Partners often find it difficult to attend to the needs of their loved one with schizophrenia and still have time to spend with their children. In an attempt to protect children from information that may upset them, some spouses don't talk to them about their parent's mental illness. Unfortunately, this avoidance can often cause children to feel even more confused and worried. They may even blame themselves for causing their parent's illness. You will find more information about handling some of the challenges related to parenting in Chapter 9.

Strategies for Coping When Your Partner Has Schizophrenia

Although having a partner with schizophrenia presents challenges, you can use several strategies to help both of you cope more effectively. As you read through and evaluate the different strategies, keep in mind that your relationship with your partner is important in its own right and needs to be nurtured and supported. At the same time, each of your needs must be addressed. It's important to choose strategies that address the needs of the relationship as well as those of the two of you as individuals within that relationship.

• *Learn about the illness.* Knowledge about schizophrenia can keep you from feeling overwhelmed and can assist you in helping your partner. Chapters 1 and 2 can help you understand the illness and the characteristic behaviors you may have observed. As you and your partner develop more of a recovery vision, as described in Chapter 3, you will also feel more confident in encouraging her to pursue personal goals.

Besides the publications listed at the end of each chapter in this book, you can find additional information about schizophrenia at libraries and from organizations such as the National Alliance on Mental Illness (NAMI).

• *Support your partner's treatment.* The course of schizophrenia can be improved by comprehensive treatment, and as a spouse or partner you are in a unique position to reinforce the message that such treatment is beneficial. Because you spend more time with your partner and know her better than any professional, you are also in a special position to notice signs of stress and early signs of relapse. You can use this knowledge to help your partner develop an effective relapse prevention plan (see Chapter 12). Your participation on the treatment team can be invaluable to your partner.

• *Support your partner in taking medication.* Medications are still the most effective treatment for schizophrenia. You can help your partner remember to take medication by working with him to set up a system that makes taking medication part of the daily routine. For example, your partner may want to take medication at breakfast and could place the pill bottle next to the coffee pot or cereal boxes. He might like to use reminders or cues, such as placing Post-It notes on the bathroom mirror, writing on the calendar, or using pill organizers. Many people with schizophrenia also appreciate being able to talk openly with someone they can trust, such as their spouse, about medication side effects and their concerns about using medication, per se. You may want to ask your partner if you can attend some of her doctor's appointments together so that you can understand more about medications. Chapter 10 provides more information about medications and strategies for using them effectively.

• *Reduce household stress.* As described in Chapter 2, stress can cause symptom relapses. Sometimes it's helpful to reduce noise and increase predictability by maintaining a schedule for meals and other daily events. You can also become more aware of how you communicate with your partner; try to minimize the stress that comes from criticism, nagging, or repeated prompting. On the other hand, extreme self-sacrificing behavior can also be stressful to your partner, even when meant to be helpful.

Finally, although disagreements are bound to occur in any relationship, your communication should be as positive as possible. Chapters 14, 15, and 16 provide specific suggestions for developing effective communication and problem-solving skills that couples can use to reduce stress.

• *Help your partner avoid drinking and using drugs.* Many couples like to drink, smoke marijuana, or use other drugs together. Using substances is part of the way many people relax or socialize and may even be part of their intimacy style and sexual relationships. Substance use in even small amounts, however, can exacerbate the symptoms of schizophrenia and increase the risk of relapse. If you and your partner usually drink or use drugs together, his efforts to avoid substance use are likely to be more successful with your support.

Openly discussing the potential problems of using substances may be a good way to begin. You can then work together to identify other, less risky sources of achieving the effects that you have been getting from substances. If you drink or use drugs to reduce stress, what are some other ways you might increase the feeling of relaxation? If you drink to feel more intimate, what else would make you feel closer to your partner? One man said, "Jeannie and I used to need a drink to relax. We both realize that alcohol makes things worse for her now, so we've started trying other things, like going for a walk or listening to music." For more information about alcohol and drug abuse, see Chapter 22.

• *Develop a fair distribution of labor.* In the course of your partner's illness, there may be times when you need to do most of the work in maintaining the household, such as when the symptoms are very strong or during a hospitalization. When your partner is not in a crisis, however, it's important to work out a fair way of dividing the labor, based on each person's abilities. For most couples, including those for whom schizophrenia is not an issue, this division does not mean that everything will be 50/50. One person may still do more of the work, but the labor for maintaining the household should not fall solely on one person's shoulders. If you do *all* the work, you may soon feel resentful and burned out, and your partner will likely feel guilty and ineffectual. Sharing the household tasks reinforces the feeling of partnership.

• *Attend to your own needs.* In every intimate relationship it's important for partners to attend to their own needs as well as those of the other partner. Some might continue their education or move forward in their careers; others might pursue friendships, interests, and hobbies they find rewarding. If you ignore your own needs and sacrifice everything for your partner, you are likely to become dissatisfied with your relationship. As one woman acknowledged, "I'm glad I continued my training as a nurse. Becoming a nurse was very important to me, and I would have felt trapped if I had given that up."

Attending to your own needs also benefits each of you individually by reducing stress. Whether it's going running as you always have, attending your book club meetings, or taking a sailing class, if it relaxes and rejuvenates you, it will renew your energies for supporting your partner in coping with schizophrenia. In the process, it will help relieve the stress your partner may feel about his needs interfering with your life. "My wife encouraged me to keep up with my friends," said one husband whose wife has schizophrenia. "She said it would make her feel guilty if I lost touch with my fishing buddies."

• *Nurture your loving relationship.* Your relationship with your partner should extend beyond helping her cope with the illness, so that you don't become more like nurse and patient or parent and child than loving partners. Look for opportunities to connect through the activities you've always enjoyed together and to share your hopes, dreams, love, and what really matters to you in intimate conversation.

Keeping the romance alive in your relationship is also critical. Some couples say they set aside time every week to go out on a "date" and agree *not* to talk about problems then. They also make sure to express affection on a daily basis, remembering to say "I love you" and giving the partner a hug or kiss. Maintaining your sexual relationship is important as well; regularly set aside time when you can have privacy and feel relaxed and open to intimacy.

• *Directly address financial issues.* It's important to prepare for potential decreases in income and increases in expenses when your partner has schizophrenia. Your income could be affected by leaves of absence from work, periods of unemployment, interruption of retirement plans, and lost opportunities for promotions. Insurance copayments for psychiatric treatment, uninsured hospitalizations or outpatient visits, prescription medications, and the need to pay for services that your partner previously provided (e.g., childcare, household repairs) can strain your budget. Careful budgeting to take these possibilities into account may be all you need to do. But you might also explore financial and insurance benefits for which your husband or wife may be eligible, such as Social Security Disability, as described in Chapter 5. In addition, you should address, perhaps with the assistance of a financial planner, the issue of long-term financial security, including adequate funds for retirement.

• *Seek support and/or therapy.* Many people find it helpful to participate in a program designed for families of persons with mental illness. See page 64 for more information. Some chapters of NAMI and some community mental health centers have support groups specifically for spouses of people with mental illness. For example, Edie Mannion, at the Mental Health Association of Southeastern Pennsylvania, developed the Spouse Coping Skills Workshop in response to the unique needs of people whose partners have mental illness.

Sometimes couples therapy is helpful for (1) developing more effective communication skills that allow partners to express feelings constructively and (2) learning how to solve problems together. Be sure to seek a therapist who is knowledgeable not only about couples counseling but also about mental illness and strategies for coping with it.

• *Find strength in spirituality/religious faith.* Many people find support and strength for their relationship from spiritual or religious sources. Spirituality means different things to different people. For some, it means going to services regularly at their church, synagogue, temple, or mosque. For others it means communing with nature, practicing meditation, or helping others. For still others, personal prayer to a higher power is most meaningful. If spirituality is important to you, make time to participate in the activities that you find comforting and supportive.

• *Seek assistance regarding parenting.* If you and your partner are deciding whether to have children and have questions about the risk of a child developing schizophrenia, talk to your partner's psychiatrist and to a genetic counselor. Generally, the risk of a child with a parent with schizophrenia developing the illness is about 1 in 10 (10%) compared to about 1 in 100 (1%) if neither parent has schizophrenia. Talking over these risks with a doctor or counselor may help you make this important personal decision. If you already have children and are experiencing challenges related to parenting, you'll find some practical strategies in Chapter 9. You should also inquire at your local community mental health center about parenting programs designed for parents who have mental illness.

• *Strengthen communication and problem-solving skills.* Effective communication is important in any relationship. When schizophrenia affects one of the partners, it becomes even more critical. The symptoms of schizophrenia (such as delusions, hallucinations, and attention problems) may interfere with your partner's ability to pay full attention to what you say and may inhibit him from responding. Schizophrenia may also cause your partner to have a flat facial and vocal expression, which makes it difficult to read how he is feeling. Your partner may appear uninterested in what you're saying, even though he really cares. In addition, your partner may have little to talk about when he is feeling demoralized and withdrawn.

If you've noticed that communication with your partner is difficult, you may benefit from Chapters 14 and 15, where suggestions include:

- Getting to the point
- Expressing your feelings directly
- Using praise
- Checking out what your partner thinks or feels
- Being clear and specific
- Solving problems using a step-by-step method

If arguments, hostility, excessive criticism, raised voices, or negative voice tone occur frequently, you and your partner might benefit from working with a therapist to develop additional communication skills training. Behavioral family therapy is one approach to couple or family counseling that involves improving communication and problem-solving skills.

Sharing the Challenge: The Way to a Deeper Relationship

Schizophrenia can have a major impact on all close relationships, especially marriage and other committed partnerships. However, by learning about the illness together and developing strategies for managing it while keeping your relationship alive, you can maintain your commitment to, and enjoyment of, each other. An old adage states that "crisis is opportunity." Schizophrenia can be viewed as a crisis, and inherent in it lies the opportunity to dig deeper into your mutual bond, gather strength together, and become closer as you forge ahead in your shared lives. Many couples who face schizophrenia together become more intimate and appreciative of one another as they learn how to cope with the illness as but one of many of life's shared challenges.

Resources

Clausen, J. A. (1986). A 15- to 20-year follow-up of married adult psychiatric patients. In L. Erlenmeyer-Kimling & N. E. Miller (Eds.), *Life-span research on the prediction of psychopathology* (pp. 175–194). Hillsdale, NJ: Erlbaum. This chapter describes a long-term follow-up study of married persons with psychiatric disorders, many of whom have schizophrenia.

Fernando, R. A. (2004). *Loving a schizophrenic: A true story of love, loyalty and courage*. Singapore: Rank Books. The back cover accurately captures this couple's triumph over schizophrenia: "A heartwarming story of the healing power of love, this book chronicles the trials and tribulations of their courtship and 30-year marriage and provides an insightful peek into caring for a loved one stricken with mental illness."

Nasar, S. (1998). *A beautiful mind: The life of mathmatical genius and Nobel laureate John Nash*. New York: Simon & Schuster. The author includes the point of view and experiences of Dr. Nash's wife.

CHAPTER 9

Parenting and Children

Many people with schizophrenia have children or would like to have children in the future. If your relative has a child or is expecting one, you may worry that the additional strain of parenting could precipitate relapses or that schizophrenia may impair your relative's ability to care for a child. This chapter offers some ideas for helping your relative and her children.

If your relative is *your* mother or father, you may have other concerns. These, too, are addressed in the following pages.

Basic Facts about Schizophrenia and Parenting

Fifty to 70% of women and about 25% of men with schizophrenia marry. The difference in marriage rates appears to be related to the fact that women tend to develop schizophrenia at a slightly older age than men, which makes it more likely that they will date and marry before the illness surfaces. The lower rate of marriage for men with schizophrenia may also be due to the fact that society expects a man to take the more active role in courtship, which is difficult if he has psychotic symptoms or negative symptoms, such as lack of initiative, low energy, and social withdrawal.

The illness often poses challenges to maintaining a close relationship, leading to higher rates of marital distress and divorce among people with schizophrenia who marry. Marital outcomes in women and men with schizophrenia appear to be different. On average, women with schizophrenia tend to have a higher rate of separation and divorce than men with the illness, which results in more women living as single parents without the support of a partner.

Women with schizophrenia are almost as likely as other women to have children. Men with schizophrenia, on the other hand, are much less likely to have children than other men. Several research studies of parents who have schizophrenia have found that their relationships with their children are very important to them. However, symptoms such as hallucinations, delusions, cognitive problems, and lack of energy and initiative can interfere with the parenting ability of even the most loving and caring person, and it is common for men and women with schizophrenia to have significant difficulties raising their children. For example, mothers show more tension and have fewer interactions with their children than other mothers. Because of the difficulties in parenting, many parents give up or lose custody of their children, who may then live with relatives or in foster homes.

If your relative with schizophrenia is a parent, you can help in many ways. Research shows that receiving support and assistance from caring individuals helps people with schizophrenia function more effectively as parents and helps their children grow up more resilient and happy.

Experiences of People with Schizophrenia Who Have Children

If your relative is rarely troubled by symptoms, he may have very few parenting difficulties related to the illness and need only the usual support appreciated by any parent, such as occasional help with childcare. If your relative has episodes of severe symptoms but functions well between episodes, he may need extra assistance during those times. If your relative has ongoing symptoms that interfere with parenting, he is likely to need regular assistance. Although each person's situation is unique, the following are typical of the challenges that your relative may face as a parent.

Interference from Psychotic Symptoms

Hallucinations or delusions can be distracting and make it difficult to judge reality. This type of difficulty is especially important when caring for small children. One parent said, "I enjoyed feeding my little boy his lunch, but sometimes voices would tell me that his food was poisoned, so to protect him I would throw away his peanut butter sandwich." Another parent said that he once believed he was a special agent of the FBI and his children were spies in disguise. "I didn't *really* think it was true, but I felt tense around my kids because of that."

Interference from Negative Symptoms

Negative symptoms such as low energy, lack of initiative, social withdrawal, and diminished emotional expressiveness can also cause difficulties. One mother with low energy often felt extremely tired and slept long hours, even though her young children woke up early and needed supervision. Low energy also interfered with her ability to take her children to the playground or respond to their requests to play games with them. One father felt uncomfortable being around people and was reluctant to take his child to a play group where conversation with other parents was expected. When parents have diminished emotional expressiveness, their children may have trouble reading their emotions and may think, for example, that their parents are angry with them even when they are not or are not interested in them when they are.

Cognitive Problems

Difficulties with attention, concentration, and memory may pose problems for parents. One mother found it hard to keep track of the many school holidays of her first grader and on several occasions walked him to school when it wasn't in session. Another mother reported having trouble staying focused when she took her child with her to the grocery store and would sometimes come home with only one or two of the many items she had intended to buy. One father with schizophrenia said, "I wanted to help my son with his math homework, but even though I knew the material, my concentration was poor, and I couldn't explain things to him." Some parents describe being disorganized about housework and putting groceries away in places that made it hard to find them later.

Dealing with the Stresses of Parenting

Parenting can be stressful to anyone, but schizophrenia may leave parents even more vulnerable. "I would get so upset when my baby daughter was crying," said one mother. "Even if it was just for a little while, it could unsettle me for the rest of the day." A father said that when his son was in the "terrible twos" stage and saying "no" to everything, "I could handle that for only a little while before calling my wife in; she didn't take it so personally."

Isolation

Many parents with schizophrenia who have young children report that they have few contacts with other adults. "I just take care of my kids all day sometimes and never see anyone else," said one mother. "I'm a single parent, and I don't have anyone to talk to about things that come up with the kids." Many times the children may feel isolated, too, because their parents find it difficult to arrange play dates or visit other families with children.

Separations Due to Hospitalizations

The hospitalization of a parent with schizophrenia has an effect on the whole family. Young children, especially, miss their parents and wonder where they are and when they are coming back. Children may even worry that *they* did something to cause their parent to leave them. Parents also suffer during separations from their children. One mother said, "I hated to go to the hospital, even though I knew I needed it, because Cindy would miss me. And I missed her terribly." If separations are frequent, it may be more difficult for the child to bond and form a trusting relationship with the absent parent. The difficulties can be compounded if children are not told where or why their parents are going, or if alternative childrearing arrangements are required such as being raised by other relatives or requiring foster care.

Behavior That May Put Their Children at Risk

Sometimes parents with schizophrenia behave in ways that could endanger their children. Severe negative symptoms may result in neglect of children, such as one mother who stayed in bed all day, unable to change her toddler's diapers or fix her lunch. Psychotic symptoms such as hallucinations or delusions can lead a parent to engage in dangerous behavior. One mother told us, "The voices were telling me that my little boy was possessed by the devil and that the only way to save him was to hike to the lake and baptize him. The voices were so convincing. I feel terrible every time I think about Aaron getting sunburned and hungry on the way to that lake."

Severe psychotic symptoms can sometimes lead to more dangerous behavior toward the child, such as when a parent believes that her child is not real or that she must kill her child to prevent her from future suffering. These situations are rare, but nonetheless they occur. Preventive steps can be taken by monitoring the parent's symptoms closely, ensuring that severe psychotic symptoms are treated rapidly and effectively, and helping the parent with childrearing responsibilities. In some situations you may need to take over your relative's parenting responsibilities, at least temporarily, to ensure a child's safety.

Concern about Losing Custody

When parents with schizophrenia experience severe symptoms and are unable to care for their children, or when they put their child at risk, the local child protection agency may become involved. This agency may provide additional support for the parent or place the child in foster care if there are no relatives to take care of him. Most parents find it very distressing to lose custody of their children, even temporarily. In fact, avoiding losing custody of their children is a powerful motivator for some parents to become more actively involved in treatment and to take additional steps to manage their mental illness more effectively. "I love my children so much," said one mother, "and it just tore me apart when they went to foster care. I vowed to do anything I could to be a better parent so it would never happen again."

Strategies for Helping Your Relative with Parenting

If your relative experiences challenges as a parent, there are several ways that you can help. Remember that this assistance can be critical in helping your relative retain custody of her children. As you read the following suggestions, keep in mind that everything you do to help your relative will also help her children.

• *Become aware of your relative's parenting strengths.* People with schizophrenia, like anyone else, have strengths and weaknesses as parents. Being aware of both in your relative will give you a balanced perspective and allow you to identify areas in which assistance may be needed. A frequently noted strength of parents with schizophrenia is their strong love for their children and the desire to be good parents. "Having children and doing a good job raising them was very important to me," one mother said. "Although it's been difficult at times, it has also brought me great joy." Let your relative know that you notice and appreciate all the positive things he does as a parent. One uncle, who was very involved in helping his niece, said, "Neisha was so surprised when I complimented her about the imaginative games she played with her son. She thought only about her short-comings."

• *Provide assistance as needed.* Like all parents, your relative may appreciate assistance with childcare and cooking or housework. You may notice, however, that your relative needs more help in certain areas during times of stress. "My son was a good father in so many ways," said one mother, "but when he wasn't sleeping well or got stressed out about something, he lost his patience with his daughter. I used to take her to my house for a few days to let him get himself back together." You may notice your relative needs help on a more regular basis. "For several years I helped Noreen with the grocery shopping and picked up Aiden from school every day," said one woman's aunt. "It was a big responsibility, but I saw that she could do well in other ways if I took those things off her mind."

• *Encourage your relative to learn how to manage her illness.* Family members often report that the desire to parent well has motivated their relative to partici-pate in treatment. "Sonia was unwilling to take medication until we had some long conversations about how it might help her control the voices that were get-ting in the way of her taking care of her baby," said the sister of one mother with schizophrenia. "She really cares about being a good mom and said she would try taking medication if it would help her do that." After talking with her brother and sister about their concerns, one mother with schizophrenia agreed to work on a relapse prevention plan with her treatment team because she realized that relapses and hospitalizations resulted in separations from her daughter.

When discussing the connection between good parenting and taking care of his illness with your relative, be supportive and encouraging and avoid criticism or blaming. You might try the *Socratic method* (described in Chapter 17), which involves asking a series of questions, to eventually lead your relative to his own conclusion. The advantage of this approach is that your relative is more likely to accept his own answers and conclusions than to accept what you tell him to do. Etta's brother used gentle questioning to help her examine how she might prevent future hospitalizations to avoid being separated from her 2-year-old daughter.

• *Monitor early warning signs and develop a relapse prevention plan.* To prevent the effects of relapses and hospitalizations on parenting, you can help your relative become more aware of the early warning signs of relapse and develop a relapse prevention plan. See Chapter 12 for more details about developing a relapse prevention plan.

• *Help your relative learn how to cope with persistent symptoms.* If your relative is troubled by persistent symptoms, you can help him learn coping strategies to minimize the effects, as described in Part V of this book. One husband helped his wife identify a strategy for coping with auditory hallucinations. By humming to herself while she changed her baby's diapers, she was able to pay less attention to the voices, and her baby seemed to enjoy hearing the melody. A father who experienced diminished emotional expressiveness worked on this problem with his sister and learned to verbally express his feelings to his children, rather than rely on his facial expression and voice tone.

• *Strengthen your relationship with the children.* Abundant research shows that children who grow up with access to good social support and a caring, loving person in their lives are more resilient to stress and lead happier and more productive lives. So, developing a strong, positive relationship with your relative's children is bound to be beneficial. And that relationship will also make your relative's children feel comfortable with you should they need care when your relative is experiencing symptoms, going to an appointment, or in the hospital. If you are the spouse or partner of the parent with schizophrenia, you naturally spend time with your children and have already developed strong relationships with them. If you are the sibling, parent, or other family member, look for opportunities to spend time with your relative's children on a regular basis, well in advance of any crisis that might arise.

• *Assist your relative in developing a childcare plan.* It's important to plan in advance for childcare should your relative suffer a relapse. You may play an important part in the plan by agreeing to care for your relative's children in case the need arises. The Parent Project Team of the Queensland Centre for Mental Health Research in Australia suggests developing a written childcare plan. Worksheet 9.1 at the end of the chapter provides a form for developing such a plan with your relative. We suggest that the people who agree to be part of the plan sign it and receive a copy and that the children be made aware of its important details.

• *Encourage your relative to take part in a parenting program.* Specialized parenting programs for people with mental illness teach specific parenting strategies. Some are group based and others are home based. Contact the Invisible Children's Project at the National Mental Health Association in Arlington, VA (see Resources at the end of this chapter) to identify selected programs throughout the United States. In the absence of a specialized program, however, you can help your relative investigate general parenting programs available in your community, such as those sponsored by the YMCA, the library, the school system, or a religious organization.

Developing an Awareness of Potential Problems for Children

Having a parent with schizophrenia does not mean that a child will necessarily develop problems. The next section of this chapter can help an adult or adolescent child understand and cope with having a parent with schizophrenia. If you are another relative of someone with schizophrenia, the section will help you become aware of potential problems for children and to take preventive steps. For example, if you realize that some children feel pressured into adopting a parental role with their younger siblings, you will be better able to help by making sure that the children get their needs met from some other source. If you realize that children of parents with schizophrenia are often isolated and understimulated, you would be alert to opportunities to get your relative's children involved in outside activities, such as sports, Scouts, dance, music, art, or programs at your place of worship.

Teamwork

Helping a loved one with schizophrenia often involves several family members working together as well as they can. The willingness of different members to pitch in becomes all the more critical when the person with schizophrenia has children, and the complications imposed by the illness are multiplied. The Thomas family illustrates how one family worked together to address the parenting needs of a young mother with schizophrenia and her husband.

Samantha developed schizophrenia in her mid-20s and married Nathaniel a few years later. Within a year of their marriage they had their first child, and a year and a half later they had a second child. The children were very much welcomed by Samantha and Nathaniel, but it was difficult to attend to their many needs. Samantha's negative symptoms often made it difficult for her to get up and take care of the children; feeding them regular meals, changing their diapers, and keeping them dressed in clean clothes were substantial challenges for her. Nathaniel worked long hours as a painter's assistant and was frequently unavailable to help with the children.

Samantha and Nathaniel together had a lot of difficulty keeping up with their children's needs. Samantha lived in the same town as, and had regular contact with, her sister, brother, and father, who all became concerned that the children were sometimes hungry and wearing dirty clothes when they arrived for visits. Samantha's case manager was also concerned with Samantha and her husband's ability to take care of their children and retain legal custody, and she discussed this issue with the couple and the rest of the family. She referred them to a clinician trained in family psychoeducation (see Chapter 5) who worked closely with them, teaching them about schizophrenia and its treatment and helping them address the parenting problems Samantha was experiencing.

Working as a team, the family members divided up the basic childcare tasks that Samantha had difficulty doing regularly. For example, Samantha's father, sister, and brother each committed to coming to Samantha and Nathaniel's house once a week to do a few loads of laundry and prepare a simple dinner. They also picked one Saturday per month when they would take the children to their own homes to give Samantha and Nathaniel some time alone and to give the children an outing. Nathaniel agreed to help more with grocery shopping and taking the children to the playground on the weekends.

Samantha said she appreciated the help with the physical care of the children but at times felt confused and stressed by certain aspects of parenting, such as how to respond to her 2-year-old saying "No" all the time. At the suggestion of the family clinician, she and Nathaniel started participating in a parenting program and got ideas from the teacher about disciplining young children in a firm but nonpunitive way. They also received support from the other parents, who were dealing with similar challenges. While they attended the 10-week program, Samantha's father and siblings took turns babysitting the children.

All was not smooth sailing. For example, on one occasion Samantha stopped taking her medication and experienced a return of auditory hallucinations. Because her family members each had weekly contact, they noticed that she was talking to herself and neglecting some childcare tasks such as changing the children's clothing and putting away milk and other perishable foods. They conferred with each other and Nathaniel and immediately called a family meeting. They presented their concerns in a supportive way, emphasizing that they knew Samantha wanted to be a good parent. At first she denied having any problems with symptoms, but gradually she came to agree that she was feeling "stressed out by these voices in my head" and admitted she had thrown out her medications. She agreed to see her doctor the next day, and her father offered to drive her there and to the pharmacy. Her sister arranged to take care of the children while she was at the appointment, and her brother offered to help out with the children in the evening. Because the medication did not take effect immediately, Samantha's relatives ended up taking turns having the children at their home for a few weeks.

Over the years, Samantha's family had regular hands-on involvement with her and her children. Although it was time-consuming and at times challenging to juggle their other responsibilities, they worked as a team and felt pride as a family that they had helped one of their members achieve her goal of being a good parent.

Having a Parent with Schizophrenia

Having a mother or father with schizophrenia can have a significant impact on your childhood and may influence the way you think and feel as a teenager or an adult. Understanding your feelings about your parent and coming to terms with how she has affected your life can help set the stage for coping more effectively.

Confusion

Many adult children describe being very confused and unsettled by the behavior of their parent with schizophrenia. Often strange behaviors were related to psychotic symptoms such as auditory hallucinations or delusions. "When I was little, sometimes I would find my mother putting away my toys, talking with the stuffed animals," said one young man, remembering his childhood. "It scared me." One teenager tells of her father watching cartoons attentively, taking pages of notes about the characters. "He said that the cartoon characters were talking in a special code and that he was going to figure it out. I sure couldn't figure him out."

Sometimes the confusing actions of your parent may have been caused by negative symptoms, such as low energy, lack of initiative, or diminished facial expressiveness. "I couldn't figure out why my mom never had the energy to push me on the swings at the playground," said one young woman, remembering her childhood. "The other moms did that with no trouble." One teenager, who currently lives with his father, finds it difficult to read his emotional state, saying, "My dad's face always looks kind of flat. I can't even tell if he's glad to see me or if he's interested in what I'm saying."

Perhaps no one told you the facts about your parent's mental illness or why she needed to go to the hospital, and you tried to figure things out on your own. "I wish someone had told me why Mom acted the way she did," said one young woman. "My theories were pretty wacky, like thinking it had something to do with what she ate, or even worse, thinking it was caused by giving birth to me or my brother."

For some children additional confusion comes from observing their parents' complicated relationships. These children often see love and affection between their parents, but also a great deal of stress and conflict. Although this kind of strain can occur in any marriage when one partner has a chronic medical illness, it can be more severe when the illness involves psychiatric symptoms. As Chantelle said about her parents' marriage, "They went through such extreme ups and downs. One day they were affectionate to each other and to us kids. The next day Mom was accusing Dad of having an affair with every woman on the block and us of 'colluding with the devil.' It took me years to believe that people could love each other and not have all that drama."

Embarrassment and Stigmatization

You may have experienced situations (perhaps many) where your parent's behavior embarrassed you. "My mother collected stones from the road sometimes," said one son. "She told the neighbors that these pieces of rock would get us all into heaven. I was mortified." You may have been asked by others to explain your parent's behavior, such as the daughter who said that her fourth-grade classmates always asked why her mother included unusual items in her lunch, such as foil-wrapped thimbles and empty candy wrappers. "I didn't understand it myself, so how could I explain it to anyone else? I started eating lunch by myself to avoid the questions."

You may have felt stigmatized by having a parent with schizophrenia, especially if you heard people in the community making negative comments about mental illness in general and even specific, critical comments about your parents. Nadia's best friend in high school stopped spending time with her because her parents told her that "Nadia's father is a psycho, and he might kill someone someday." Children may avoid being with their parents away from home so they don't have to deal with embarrassment or stigma. This avoidance deprives children of opportunities to be with other people and learn skills for socializing.

Even as an adult you might find yourself in embarrassing situations. "I guess I'm pretty used to being in awkward spots with my dad by now," said one man. "Although when he starts to talk to the waitress about which menu items have been blessed by the pope, I still get self-conscious."

Instances of Neglect

Severe symptoms may have caused your parent to neglect you at times. "I'm old enough to take care of myself now," said one teenager, "but it was a real problem when I was younger and Mom used to say she'd be back in a minute, but my sister and I were alone for hours. I learned that I couldn't count on her." Another teenager said he remembered times when there was nothing to eat but cereal for several days.

Getting Pulled into a Caregiving Role

You may have experienced being pulled in, at a young age, to help or take care of your parent. "I remember going to the store for my mom when I could barely carry the grocery sack by myself," said one young adult. "Lots of times she was either too worn out or too scared by the voices to face the outside world. So I ended up doing many of the errands." One teenager said he often had to seek help when his mother was experiencing severe symptoms. "One of the first things I remember doing when I got my driver's license was taking my mom to the psychiatric emergency room." Older children may assume the role of taking care of younger siblings when their parent can't do so. "I used to miss school sometimes to take care of my little brother and sister," says one young woman. "Somebody had to do it." Other children find themselves consoling their other parent over "losing" a spouse to schizophrenia. "My poor father," said one young woman. "He was lost without my mother, and I used to make his dinner and keep him company so he wouldn't be so sad."

If you were asked to take on a "parentified" role at a young age you may feel as if you were cheated out of your childhood. Furthermore, as adults, many people who had a parent with schizophrenia say they are reluctant to have children of their own. "I had more than enough of being a mom when I took care of my younger brother and sister all those years," said one woman. "I just want to be responsible for myself." Some adults may still be taking care of their parent with schizophrenia, which takes away time and energy from developing relationships and careers. "I want to meet someone and get married," said one man, "but I always seem to be getting crisis calls about Dad. When do I have time for myself?"

Additional problems can arise as the parent with schizophrenia gets older. Although many people with schizophrenia have less severe symptoms later in life, their general health may be poor. Declining health is often a natural consequence of aging, but it may be magnified for many people with schizophrenia because they did not receive good health care. In addition, many people have health problems related to smoking, lack of exercise, and obesity. Adult children who have an aging parent with schizophrenia must often question anew how involved they should be and how they can balance their own needs with those of their parent.

Keeping Family Secrets

Stigma often motivates people with schizophrenia and their families to keep that information very private. Unfortunately, this stance often puts children in the awkward position of having to keep secrets. "From a very early age I was told not to tell anyone at all about my dad's hearing voices and having to go to the psychiatric hospital," said one man. "I used to lie when the minister asked why he wasn't at church and say that he broke his leg or he was visiting his cousin in Atlanta or that he was fixing the roof. I got almost too good at lying, which caused me trouble later in life." Sometimes children begin to feel that *any* personal information is dangerous to reveal and become habitually secretive. "It was hard to make friends because I never told them anything about myself or my home life," said one teenager. "Other kids thought I was stuck up and just gave up on me."

Some people continue to keep the secret of their parent's mental illness into adulthood. "Even now none of my friends realizes that my mother has schizophrenia," said one woman. "I've been dating a guy for a whole year now, and we've gotten pretty serious. He has asked to meet my parents, and I keep putting him off. I'm afraid he won't understand or it will hurt our relationship."

Isolation

Like many people whose parents have schizophrenia, you may have felt isolated as a child and continue to feel alone in many respects as an adult. "No one understands what I'm going through," said one teenager. "The other kids are worrying about cell phones and wearing the latest clothes. Not me. I'm the one who's worried about whether it's safe to leave his mom alone at home while he's at school. I feel like I'm the only one who has to go through this." Many children find it difficult to share with others or to form close relationships even as adults.

Concern about Genetic Vulnerability to Schizophrenia

You may worry that whatever caused your mother or father's schizophrenia will cause you to develop the illness. This is not a completely unrealistic concern, because having a close relative with schizophrenia (such as a parent) does increase the risk of developing it. One man said that as a teenager he finally asked his mother's psychiatrist about his level of risk. "He could have emphasized that I have a 10% chance of developing schizophrenia, but I'm glad he put it a different way. He said I had a *90%* chance of *not* getting it."

You may also worry that even if you do not develop schizophrenia yourself, your children would have an increased risk of developing it because their grandparent has the illness. For some adult children of parents with schizophrenia, this factor enters into their decision to have children. Although the risk of developing schizophrenia is less if a person has a grandparent rather than a parent with the illness, it is still slightly higher—about 3%—than for someone who has no relatives with schizophrenia. If this issue concerns you, talk to a genetic counselor.

In the past, people with schizophrenia typically spent much of their lives in institutions, but today they are much more likely to live in the community and to have contact with extended family, including grandchildren. You may find yourself needing to answer your own child's question, "Why does Grandma behave that way?"

Strategies for Coping with a Parent with Schizophrenia

- *Learn about schizophrenia.* Becoming knowledgeable about your parent's illness will help you understand what you've been observing over the years and to recognize some of the challenges with which your parent has been dealing. Chapters 1 and 2 contain basic information about schizophrenia. You'll find additional information about schizophrenia in the books listed in the Resources section at the end of this chapter, at the public library, or at the local chapter of the National Alliance on Mental Illness (NAMI). If you have a younger brother or sister, or a child of your own, you may want to share some of the books appropriate for the child's age. Reading Chapter 3, which discusses recovery from schizophrenia and the fact that the illness often improves over time, will also help you develop a more optimistic view of your parent's future.

- *Take care of your own needs.* Avoid becoming so involved in helping your parent that you miss out on pursuing your own interests and ambitions. If you're a teenager, it's especially important not to neglect school and friends. Try to find outlets for your talents, such as music, dance, sports, and art. Look for organizations where you can meet a wide range of other people, such as scouting programs, religious groups, or volunteer and advocacy programs (such as Habitat for Humanity or the Sierra Club). One teenager said, "Being on the high school volleyball team was a lifesaver for me. I got to meet other kids, and we had sports in common. The other parents were happy to give me rides to the games, too. It was a chance to get away from some of the stresses of home and to do something for myself for a change." If you're an adult, be sure to pursue educational, career, and family goals and to balance your own needs with those of your parent. "I have my own family," says one man, "but I take turns with my brothers and sisters in helping out when my mom has troubles."

• *Get support.* If you've felt alone in having a parent with schizophrenia, you may be interested in meeting others who can share your experiences. Some CMHCs offer special programs for people of different ages who have mental illness in their family, and new programs are currently being developed. For example, the Mental Health Association of Southeastern Pennsylvania in Philadelphia has developed a 6-week coping skills program for children ages 7–10, an interactive website for adolescents, and a workshop and support group for adult children of parents with mental illness (see the Resources section at the end of this chapter).

Many adults benefit from support groups such as the Sibling and Adult Children Network, which is part of NAMI. This group brings people together to talk about their experiences and to share strategies and information about resources. If you attend a support group, either as a teenager or as an adult, you are not required to talk about yourself. But whether or not you speak in a support group, you will find that you are not alone, that others share your experiences, *and* that others care. You may also benefit from talking to a counselor or therapist who can provide support and help you develop strategies for responding to particular problems.

• *Decide how involved you want to be.* How involved you are with your mother or father depends a great deal on your age, your relationship with this parent, other responsibilities, and additional sources of support available to you. Some teenagers are closely involved in their parent's day-to-day affairs, whereas others feel comfortable keeping more of a distance. One teenager said, "My dad handles most of the things that have to do with Mom's schizophrenia, but my sister and I pitch in around the house when she's having a bad day." Another teenager said, "My mom is a single parent, so I end up taking up a lot of the slack. My uncle is real helpful, though, and I call him a lot." Adults also find different levels of involvement comfortable. Some adults have minimal contact with their parent, whereas others are closely involved with their care on a regular basis.

Issues of level of involvement also arise as the parent ages. The parent may have fewer or less severe symptoms as she gets older, and a closer positive relationship may be possible. However, the parent may also have significant physical problems related to aging and may require a great deal of assistance. Like the rest of the population, adult children of aging parents vary widely as to how much care they provide directly and how much they help their parents get the help they need from public and private agencies. As one adult daughter said, "I have young children, and both my husband and I need to work to make ends meet. It took a long time, but my sister and I found a nursing home that understands Mom's mental illness and her physical problems. We visit her once a week and keep an eye on her care."

At a minimum, we recommend trying to remain informed about how daily life is going for your mother or father and how treatment is progressing.

• *Identify your strengths and those of your parent* Depending on the experience you've had with your parent, you may be troubled by bad memories and negative feelings. It's natural to focus on the downside of things when you've had a difficult time, but it's important to balance this view with an awareness of your personal strengths, those of your parent, and the strengths of your entire family. Many people who have a parent with schizophrenia feel that because of their experience, they developed certain strengths such as perseverance, ingenuity, resilience, and compassion. Others say that, as they learn more about the illness, they begin to recognize the struggle that their parent endured and the strength and courage it took to survive. You may become more aware of the strengths of your family, working collectively, as reflected by their love and support for one another, their ability to endure the hardships imposed by schizophrenia, and their commitment to each other. Thinking more positively does not take away the difficulties you've experienced, but it may help you move beyond the events of the past and develop more optimism about what you (and your parent) can experience in the future.

Family Strengths

Helping a person with schizophrenia who has children can be a great challenge. Whether you are the relative of someone with schizophrenia who is a parent or you are the child of a parent with schizophrenia, you know firsthand that the illness affects many aspects of family life, especially the parent–child relationship. Learning about schizophrenia and sharing your thoughts, feelings, and concerns with other family members and friends are important steps toward coping with the illness and appreciating the strengths of everyone in your family. If your loved one is a parent, you can also support him and form nurturing relationships with the children. If you're the child of someone with schizophrenia, you may benefit from the assistance of other family members and from meeting others who can share your experiences. With time and support, your relationship with your parent can be positive and rewarding.

Resources

Alda, A. (2005). *Never have your dog stuffed and other things I've learned* New York: Random House. In this poignant, amusing memoir actor-writer-director Alan Alda reminisces about his life, including growing up with and learning to understand his mother with schizophrenia.

Brown, M., & Parker Roberts, D. (2000). *Growing up with a schizophrenic mother.* Jefferson, NC, and London: McFarland & Company, Inc. Research into the experience of having a mother with schizophrenia found many children had unpleasant experiences, but the authors are careful to blame the illness and describe positive experiences and close mother–child bonds as well.

Gopfert, M., Webster, J., & Seeman, M. V. (Eds.). (2004). *Parental psychiatric disorder: Distressed parents and their families.* Cambridge, UK: Cambridge University Press. An international multidisciplinary team of professionals reviews the most up-to-date interventions for children whose parents have a psychiatric disorder. Some chapters are aimed at clinicians, but others, such as Chapter 1, will be useful to family members who wonder how much to tell children.

Holly, T. E., & Holly, J. (1997). *My mother's keeper: A daughter's memoir of growing up in the shadow of mental illness.* New York: Avon Grove. The author was primarily raised by her relatives but assumed guardianship at age 16 for her mother.

Mack, M. (2004). *Homework.* 33 Harding Street, Suite 2, Cambridge, MA: Big Twig Press. *Homework* is a booklet of selections from a one-man play about Mr. Mack's experiences growing up with a mother who had schizophrenia, which he presents to a variety of audiences, including the general public, consumers, family members, and providers of mental health services. E-mail address: *mmack@alum.mit.edu*.

Olson, L. S. (1994). *He was still my daddy: Coming to terms with mental illness.* Portland, OR: Ogden House. A teenager's account of growing up with a father who has schizophrenia.

Secunda, V. (1998). *When madness comes home: Help and hope for families of the mentally ill.* New York: Hyperion. Focuses on the experiences of children, siblings, and spouses of persons with mental illness.

For Younger Readers

Adler, C. S. (1983). *The shell lady's daughter.* New York: Fawcett Books. A 14-year-old girl goes to live with her grandparents in Florida after her mother has an episode of mental illness. (Available from *www.backinprint.com*)

Alma, A. (2000). *Summer of changes.* Victoria, BC: Sono Nis Press. Tells the story of an 11-year-old girl who spends some time living with foster parents because her mother has schizophrenia.

Campbell, B. M. (2003). *Sometimes my mommy gets angry.* New York: Putnam. In this illustrated book for young children, a grandmother helps her granddaughter see that her mentally ill mother loves her.

Diner, S. (1989). *Nothing to be ashamed of: Growing up with mental illness in your family.* New York: Lothrop. This book is written for youngsters ages 10–15.

McDonald, B. (1994). *Helping each other.* Available through NAMI, this is a coloring book to help young children understand that families can work together on challenges presented by illnesses.

Riley, J. (1982). *Only my mouth is smiling*. New York: William Morrow. Three siblings move away from their home in Chicago with their mother, who has mental illness. For young adults.

Websites with Information for Children, Teenagers, and Adult Children

www.aicafmha.net.au/copmi. The Australian Infant, Child, Adolescent and Family Mental Health Association has a special section for children at its website.

www.copmi.net.au. Children of Parents with a Mental Illness. This Australian resource center for information relating to families where a parent has a mental illness offers helpful booklets, such as "The Best for Me and My Baby," "Family Talk," and "Baby Care Plan" (click on "Education," then "Downloadable Booklets").

www.itsallright.org. SANE of Australia has a website for teenagers with a relative with mental illness that provides information and suggestions specifically aimed at young people.

www.mhasp.org. The Mental Health Association of Southeastern Pennsylvania has an interactive website for children of parents with mental illness, including separate sections for adolescents, family members, teachers, and professionals.

www.nami.org. NAMI's website includes a section called "Coping Tips for Siblings and Adult Children of Persons with Mental Illness."

www.nmha.org/children/invisible.cfm. The Invisible Children Project's website contains information about services for children whose parents have mental illness.

www.outoftheshadow.com. Susan Smiley filmed a documentary, *Out of the Shadow*, about growing up with a mother with schizophrenia. The website has information on how to purchase copies of the film, or you can call (310) 636-0116.

www.vicnet.net.au (search for NNAAMI). The National Network of Adult and Adolescent Children Who Have a Mentally Ill Parent (NNAAMI) website has first-person accounts and relevant articles.

www.youngcarers.net. The Princess Royal Trust for Carers in the United Kingdom has a special website for teenagers caring for a relative with mental illness. It addresses feelings, provides referrals to helpful agencies, and offers personal stories of others going through the same problems.

Parenting Resources

Brunette, M., Richardson, F., White, L., Bemis, G., & Eelkema, R. (2004). Integrated family treatment for parents with severe mental illness. *Journal of Psychiatric Rehabilitation, 28*, 177–180. The authors describe a home-based parenting training and family support program for parents with severe mental illness.

Dinkmeyer, D., McKay, G., & Dinkmeyer, D., Jr. (1997). *The parent's handbook: Systematic training for effective parenting (STEP)*. Pines, MN: American Guidance Service. Teaches ways to communicate with children, to encourage them, and to use nonpunitive discipline when necessary.

The Institute for Health and Recovery in Cambridge, MA, offers a publication (*Nurturing Families Affected by Substance Abuse, Mental Illness and Trauma*) containing parenting curriculum with guidelines for one-on-one mentoring sessions, psychoeducational groups for parents, and parent–child activity sessions. It can be found by going to their website (*www.healthrecovery.org*) and clicking on "Products."

Nicholson, J., Henry, A., Clayfield, J., & Phillips, S. (2001). *Parenting well when you're depressed: A complete resource for maintaining a healthy family.* Oakland, CA: New Harbinger. Contains practical suggestions for parents who have depression; many of the suggestions are applicable to parents with schizophrenia.

The Parents Leadership Institute has a variety of parenting videotapes (such as *Setting Limits with Children*) listed at their website: *www.parentleaders.org*.

Queensland Centre for Mental Health Research. *The needs of parents with psychotic disorders: A kit for service providers*. (Available from *www.qcmhr.uq.edu.au/pdfs/full%20parent%20kit.pdf*) Written for professionals, this book contains a wealth of practical information useful to anyone, including family members, involved in helping parents with a serious mental illness. A free hard copy of the kit can be obtained from:

> Duncan McLean, Research Scientist
> QCMHR
> The Park-Centre for Mental Health
> Locked Bag 500
> Richlands, Queensland, 4077
> Australia
> +61 7 3271 8686
> +61 7 3271 8698 (fax)
> *duncan_mclean@qcmhr.uq.edu.au*

Childcare Plan

Name of parent: _____ Date of plan: _____

Names and ages of children: _____

_____

Name, address, and phone numbers of two people who agree to look after the children	1. 2.
Who will contact these people?	
How will the children get to their houses?	
What do the children need to take with them, such as clothing, toiletry items, special stuffed animals or toys, medications, or medical supplies?	
Describe any special routines that would help the children feel more comfortable away from home.	

Signature of parent: _____

Signature of contact person 1: _____

Signature of contact person 2: _____

PART III

Preventing Relapses

CHAPTER 10

Medication

*A*ntipsychotic medications, also called *neuroleptics* or *major tranquilizers*, are an enormous benefit to the vast majority of people with schizophrenia. Medication is not a *cure* for schizophrenia, and most people need other treatments as well, but it is an important foundation that should be used in combination with psychosocial treatments. This chapter provides you with practical information about the medications used to treat schizophrenia, their benefits and side effects, how to handle common problems (e.g., your relative stops taking his medication), and how to evaluate the quality of your relative's pharmacological treatment.

The Discovery of Antipsychotic Medications

Like many other medications, antipsychotic medications were discovered accidentally. In the 1950s scientists synthesized a new medication intended for the treatment of high blood pressure, *chlorpromazine* (brand name *Thorazine*). Laboratory tests on animals found that chlorpromazine was safe, and although it had limited effects on blood pressure, scientists noted that it had a mildly tranquilizing effect. Researchers began to explore whether chlorpromazine might be useful in people with psychiatric disorders. Their most astonishing discovery was that it dramatically reduced psychotic symptoms such as hallucinations and delusions in people with schizophrenia. Following these initial experiments, numerous controlled studies confirmed its effectiveness in treating schizophrenia.

As the remarkable effects of chlorpromazine were recognized, it became widely used to help many people move out of state hospitals and back into the community. With the success of chlorpromazine, scientists developed other anti-

---

We appreciate the helpful comments of Mary Brunette, MD, and Douglas Noordsy, MD, on this chapter.

psychotic medications that had similar positive effects in the following decades. The development of new antipsychotic medications for schizophrenia continues.

How Do Antipsychotic Medications Work?

Scientists believe that antipsychotic medications are effective because of their impact on a chemical in the brain, *dopamine*, which functions as a *neurotransmitter*—a substance that transmits nerve impulses across a synapse. Research conducted on laboratory animals has shown that the potency of different antipsychotic medications can be explained almost perfectly by the amount of dopamine in the brain that is *blocked* by that medication. Drugs that increase dopamine, such as stimulants (e.g., cocaine, amphetamine), tend to worsen the symptoms of schizophrenia, whereas drugs with no effect on dopamine tend not to affect the symptoms of the disorder.

The role of dopamine in the regulation of mood, thinking, and behavior is complex. For example, there is more than one type of dopamine receptor, and different antipsychotic medications have different effects on each type. Furthermore, dopamine serves different functions in different parts of the brain. Some theories state that people with schizophrenia have too little dopamine in the *prefrontal cortex* (a part of the brain involved in attention and processing information) and too much in the *mesolimbic area* of the brain (involved in imagery, perception, and emotion). To complicate matters, some antipsychotics influence other important neurotransmitters, such as *serotonin*. Every day scientists are learning more about how the brain works (both in people without a psychiatric disorder and in those with a disorder), and this knowledge is gradually being translated into better treatments for those with schizophrenia.

How Antipsychotic Medications Affect Schizophrenia

Antipsychotic medications can reduce the severity of symptoms and also prevent relapses.

Symptom Reduction

Antipsychotics can dramatically reduce the most prominent psychotic symptoms of schizophrenia (such as hallucinations, delusions, bizarre behavior, and odd speech) but more modestly reduce negative symptoms (such as poverty of speech, apathy, and difficulty concentrating). Antipsychotic medications can take rapid effect, sometimes producing noticeable changes within a few hours, but more often several days or weeks are required, and several months may be needed to achieve maximum benefit.

Although antipsychotic medication can substantially reduce the symptoms of schizophrenia, some symptoms typically persist. Most people continue to experience some negative symptoms and cognitive difficulties. Between 20% and 40% continue to have hallucinations or delusions, although these symptoms may be significantly reduced by medication. These *residual symptoms* are often troublesome and interfere with day-to-day functioning, which is one reason antipsychotics alone are usually not a sufficient treatment for schizophrenia.

Relapse Prevention

In addition to reducing the severity of symptoms, antipsychotics significantly lower vulnerability to symptom relapses and rehospitalizations. In the year after leaving the hospital, about 7 out of 10 people with schizophrenia (70%) *not* taking medication will have a relapse, compared to only 3 out of 10 people (30%) who take medication regularly. Thus, even after symptoms have been effectively reduced, continuing to take antipsychotics on a regular basis can stabilize the illness. If a relapse does occur despite the beneficial effects of the medication, it tends to be milder and to occur less often; temporarily increasing the dosage of antipsychotic medication will effectively treat it. To keep your relative's symptoms to a minimum and to avoid relapses, it is therefore important that she take medication on a regular basis.

How Are Antipsychotics Taken?

The most common way of taking antipsychotics is in pill or liquid form between one and three times a day. Some antipsychotics are available in tablets that dissolve in the mouth (to assure that the medication is swallowed). Some can be taken in the form of short-acting injections, which may be used in emergency situations to help a person calm down. Long-acting injections, given once every 2–4 weeks, are also available for some antipsychotic medications and may be used for people who do not want to take pills. These injections distribute the medication throughout the body on a constant basis over the following weeks, similar to time-release medications available for colds and allergies, and then gradually leave the body after the 2–4 weeks have passed. Between the injections, the person need not take any more antipsychotic medication, although occasionally additional oral medication may be prescribed temporarily.

Specific Types of Antipsychotic Medication

Since the discovery of chlorpromazine (or Thorazine), many other beneficial antipsychotics have been developed. You and your relative may be familiar with several different medications. The *potency* of these medications differs, which means that higher doses of a less potent medication are given to achieve benefits similar to those of a more potent one. To understand the differences between various types of antipsychotic medication, it may be helpful to look at two broad categories: *novel* (also called *atypical*) *antipsychotics* and *conventional* (also called *traditional*) *antipsychotics*. Although conventional antipsychotics were discovered first, over the past decade novel antipsychotics have become the first line of treatment for many people with schizophrenia, so we'll discuss them first.

Novel Antipsychotics

The term *novel* is used to describe antipsychotic medications that have different side effects and operate in different ways from conventional antipsychotics. One novel antipsychotic medication, clozapine, was discovered in the late 1950s, although it wasn't available for use in the United States until 1989. The others became available in the 1990s or after 2000. With the exception of clozapine, the novel antipsychotics were developed following years of scientific research aimed at understanding how conventional antipsychotics work and trying to make even more effective medications with fewer and less serious side effects. Novel antipsychotic medications and their side effects are presented in the following table.

Novel antipsychotics differ from conventional antipsychotics in their effec-

Novel Antipsychotics and Their Side Effects					
		Common side effects			
Chemical name	Brand name	Motor	Anticholinergic	Sedation	Weight gain
Aripiprazole	Abilify	+	0	+/−	0
Clozapine[a,b]	Clozaril, Fazaclo	0	++	+++	+++
Olanzapine[a,c]	Zyprexa, Zydis, Symbyax	+	+	++	+++
Quetiapine	Seroquel	0	+	++	++
Risperidone[a,b,d]	Risperdal, M-tabs, Consta	++	0	+	++
Ziprasidone[c]	Geodon	+	0	+/−	0

Note. 0 = little or no effect; the number of +s denotes the strength of the side effect. Common *motor side effects* include tremors, muscle stiffness, akathisia (inner feeling of restlessness or agitation), and akinesia (reduced spontaneous expressiveness, such as flat facial expression). Common *anticholinergic side effects* include dry mouth, blurry vision, constipation, difficulty urinating, and memory problems.
[a]Available in orally disintegrating tablets.
[b]Available in generic (risperidone, effective 2006).
[c]Available in short-acting injection.
[d]Available in long-acting, injectable preparation.

tiveness and side effects. (Because clozapine is quite different from the other novel antipsychotics in these two categories, we discuss it separately.)

Effectiveness in Treating Symptoms and Preventing Relapse

Novel antipsychotics tend to be more effective at preventing symptom relapses than conventional antipsychotics. There is also some evidence that novel antipsychotics are more effective treating negative symptoms and cognitive impairment, although research continues to examine this question.

Side Effects

Both the novel and the conventional antipsychotic medications vary tremendously. In general, novel medications are much less likely to cause *motor* (or *extrapyramidal*) side effects such as muscle stiffness, tremors, *akathisia* (feeling of restlessness), and *akinesia* (decreased spontaneous expressiveness) than conventional antipsychotics. Because these side effects cause significant discomfort, minimizing them is an important advance.

Another type of side effect often caused by conventional antipsychotics is *anticholinergic* side effects. *Choline* is a brain neurotransmitter that is blocked by some antipsychotics, leading to anticholinergic side effects such as dry mouth, blurry vision, constipation, difficulty urinating, and memory problems. Although anticholinergic effects can occur with some novel antipsychotics, they tend to be less severe than with most conventional antipsychotics.

One side effect of conventional antipsychotics that is of particular concern is *tardive dyskinesia*, a neurological syndrome involving abnormal involuntary movements, usually in the hands, feet, tongue, or lips. The term comes from the Latin words *tardive*, meaning "appearing late," and *dyskinesia*, meaning "involuntary, nonrhythmic movement," because the syndrome develops only after a person has been taking antipsychotics for an extended period of time—usually several years, although it can develop sooner. Unlike the other side effects, tardive dyskinesia is permanent for most people and usually does not cease or improve when the medication is stopped. Fortunately, novel antipsychotics are less prone to causing tardive dyskinesia, and clozapine (discussed below) does not cause it at all.

Although novel antipsychotics have advantages over conventional antipsychotics in some side effects, they also tend to have metabolic effects, including greater weight gain and changes in blood sugar (leading to diabetes) and lipid levels (increasing risk of coronary artery disease). Because many novel antipsychotics are different from each other and may produce different side effects, you should get information about a particular medication by asking your doctor, consulting the *Physicians' Desk Reference*, or going to *www.pdrhealth.com* or *www.healthsquare.com*.

Clozapine

Clozapine is a novel antipsychotic medication that is unique compared to all other antipsychotic medications, both conventional and novel. Clozapine is more effective than other antipsychotic medications for the treatment of a variety of persistent symptoms and problem behaviors in schizophrenia, including severe psychotic symptoms, negative symptoms, suicidal thinking and behavior, and aggression. There is also some evidence that clozapine is more effective than other antipsychotics in treating alcohol and drug use problems in those with schizophrenia. In numerous research studies, people with schizophrenia who had not benefited substantially from conventional antipsychotics showed significant improvements after receiving clozapine.

As mentioned earlier, another remarkable feature of clozapine is that, unlike other antipsychotics, it does not cause tardive dyskinesia. It can even improve the condition in those who already have tardive dyskinesia, although it does not eliminate it altogether. For this reason, clozapine is recommended for people with severe tardive dyskinesia.

Clozapine also has some unique side effects, such as increased salivation (drooling). The most serious side effect unique to clozapine is *agranulocytosis*, a reduction in the number of white blood cells (necessary to fight disease), in somewhat less than 1 in 100, or 1%, of those who take it. Those who take clozapine must therefore have their white blood cell count checked regularly with a simple blood test (performed weekly for the first 6 months, then every 2 weeks, and then monthly). This monitoring allows doctors to respond immediately with a lower dose or switch to another medication, so clozapine is nearly always safe.

Conventional Antipsychotics

Conventional antipsychotics such as chlorpromazine were the most widely available antipsychotic medication throughout the world from the 1960s until the 1990s. These medications are effective for many individuals and they continue to be used, although in many instances they have been replaced by novel antipsychotics. Conventional antipsychotics and their side effects are summarized in the following table. The effects of different conventional antipsychotics on reducing symptoms and relapses are similar, although their side effects may differ significantly. For example, whereas chlorpromazine is quite sedating, haloperidol (Haldol) is not.

In addition to the side effects listed in the table (and tardive dyskinesia, discussed on p. 151), conventional antipsychotics can cause slowed thinking, dizziness, sexual dysfunction (such as difficulty getting an erection), and sensitivity to sunlight. These problems can also occur with some novel antipsychotics, although they tend to be less severe. Some of these side effects are temporary and will improve on their own as your relative becomes used to the medication.

Conventional Antipsychotics and Their Side Effects

Chemical name	Brand name	Common side effects			
		Motor	Anticholinergic	Sedation	Weight gain
Chlorpromazine	Thorazine	+	+++	+++	++
Fluphenazine	Prolixin[a]	+++	0	+	+
Haloperidol	Haldol[a]	+++	0	+	+
Loxapine	Loxitane	++	++	++	+
Mesoridazine	Serentil	+	+++	+++	++
Molindone	Moban	++	++	++	0
Perphenazine	Trilafon	+++	+	+	++
Pimozide	Orap	+++	0	+	0
Thioridazine	Mellaril	+	+++	+++	+++
Thiothixene	Navane	+++	+	+	++
Trifluoperazine	Stelazine	+++	+	+	0

Note. 0 = little or no effect; the number of +s denotes the strength of the side effect. Common *motor side effects* include tremors, muscle stiffness, akathisia (inner feeling of restlessness or agitation), and akinesia (reduced spontaneous expressiveness, such as flat facial expression). Common *anticholinergic side effects* include dry mouth, blurry vision, constipation, difficulty urinating, and memory problems.
[a]Available in long-acting, injectable preparations.

Others may persist and improve only when the dosage is reduced or your relative is switched to another medication. It's rare for people to have all of these side effects from conventional antipsychotics, and many people have few or no side effects. Prescribers monitor for these side effects and adjust or switch medications, if necessary, to eliminate or minimize them.

Weighing the Pros and Cons of Novel versus Conventional Antipsychotics

Novel antipsychotics are a significant advance in the treatment of schizophrenia and have notable advantages over conventional antipsychotics, including less severity of some of the most troubling side effects typical of conventional antipsychotics. They may also be more effective at addressing the more stubborn symptoms of schizophrenia, including negative symptoms and cognitive impairment. Clozapine is especially helpful for people with treatment-resistant psychotic symptoms, and it is the only medication that doesn't cause tardive dyskinesia. It also may be helpful in treating suicidality, substance abuse, and aggression.

Despite such clear advantages, novel antipsychotics have some distinct disadvantages as well. As noted, many of the novel antipsychotics are associated with metabolic problems such as weight gain, increased lipid levels, and a higher chance of developing diabetes. Clozapine has a number of unique side effects, one (agranulocytosis) that is serious and requires special monitoring. Each of the novel antipsychotics also has unique side effects that merit consideration. For example, quetiapine (Seroquel) can increase the risk of developing cataracts, and ziprasidone (Geodon) can cause heart rhythm abnormalities.

Furthermore, although novel antipsychotics have some clinical and side effect advantages over conventional antipsychotics, many individuals respond very well to the conventional antipsychotics and experience few or no problematic side effects. For these people, conventional antipsychotics are an excellent choice, and the novel antipsychotics offer no advantage. In addition, although conventional antipsychotics carry a greater risk of tardive dyskinesia, this risk can be minimized by prescribing the lowest possible dosage of medication.

Another consideration is cost: Few novel antipsychotics are available in generic formulations at this time, and therefore are much less affordable for people who must pay some or all of the costs. Please be aware, however, that all of the manufacturers of novel antipsychotics have "compassionate care" programs that offer the drugs at reduced (or no) cost to those with limited financial resources.

To help you weigh all these considerations, the table on page 153 summarizes the pros and cons. Which medication to use is a very personal decision based on your relative's response—the positive effects of the medication as well as the side effects. Each person's response to a medication is unique, and the wide selection of medications available increases the chances of finding the right medication for your loved one.

How to Recognize Medication Side Effects

Side effects occur when the actions of a medication that help treat an illness in one part of the body have undesired effects on other parts of the body, where the medication is not needed. It's important to be able to recognize possible medication side effects in your relative for two reasons. First, your relative might not be aware that medications are causing these unpleasant sensations or changes and may suffer needlessly. Second, some people with schizophrenia *are* aware of medication side effects but deal with them by skipping doses or refusing to take their medication. Monitoring your relative's side effects and taking action when necessary can prevent problems with adherence that may lead to relapses and rehospitalizations.

To evaluate whether your relative is experiencing medication side effects, complete the Side Effects Checklist (Worksheet 10.1) at the end of this chapter. This checklist will help you identify *possible* side effects of antipsychotic medications, but be aware that some of these side effects overlap with the symptoms of schizophrenia. For example, schizophrenia and medications can cause drowsiness and diminished emotional expressiveness. Discussing your impressions with

Comparison of Conventional and Novel Antipsychotics	
Conventional	Novel
Treatment effects	
• Effective in treating symptoms and preventing relapse for many people	• Clozapine more effective for psychotic and negative symptoms, prevention of suicide, reduction of aggression • Other novel antipsychotics possibly more effective for negative symptoms and cognitive impairment • Novel antipsychotics more effective at preventing relapses
Side effects	
• Less severe weight gain and related metabolic problems (such as diabetes, lipid levels)	• Less severe motor side effects • Less severe anticholinergic side effects (except clozapine) • Lower risk of tardive dyskinesia (no risk for clozapine) • For clozapine, need for regular blood tests to monitor white blood cell count
Other considerations	
• Less costly	• Restricted availability of some medications in some insurance plan formularies

your loved one or talking to her doctor may help you fill in the picture of her side effects. Identifying possible medication side effects is the first step toward reducing them or helping your relative cope with them more effectively.

Generally, side effects can be managed using medication and coping strategies.

Managing Side Effects through Medication

Medication side effects can often be addressed by modifying some aspect of the person's medication regimen: (1) changing the timing of taking the medication, (2) reducing the dosage, (3) prescribing another medication for the side effects, or (4) switching to another medication.

1. Some side effects can be managed strategically. For example, many people with schizophrenia have difficulty sleeping. A medication that causes sedation may be given before bedtime so that the sedation can help the person fall asleep and stay asleep through the night. Stimulating medications can be given in the morning.

2. Many side effects are "dose-related," meaning that as the dose is increased, the side effects worsen. Reducing the dosage of antipsychotic medication can be one way of dealing with unpleasant side effects. Naturally, however, dosages should be lowered cautiously so that the positive, desirable effects of the medication aren't lost to the point of worsening symptoms or leading to a relapse. If your relative and his doctor agree to try dosage reduction, careful monitoring will allow the dosage to be upped in time to prevent a relapse should symptoms worsen.

3. Another method for reducing side effects is to prescribe additional medications. A range of different side effect medications can be used; *anticholinergic medications* (such as *Cogentin*) are frequently prescribed for parkinsonian side effects such as stiffness and tremor or the muscle stiffness or spasms called *dystonic side effects. Parkinsonism* is a syndrome that includes stiff muscles, slowed movements, and a "pill rolling" tremor (a fine tremor in the hands that resembles rolling a pill between the thumb and forefinger). When it is a side effect of a medication that impacts a particular dopamine center in the brain, it can be treated effectively by anticholinergic medications such as Cogentin. Other types of medication are also used to treat movement-related side effects, such as benzodiazepines (such as *Klonopin*), beta-blockers (such as *Tenormin*), and dopamine agonists (such as *Symmetrel*). In almost all cases, side effect medications are taken orally, in the form of pills. However, anticholinergic medications are sometimes given by injection to treat an *acute dystonic reaction*—a dramatic stiffening of muscles or a muscle spasm affecting such areas as the jaw, tongue, eyes, spine, and neck—most often caused by a conventional antipsychotic medication. These reactions are uncomfortable and can be frightening, but they can be treated quickly and effectively.

Side effect medications can produce their own side effects. For example, anticholinergic medications used to treat parkinsonism (stiff muscles and tremor) can cause dry mouth, constipation, drowsiness, blurred vision, or memory loss. Prescribers use medications carefully to avoid giving two medications with the same side effect profile.

4. If all these efforts fail, your relative's doctor may recommend switching to another type of antipsychotic medication. A different medication can be just as effective or more effective for treating the symptoms of schizophrenia.

Coping Strategies for Medication Side Effects

Even with the best possible medication regimen, your relative may experience some side effects, but coping strategies can reduce their discomfort.

Drowsiness

If sedation makes it difficult for your relative to pay attention and interact with others, scheduling a brief nap may help. Or, if your relative is taking some medication in the morning, discuss with the doctor whether taking all of it in the evening, before bed, might help.

Increased Appetite and Weight Gain

Increased appetite and weight gain are common problems with some antipsychotic medications that may interfere with accurately perceiving hunger and fullness. Planning meals and portions, rather than eating whenever hungry, is the recommended solution. In addition, cutting out one or two high-calorie foods, such as sweets, sodas, fried foods, butter, or fast food, and instead eating fresh fruits and vegetables and using sugar substitutes, can be helpful. Regular exercise, such as brisk walking, jogging, aerobics, or bicycling, can also minimize weight gain. Special weight loss classes may be available at your relative's community mental health center or elsewhere in the community.

Akathisia

Some people find that exercise or vigorous work activity reduces the discomfort and restlessness caused by akathisia. For moderate to severe akathisia, however, switching to another type of antipsychotic, preferably a novel antipsychotic, is usually advisable.

Muscle Stiffness

Antipsychotics are most likely to cause muscle stiffness in the shoulders and neck. Physical exercise or muscle stretching and isometrics (tensing muscles tightly, counting to 5, then slowly relaxing) can help, but if muscle stiffness is significant, side effect medication or an alternative medication should be considered.

Dizziness

Dizziness usually occurs upon rising quickly from a prone or sitting position or from a bathtub. The simplest solution is to avoid dizziness by first moving from a prone to a sitting position and then rising slowly. In addition, your family member should make sure he drinks enough water (6–8 glasses a day). If your family member has this type of dizziness, the doctor should take his blood pressure in the sitting and then standing position. If this type of problem is moderate to severe, a medication change should be considered.

Blurred Vision

This side effect can result from either anticholinergic or antipsychotic medications. Often vision improves spontaneously as the person becomes accustomed to the medication. Reading glasses available from a drugstore may improve vision. If this side effect persists, a medication change should be considered.

Tremor

Mild tremors of the hands or other extremities are most common soon after the person has begun to take antipsychotics or after the dosage has been increased, and improvement often occurs spontaneously. If your relative has hand tremors, avoid filling cups and glasses to the brim to prevent spilling. Some types of tremors will go away with a side effect medication.

Tardive Dyskinesia

This syndrome can be bothersome to some people. However, many others are unaware of the movements in their hands, feet, tongue, or lips. Some evidence suggests that vitamin E or a benzodiazepine medication may reduce the severity of this side effect. The most clearly effective treatment is the antipsychotic clozapine (as noted on p. 150). Often the movements will worsen transiently if the medication dose is lowered or stopped. Sometimes the syndrome goes away on its own, and sometimes it does not. Tardive dyskinesia symptoms remain mild and stable over time for most people, but occasionally they progress and become severe. For unknown reasons, tardive dyskinesia develops more commonly in women, in older people, and in those who have a mood rather than a psychotic disorder.

Other Medications

People with schizophrenia are commonly treated with numerous medications to address problems such as depression, anxiety, and mood instability, as well as more than one type of antipsychotic. In fact, the number of medications prescribed can be staggering, with some people taking as many as 5–10 medications. Remembering when to take each medication can be a formidable task, and the cost of medications can be high, so you may wonder whether all of these medications are helpful and necessary. Knowing something about the research into the effectiveness of different medications for schizophrenia can assist you in evaluating the effects in your relative.

Multiple Antipsychotic Medications

In recent years doctors have increasingly begun to prescribe more than one type of antipsychotic medication for people with schizophrenia. It is important to know that very little scientific evidence supports this practice. A few studies, most of them flawed, have found multiple antipsychotic medications beneficial, but better-designed studies have not supported these findings; furthermore, research suggests that taking multiple antipsychotics increases side effects.

Antianxiety and Sedative–Hypnotic Medications

Because anxiety is one of the most common and debilitating symptoms of schizophrenia, antianxiety and sedative–hypnotic medications are sometimes prescribed. The type most commonly prescribed is the *benzodiazepine* class. Little research supports the benefits of antianxiety medications for people with schizophrenia, but some people seem to find them helpful.

The side effects of benzodiazepines are generally mild—they may reduce muscular coordination, especially early in treatment, and are nearly always sedating—but the most important concern is that these medications can be addictive. People can develop *tolerance* to benzodiazepines, which means that they require higher doses to achieve the same effects. Discontinuation of high doses of medications can also cause uncomfortable and sometimes dangerous withdrawal symptoms. Nevertheless, most people who take these medications do not become addicted to them. Chapter 20 describes non-medication-related coping strategies for dealing with anxiety.

Antidepressant Medications

Depression is very common in schizophrenia and can be either a sign of returning psychosis or an emotional reaction to having a psychotic illness. A wide range of antidepressant medications have been found to improve depression in people with major depression. Although the research evidence is mixed, some data show that antidepressant medications can reduce depression in some people with schizophrenia. People who are depressed and have a schizoaffective disorder (see next section) are most likely to benefit from antidepressants. In addition, many antidepressant medications are effective for managing anxiety. Chapter 21 describes non-medication-related coping strategies for dealing with depression.

Mood-Stabilizing Medications

Mood-stabilizing medications are frequently prescribed for those with a bipolar disorder or for people who have manic and depressive phases with their schizophrenia, called *schizoaffective disorder*. These medications tend to reduce both manic symptoms (such as grandiosity and decreased need for sleep) and mood instability in people with this disorder. Three mood-stabilizing medications are used most often: lithium, Tegretol, and Depakote (or Depakene). Little scientific research supports the effects of mood-stabilizing medications on schizophrenia, although there is some evidence that they may be helpful for some individuals with schizoaffective disorder. There is also some evidence that these medications may help control psychotic symptoms when used with antipsychotic medications.

Nutritional Supplements

Several nutritional supplements have been proposed as helpful in schizophrenia, but there is little evidence to support these claims. One of the better studied is omega-3 fatty acids—fish oils. In some studies these supplements have been shown to help control symptoms of schizophrenia, when used with antipsychotic medications. Other studies have not found this effect. Nutritional supplements can be expensive and their manufacture is not closely regulated. Although most supplements have few side effects, some can be dangerous for your health. It is important to carefully research a nutritional claim and discuss it with your relative's doctor before adding a nutritional supplement to the medication regimen.

Other Medical Treatments for Schizophrenia

In the history of modern medicine, many different medical treatments have been tried to help people with schizophrenia, but few have been proven effective in a series of carefully conducted scientific studies. A few of the unsuccessful treatment strategies you might have heard about include *orthomolecular approaches* (such as megavitamins), *hemodialysis* (kidney dialysis), *psychosurgery* (surgery on parts of the brain, including the frontal lobes or *lobotomy*), and *insulin shock* (giving a person high doses of insulin to induce a temporary state of coma). We advise you to remain skeptical about new treatments for schizophrenia until they have been scientifically evaluated.

However, one nonpharmacological medical treatment for schizophrenia deserves special mention: electroconvulsive therapy.

Electroconvulsive Therapy

Electroconvulsive therapy (ECT) is a treatment in which a mild electrical shock is given to a person's brain to induce a controlled seizure. During a seizure, all of the brain cells fire vigorously at once, which may allow brain circuits to reset themselves. ECT is used primarily for people with severe major depression, especially when they have experienced little benefit from antidepressant medications, where it can be an effective, even a lifesaving, intervention. ECT is used much less frequently for schizophrenia, but there are occasions when it can be helpful, such as to improve movement in people who are *catatonic* (in a stuporous state or rigidly maintaining a particular position) and to calm people who are in a state of severe, uncontrolled agitation or excitement. Fortunately, such cases tend to be rare. Finally, ECT is sometimes effective for people with schizophrenia who have severe depression and do not respond to medications. ECT has a frightening reputation thanks to early misuse and depiction in movies, but it can be a safe and potent treatment in some cases. Your relative's doctor will consider the pros and cons carefully and answer any questions you have should this treatment seem worth considering.

The Importance of Taking Medication as Prescribed

Antipsychotic medications are the most potent treatment currently available for schizophrenia, but they are effective only when taken on a regular basis. When taken irregularly, the medication level in the body fluctuates, reducing its effectiveness. Also, side effects such as tardive dyskinesia are more common in people who go on and off their medication. Unfortunately, 50–75% of those with schizophrenia depart from their prescribed medication regimen at some point. To help your relative stick to his medication regimen, start by understanding why so many people don't do so.

Why People Don't Take Their Medication Regularly

People with all kinds of medical problems may fail to take their medication as prescribed, either because they don't like the side effects or because the symptoms it is intended to address aren't that bothersome. The same is often true for people with schizophrenia. Antipsychotics can cause troubling side effects that may prompt your relative to stop taking her medication. In addition, although medications may prevent relapses in the long run, stopping medication is often not associated with an immediate increase in symptoms, so your relative may feel she can stop taking her medication without negative consequences.

People who don't think they have schizophrenia often refuse to take medications, and some also deny that that they have any problems at all. This denial may help these people not to think of themselves as failures in their family or society. Ironically, *not* believing that one has schizophrenia can worsen the illness because of the belief that it is not necessary to take medications. Nevertheless, kind and persistent doctors and families can persuade people who don't have insight to take medication regularly.

Taking medication regularly can be an unpleasant reminder of their difficulties for people who do have insight into their illness or some awareness of the problems they experience. Forgetting to take medication means avoiding the negative thoughts associated with the illness and the limits it imposes. The problem of forgetting to take medication is often compounded in schizophrenia because so many people with the disorder have memory problems.

Other symptoms of schizophrenia can also foster a refusal to take medications. People with schizophrenia often experience *negativity*, a sense of defeat, hopelessness, and unwillingness to try to change. People who are negativistic often believe that change is impossible or not worth the effort, and they resist attempts to get them to take medication and resent efforts to personally engage them, preferring to be left alone. Improving medication adherence can be very difficult with these individuals because they experience any interaction as an intrusion into their world.

Psychotic symptoms can also interfere with medication adherence. Your relative may be suspicious or hostile toward others based on delusional beliefs that they want to hurt him. We've known people who believed that their parents were trying to "poison" them by convincing them to take antipsychotic medications. These beliefs can be difficult to counter because often there is a grain of truth to them; relatives and mental health professionals *are* trying to control the person (or at least the symptoms of her illness) with antipsychotic medications, and these medications *can* produce unpleasant side effects and subjective states. Most people use the word *poison* to refer to substances that kill people or have toxic effects without any benefits. If your relative does not acknowledge any benefits of medication and is aware only of its negative side effects, viewing it as poison may not seem so farfetched.

Clues That Your Relative Is Not Taking Medication

You may already know whether or not your relative adheres to his prescribed medication. For example, you may have seen him take medication regularly, or you may have had arguments in which your relative has adamantly refused to take medication. On the other hand, you, like many other people with a relative who has schizophrenia, may be unsure whether he is taking medication.

One way of finding out whether your relative is taking medication is simply to ask. Many people will honestly and directly answer this question, even when they are not taking their medication as prescribed. If your relative says that he is not taking medication regularly, chances are it is true and you can begin to take steps to deal with that situation. If your relative assures you that he is taking medication, it is not necessarily true—but it may be.

One important way to tell is to watch for worsening symptoms. Although the symptoms of schizophrenia can vary in severity over time, especially with major changes or new sources of stress, they usually are relatively stable when people are taking medication. If you notice a worsening in your relative's symptoms but cannot think of any recent stressors she has faced (such as beginning a new job, changing residences, or a physical illness), she may have discontinued her medication. It's critical to detect increases in the symptoms (such as social withdrawal, hallucinations, or delusions) or early warning signs of relapse (such as anxiety, depression, or concentration problems) as soon as possible so you can take corrective action. Chapter 12 discusses how to recognize and respond to the signs of an impending relapse.

Another way of evaluating whether your relative is taking medication is to do *pill counts*: Count the number of pills in the bottle every day or every week. If too few pills are missing (or too many), your relative has not taken the correct number. The method is certainly not foolproof, because people can simply remove pills from the bottle and throw them away, especially if they know that the pills are being counted. However, this is a useful starting point for evaluating whether your relative is taking medication.

Observing your relative taking medication often provides very accurate information about her adherence. Although it's possible to hold a pill in one's cheek instead of swallowing it ("cheeking it"), spitting it out later, this does not happen often. The following strategies may increase your relative's ability to take medication on her own.

Strategies for Helping Your Relative Stick with Medication

Start by trying to establish a dialogue. During this discussion, strive to maintain an open, nonthreatening atmosphere. Explain your concerns, don't blame or threaten. Listen to your relative and try to understand the situation from his perspective, then attempt to find a common ground that includes both viewpoints.

• *Highlight the benefits*. Helping your relative understand the benefits of medication can motivate her to take it, especially benefits that match your relative's needs or desires. In our experience, people with schizophrenia respond most positively to the message that antipsychotic medications prevent rehospitalizations. Many people also benefit from knowing that medication can reduce or eliminate distressing symptoms or help them achieve personal goals, such as more independent living, holding down a job, returning to school, or having a close relationship. Think about who might be the best person to discuss these advantages with your relative—you, another family member, a friend, or someone on your relative's treatment team?

One way to help your relative decide whether medication will be beneficial is to make a list of all the pros and cons, using Worksheet 10.2. Considering both advantages and disadvantages shows that you want to help your relative make a balanced and fair decision, not a one-sided decision based only on the positives. Be sure to include the role medication may play in helping your relative achieve personal recovery goals, such as those mentioned above and discussed in Chapter 3. If this exercise reveals that your relative does not want to take medication because of side effects, work together on addressing those side effects before coming to a final decision.

Barbara took her clozapine only erratically. Her sister, with whom she had a close relationship, was very concerned because Barbara seemed to have many symptoms and had been hospitalized twice in the past year because of relapses. Of greatest concern to Barbara's sister was that she didn't seem happy, spent most of her time sleeping, and had not worked since a part-time job at a flower shop that had ended a couple of years ago. Barbara seemed to be doing worse recently than a few years ago, when she had been taking her medication more regularly. Barbara's sister suggested that they explore together the advantages and disadvantages of her taking her medication.

With her sister's help, Barbara was able to identify several advantages of taking the medication, including the fact that it had helped her stay out of the hospital and remain employed in the past as a florist. Barbara also said that she wanted to return to school to get an associate's degree and that she would like to make some new friends. In talking with her sister, Barbara realized that staying out of the hospital would, in part, help her achieve those goals. She also listed several disadvantages to taking the medication, including drowsiness and having to remember to take it.

After reviewing the pros and cons of taking medication, Barbara decided in favor of taking it but wanted help in dealing with the problems she had identified. Barbara talked over the problem of drowsiness with her doctor, who told her she could take her entire dosage at night. She also worked out a plan for remembering to take her medication by fitting it into her morning and evening routine. Through this collaborative process Barbara concluded that taking medication was feasible and helpful. As a result of taking her medication more regularly, her apathy decreased, and she applied for and got a job working as an assistant to a florist.

Address the problem of side effects. By now you're familiar with the side effects of antipsychotics and the possibility that these problems can contribute to nonadherence, so you may be in a good position to help if your relative has stopped taking medication due to side effects. You can start by encouraging him to discuss the side effects with his doctor but also help him develop coping strategies.

For your relative's conversation with the doctor to be as effective as possible, she needs to be prepared to describe the specific side effects, how often they occur, how long they've been a problem, and the degree of discomfort they cause. Your relative may find it helpful to practice the conversation with you before talking with the doctor to allay any anxiety she has, and she may also find it helpful to write down her concerns about the side effects and to check her list during the conversation with the doctor.

If your relative is still reluctant to talk over his concerns with the doctor, ask if it would help if you joined the meeting with him and the doctor. If you both agree that this option is worth pursuing, set up an appointment for you and your relative to meet with the doctor. It's best for your relative to arrange this appointment so that it's clear to the doctor that he supports the plan. In this meeting, review the problematic side effects, including how they have contributed to your relative's discontinuance of the medication, and discuss options for dealing with the problem.

As to coping strategies, the easiest way to begin is to review with your relative the specific strategies described earlier in this chapter and pick one or two.

For each particular strategy, talk it over, practice it, and then make a plan to put the strategy into action. You may need to be involved in reminding your relative to use the coping strategy or identifying other ways that she can remember to use it.

Sarah's son, Zeke, had a terrible time with akathisia (feeling restless), even when his doctor prescribed the lowest possible dosage of his antipsychotic medicine. He said, "Sometimes I feel like jumping out of my skin." Zeke was often restless and paced frequently. Because of his akathisia, Zeke began skipping doses of his medication, and some of his symptoms began to worsen. After Sarah talked over her concerns with Zeke, they decided to explore some coping strategies. Zeke came up with the idea of taking a walk every day to relieve some of the tension and feelings of restlessness. Sarah also thought this would be a good idea. She suggested they take a walk around the block together to see how it went. They did this, and Zeke reported that it helped him relax a little. They agreed on a plan that Zeke would take a walk every day around 3:00 P.M. Zeke and Sarah decided to meet the following week to see how the plan was going. At this meeting, Zeke reported that his akathisia had decreased and that he had resumed taking his medication.

• *Build medication into the daily routine.* For most people, daily living activities such as tooth brushing, showering, and going to work are so routine that they become automatic and require no planning or forethought. Making medication part of the daily routine therefore can decrease the chance of forgetting. Though establishing daily routines can be difficult for those with schizophrenia, they can do it with assistance. Rather than attempting to establish a new daily routine for your relative, try to determine what his current routine actually *is* and how taking medication could be incorporated into it.

Look for convenient times to add medication—and a reminder to take it—to your relative's daily activities. In the morning at breakfast is a good time to take medication because of easy access to beverages. If your relative eats cereal, you might put her medications close to the cereal box or where the bowls are stored. Another good time to take medication is when brushing teeth. One strategy for helping your relative remember to take medication is to put a rubber band around her medication bottle (or other type of dispenser) and then attach the toothbrush to the bottle with the rubber band. If your relative watches TV on a daily basis, taking medication could be combined with this activity, such as by putting the medication on the TV set.

• *Simplify the medication regimen.* Simplicity is golden when it comes to medication regimens. The fewer medications taken the fewer times per day, the easier it will be for your relative to adhere to the regimen. Taking medication more than once a day requires more effort and provides more opportunities for missed doses. Encourage your relative to talk to his doctor about this, because many medications prescribed for schizophrenia can be taken once a day, such as at night.

• *Use pill boxes to organize medications.* Pill boxes provide a space for each day (or multiple spaces per day) for medications to be stored, so that all the medications that need to be taken at one time are together in one place. One advantage of using a pill box is that if your relative takes more than one kind of medication, she does not have to open many different bottles each time she takes medication. Another advantage is that your relative can tell at a glance if she has taken the medication that was placed in the box for a specific day or time of day. Most drugstores carry a variety of different pill boxes, and they can also be found on the Internet. Some pill boxes contain alarms to remind people when it's time to take medication. Your relative may need help learning how to put her medications into the pill box, usually every week. Some pharmacies and mental health centers will prepare pill boxes for people so that they don't have to do it themselves.

• *Use incentives. Contingencies* are the consequences of behaviors. Behavior is shaped by the naturally occurring consequences in the environment. When you're late for work, your boss may glare at you or your pay may be docked, which may prompt you to be more punctual next time. When you cook a nice meal, family members or guests may smile and compliment your cooking, which encourages you to do it again. By systematically providing positive consequences for taking medication, or by removing privileges for not taking it (negative consequences), you can improve your relative's adherence to medication.

Adherence can be promoted most effectively when contingencies are provided for both taking and not taking medication. The best consequences to select are those that are readily available that you can control, and that your relative values. Examples of positive consequences for taking medication include receiving spending money, going on a trip or an outing, renting a video, having a special meal cooked, using the family car, spending time with someone special, and engaging in a recreational activity. The negative consequences for not taking medication can include the loss of the same activities.

If your relative lives in your home and does not take medication, the ultimate contingency (condition) that you may need to use is the privilege of continuing to live at home. As the person who pays the bills, you have the right to live in a peaceful, safe environment and to insist that your relative meet certain reasonable standards of behavior. You may choose to include medication adherence as one of those standards. However, we encourage you to use this contingency *only* if you are willing to follow through on it and insist that your relative live elsewhere if he chooses not to take medication.

To use contingencies to enhance adherence to medication, you need to write down the specific consequences of taking and not taking medication, discuss them with your relative, and post them somewhere. You also have to decide how to evaluate your relative's adherence to medication (such as observing her taking medication or counting pills). Establishing clear, meaningful, and enforceable contingencies can be a very potent strategy for enhancing adherence to medication. But, it takes time to work, and you need to be open to modifying the specific contingencies you've set.

• *Consider injectable medications.* Antipsychotic medications that can be taken in the form of long-acting injections (such as Prolixin Decanoate, Haldol Decanoate, or Risperdal Consta) can relieve you of worrying about adherence. You'll know when your relative has chosen not to adhere to her injectable medication regime, allowing you or the treatment team to intervene. They also produce a very steady blood level of the medication (more so than oral medication), which can result in better symptom reduction or fewer side effects. In addition, they relieve your relative of the need to remember to take medications and of being reminded so often about her illness.

Many people with schizophrenia readily agree to take injectable medications, but others object, usually for one of two reasons. First, they may have experienced problematic side effects from injectable medications in the past. Second, they may dislike or fear needles. The side effects of injectable medications are the same as for oral medications. However, sometimes a person is given too high a dosage the first time he is given an injectable medication, and this leads to unpleasant side effects, such as muscle spasms. If your relative has had this experience in the past, he is still a candidate for injectable medication as long as the medication is initiated at a very low dose, which can be supplemented with oral medication until the appropriate dosage of injectable medication has been determined.

People who dislike or fear needles may be more difficult to persuade to try injectable medications. Your relative may be relieved to learn that the size of the needle used to inject the medication is quite small and causes little pain. The *idea* of injectable medications may be scary to your relative, however. As people learn more about it, such as by having a conversation with a doctor, nurse, or another person who has regular injections, they sometimes warm to the idea. When talking over this option with your relative encourage her to *try* it and see how it goes. Many people who are reluctant to try injectable medications soon find out that they are not as bad as expected and agree to continue taking the medications in this form.

What If Your Relative Still Refuses to Take Medication?

You may find that no matter how hard you try, you can't persuade your relative to take medication. Because you want what is best for your relative, this can be a very frustrating and painful experience for you. Dr. Xaviar Amador, a psychologist whose brother has schizophrenia, has written about the problem of lack of insight in people with schizophrenia in his book *I Am Not Sick I Don't Need Help*. Although this is a difficult situation, remember that it's not your relative's fault and that lack of insight and negativity in response to treatment and others' efforts to help are cardinal features of this disorder. Two general recommendations may make it easier for you and your family to manage this situation.

First and foremost, try to retain or develop as positive a relationship with your relative as possible to minimize the tension that may arise from her not taking her medication. Although it may be difficult to do, you need to accept your relative's right to decide whether to take medication, even if you think it would be helpful. Showing and telling your relative that you accept and love her regardless of whether she takes medication conveys the powerful message that you share a bond that can't be destroyed, even by schizophrenia. Looking for ways of enjoying time together, sharing interests, and highlighting areas of agreement can accentuate the positive and make both of you feel better about your relationship. It may also be important to strategize ways of preventing your relative's symptoms from interfering with your relationship; this topic is addressed in Part V in this book.

Second, consider whether you and other family members are protecting your relative from the natural consequences of not taking medication and are therefore "enabling" his medication nonadherence. Not taking medication is associated with threatening, aggressive, violent, odd, or bizarre behavior as well as being unable to manage money, refusing to eat or care for oneself, and getting into trouble with the law. Family members often respond to these behaviors in the way most natural for them—by trying to protect their loved one with schizophrenia. For example, they may give their loved one money to get basic needs met, bail him out of jail when inappropriate or illegal behavior gets him into trouble, refuse to press charges when they've been assaulted, or allow him to live at home despite repeated threats and violence. Despite the fact that these acts of love are well intentioned, they may have the unintended effect of making it easier for your relative to continue not to take medication and, as a result, to function poorly.

Without the protective measures of family members, not taking medication often results in either legal problems (such as when charges are pressed in response to illegal behavior) or involuntary commitment to psychiatric treatment (when the person poses a grave threat to self or others). In either case, medication may sometimes be administered against the person's will, or the person may be compelled to take medication as a condition of returning to the community. Although it's a difficult decision to make, you may decide it's in your relative's long-term best interest not to protect her from the consequences of illness-related behaviors. The hope is that either legal consequences will force the person into treatment or her behavior will be grounds for involuntary commitment to psychiatric treatment.

If you and your family decide to allow your relative to experience the natural consequences of not taking medication, you can still let him know that you love him and want to maintain as good a relationship as possible. It is also important to know the exact laws in your region concerning committing a person to a hospital for involuntary treatment, because you may be in the best position to file the necessary papers. Chapter 13 contains more information about involuntary commitment.

The Jones family had a very difficult time with their son Matthew who steadfastly refused to take medications for his schizophrenia. Matthew's illness was out of control. He lived at home sometimes but would then go off for weeks at a time, traveling. When home, he drank frequently and used copious amounts of drugs; on several occasions he assaulted his parents when they confronted him. His parents were afraid of him and gave him money to go on trips. They often felt relieved when he left, knowing they would have a few days of peace, but worried about what he might do on his travels. He had free access to a family cabin several hours away, which he trashed regularly with parties he held there. He also frequently got into trouble with the law for speeding (with the family car), being drunk in public, and getting into fights. Matthew's parents always faithfully bailed him out of jail and tried to smooth things over with local law enforcement officials.

On the advice of a mental health professional, Matthew's parents decided to stop supporting his destructive and self-destructive behaviors. They stopped giving him spending money and informed him that he was not allowed to live at home as long as he refused to go to the local mental health center and take medication. They also told him he was not allowed to use the family cabin, and that if he did, they would press charges for trespassing. Finally, they informed Matthew that they would not bail him out of jail again. They told him that they still loved him and always would, but they needed to feel some comfort and safety in their own lives.

Matthew was angry with his parents but did not change his behavior. He left home to visit a friend and, while using alcohol and drugs, got into trouble with the law over a fight he was involved in. Matthew's parents did not bail him out of jail; he was given a suspended sentence and placed on probation with the condition that he comply with treatment at his local community mental health center. At first Matthew refused to take medication. When his doctor at the center informed his probation officer about this nonadherence the officer told Matthew that he would be sent to jail if he did not cooperate. Matthew began taking medication. Within a few weeks Matthew's symptoms had decreased dramatically; his parents said that "he was a like a new person." At last, Matthew and his parents began the process of reestablishing a positive relationship.

Evaluating the Quality of Medication Treatment

How do you know if your relative is receiving the best pharmacological treatment possible? Because medications usually don't eliminate all symptoms, you can't know whether your relative is receiving the best treatment strictly by evaluating the severity of her symptoms. Nevertheless, certain guidelines for judging your relative's care may help you decide whether steps need to be taken to improve it.

As a first step, begin a medication log that will serve as an ongoing record. It should include all the medications your relative is taking, their dosage levels, and the reasons for each medication. When changes are made in your relative's medications, note these changes and the reasons in the log. Feel free to make copies of the Medication Log in Worksheet 10.3.

If your relative is in his first episode of psychosis and is just beginning an antipsychotic medication, encourage the doctor to do the following: suggest two or three medication options, discuss the advantages and disadvantages of each, and then allow your relative to choose the medication. In many cases, novel antipsychotics are considered the first choice over the typical agents. Because those in their first episode of psychosis tend to respond very well to novel antipsychotic medications a medication is often chosen based on potential side effects. For example, if your loved one is agitated and not sleeping, it makes sense to choose an antipsychotic that tends to be more sedating. If your loved one is apathetic and sleeping too much, a more stimulating antipsychotic could be chosen. If your loved one already has a weight problem, medications associated with weight gain should be avoided. Achieving a good match and avoiding intolerable side effects are important in creating a positive first experience of antipsychotic medication treatment. When people choose a medication with full knowledge of its potential side effects, as well as those of other options, they are more prepared to follow through with treatment.

In some states and some treatment systems, insurance providers, including state Medicaid payors, will pay only for certain antipsychotic medications, so the doctor may offer choices that are limited in this way. For example, the novel antipsychotics are generally much more expensive than the conventional medications. For some people, cost is a major factor in the choice of medication. You can help your relative figure out how the medication will be paid for (by private insurance, Medicaid, or out of pocket) and use this information when choosing a medication. More options may be available to your relative if she is willing and able to pay for her prescriptions, at least initially. Often a doctor can provide samples so that your relative can try various medications to find out if she tolerates them well prior to paying for a prescription. Once a good match is found, the doctor may be able to advocate on her behalf with your relative's insurer to pay for a medication that is not on their preferred list.

Following are different criteria you can use to evaluate your relative's treatment. No one criterion should be the deciding factor, but in combination they will give you the information you need to make informed decisions.

Multiple Medications

Again, prescribing multiple types of medication has become increasingly common even though most research does not support this practice. Specifically, no strong evidence supports the use of more than one type of antipsychotic medication. The use of antidepressant and mood-stabilizing medications in addition to the antipsychotics *can* be helpful for some people with schizoaffective disorder, although people with schizophrenia are less likely to benefit. Doctors may prescribe additional medications in well-intentioned attempts to treat symptoms that have not responded well to the initial medication. Sometimes medication is added when another problem (e.g., nonadherence or substance abuse) that is interfering with the effectiveness of the original medication treatment is not detected. Sometimes an additional medication produces a temporary benefit that then wanes, but the prescriber continues to provide it. Too often, the longer a person is receiving services in the mental health system, the greater the number of different medications she is prescribed. The risk is that a person may accrue increasing side effects (and cost) without gaining additional benefit. In many cases, people can be gradually taken off different medications and monitored to evaluate changes in symptoms. In general, use of one antipsychotic medication is preferable to taking multiple antipsychotics. If you discover that your loved one has prescriptions for two or more antipsychotics, arrange for a consultation with the primary prescriber (e.g., her psychiatrist) to discuss the pros and cons of this course.

Overmedication

Since the 1980s, a wealth of information has established that people with schizophrenia can be treated effectively with much lower doses of antipsychotics than was previously thought. Most doctors are aware of this shift in practice, but your relative may still be receiving higher than the optimal dosage. One reason overmedication occurs is that the dosage required to treat acute symptoms (e.g., during hospitalization) is usually higher than the dosage required during a period of stabilization. If your relative has been maintained on the same amount of medication for a long period of time following his last hospitalization, he may benefit from a reduction in dosage.

Overmedication often results in more side effects. However, it's difficult to know for certain that your relative is being overmedicated without changing the dosage. If a decision is made to reduce dosage, it is best to decrease it very gradually over weeks or months and to closely monitor symptoms for signs of worsening.

Frequency of Evaluations

Your relative needs to see his doctor (or nurse) regularly to have symptoms and dosage levels checked. There is no absolute rule for how frequent such visits need to be, but more frequent appointments are generally preferable to less frequent ones to detect changes in your relative's condition more rapidly. The optimal frequency of doctor visits may depend on the stability of his symptoms. If he has recently had a relapse or been hospitalized within the past 6 months, more frequent doctor's visits are advisable.

We recommend that people see their doctor or nurse every 2 weeks for at least 6 months to a year after their last relapse or hospitalization. If symptoms are severe, especially immediately after discharge, weekly appointments may be needed. After a year of stable symptoms monthly medication visits work for most people, whereas others can be seen less often, such as every 2 months. Anyone being seen less often than every month should be in contact with someone who can monitor symptoms and alert the doctor in the event of a change. Although it's common practice for people at community mental health centers to see their doctor once every 3 months, or even longer, we believe optimal pharmacological treatment depends on seeing a doctor or nurse more often.

Duration of Medication Visits

As with frequency, there is no hard and fast rule for how long a visit should last. A doctor who has never met your relative will need to spend at least a half hour to an hour getting acquainted—more if a careful diagnostic interview is conducted. After the initial meetings, checkups should take at least 15 minutes; the necessary monitoring of symptoms and side effects can't be accomplished in much less. Not every checkup needs to involve the doctor, however; often a nurse will be more familiar with the person's symptoms and level of functioning.

Availability and Responsiveness

Because quick action must be taken when symptoms change, it's important that the doctor be responsive to concerns raised about symptoms and available for special appointments when necessary. Ideally, the doctor will be responsive to concerns raised by you as well as your relative. Whether your relative lives with you or you have daily to weekly contact, chances are you are more aware of changes in symptoms than the doctor. A doctor who does not value your observations will limit your ability to work together on behalf of your relative and may compromise her overall treatment.

Doctors must protect client confidentiality, however, so your relative will have to give written permission for open communication between you and the doctor. Once permission is granted, you will be able to evaluate whether the doctor is interested in your observations and appears responsive to your concerns. If your relative refuses to give permission for your doctor to talk with you, you are still allowed to give information to your doctor (especially if it is about a vital health or safety concern), but naturally he cannot give you any information about your relative.

Advocating for Better Medication Treatment

Once you have evaluated the quality of your relative's pharmacological treatment, you should not be surprised to find that it does not meet all of our criteria. Visits at a local community mental health center are likely to be less frequent and shorter than is ideal—not because the doctor doesn't care but because public funding for mental health care is typically low and doctors often have very large caseloads. One strategy to compensate for this limitation is to supplement the evaluation conducted by the doctor with your own evaluation (Chapter 12 addresses this topic). In addition, if your relative is involved in other activities at the mental health center, such as a vocational program, her symptoms can be monitored by other staff members there. You and your relative can meet with program staff to discuss whether this monitoring is already taking place.

Any concerns that you and your relative have discussed about multiple medications or overmedication can be raised directly with the doctor in a concerned, up-front manner. Obviously, you don't want to put the doctor on the defensive by sounding accusatory or providing a specific solution and looking as if you're trying to do the doctor's job. Rather, describe the basis of your concern as specifically as possible and let the doctor suggest a solution. If you are concerned about the number of different medications your relative is taking, for example, you may want to focus on the complexity of the medication regimen. If you're concerned about overmedication, focus on the possible signs of overmedication, such as side effects. Above all, communicate with the doctor in a cooperative spirit so that you and your relative are seen as allies in the overall treatment process.

If the psychiatrist is not responsive or is underresponsive to concerns raised by you and your relative, and you continue to be dissatisfied with treatment, your next step will depend on where the treatment is provided. If treatment is provided at a community mental health center and private treatment is not an option, you may need to work within the system to try to get your concerns addressed. This may involve talking with other professionals at the center to get ideas about how to approach the problem. Sometimes these professionals can act as advocates for your relative in a manner in which you cannot. Another possible option is to explore other treatment providers who accept your relative's insurance. Many university hospitals provide high-quality pharmacological treatment and accept commonly available insurance. Similarly, some private organizations provide mental health treatment and accept insurance.

When seeking a private practice doctor, look for someone who works regularly with people who have schizophrenia (such as a psychiatrist), has access to rehabilitation interventions such as vocational services, and (if possible) has a reputation for working collaboratively with family members. Referrals can be obtained from mental health professionals, other families, and local affiliates of the National Alliance on Mental Illness (NAMI). When selecting a doctor, you will need to strike a balance between "shopping around" to get the best care and striving for the continuity that can be established by working with one professional over an extended period of time.

Common Questions about Antipsychotic Medications

• *Are antipsychotic medications addictive?* Antipsychotics are *not* addictive. Common properties of addictive drugs are that they cause pleasurable feelings, can lead to physical tolerance, and can cause withdrawal effects if the drug is stopped. Antipsychotic medications have none of these properties. Addictive drugs include alcohol, nicotine, stimulants (e.g., cocaine), and opiates (such as heroin). However, if your relative stops taking antipsychotics, his or her risk of relapse will increase.

• *Do antipsychotics interact with other drugs?* It's safe to take antipsychotic medications with other medications used to treat physical conditions such as allergies, diabetes, epilepsy, or bacterial infections, but the prescriber should be made aware of all the medications used by your relative. The doctor should be consulted if you or your relative has questions about the safety of taking specific medications. Alcohol should be used as little as possible because it can interfere with the therapeutic effects of antipsychotics. Street drugs, such as marijuana or cocaine, should be avoided. If your relative uses these substances, he should also continue to take the medications, but the prescriber needs to be made aware of your loved one's substance use.

• *What should be done if a dose of antipsychotic medication is missed?* Consult your relative's doctor regarding this question, since the answer varies from one medication to another. In some cases the doctor will inform your relative to take the next dose at the recommended time (*not* to double the dose); in other cases she will be instructed to take the missed dose as soon as she remembers.

• *For how long must an antipsychotic be taken?* If a person develops a first episode of schizophrenia (referred to as *schizophreniform disorder* if the duration is less than 6 months) and then receives medication that successfully eliminates all the symptoms, most experts agree that the person should continue to take medication for at least 1 more year. At that point, the doctor is likely to gradually taper the medication while monitoring the person to see whether he can stop the medication altogether. If symptoms begin to reappear, the medication is increased or restarted.

Experts agree that most people who have had several episodes of psychotic symptoms or who continue to experience symptoms despite taking medication will need to take antipsychotics throughout their lives. Research has evaluated whether people with schizophrenia can take medications only when their symptoms begin to worsen and not between episodes. The results of these studies suggest that this is *not* as effective a strategy for preventing relapses as taking regular, low doses of medication between episodes.

Mastering the Medication Maze

We can't say this too often: Medication is the single most powerful tool for the treatment of schizophrenia. However, like all potent interventions, it has its drawbacks. Each person responds differently to medication and finding the right one at the right dosage can be difficult, exacting work. To complicate matters further, all medications have some undesirable side effects, and many people with schizophrenia don't take their medications regularly, due to side effects, lack of insight into their illness, or just forgetting to take them.

Because of the complexities of medication and its importance in the treatment of schizophrenia, family members must become experts in it—and in negotiating medication issues with their relative and with treatment providers. To be sure, this is not an easy task. However, with information about the nature and role of medications and a close relationship with your loved one, you are in an ideal position to help her master the maze of medications and experience the tremendous benefits of doing so.

Resources

Books on Medication for Families

Diamond, R. J. (2002). *Instant psychopharmacology: A guide for the nonmedical mental health professional* (2nd ed.). New York: Norton. Highly readable and accessible to family members.

Gorman, J. M. (1998). *The essential guide to psychiatric drugs* (3rd ed.). New York: St. Martin's Press. This book includes practical information about a wide variety of medications and their side effects.

Preston, J., O'Neal, J. H., & Talaga, M. C. (2005). *Handbook of clinical psychopharmacology for therapists* (4th ed.). Oakland, CA: New Harbinger. Similar to Diamond's book, although aimed at professionals, family members will find it accessible, comprehensive, and up to date.

Weiden, P. J., Scheifler, P. L., Diamond, R. J., & Ross, R. (1999). *Breakthroughs in antipsychotic medications: A guide for consumers, families, and clinicians.* New York: Norton. This book provides a very readable account of the major progress that has been made in developing antipsychotic medications for schizophrenia over the past decade.

Websites with Information about Medication

www.dshs.state.tx.us/mhprograms/PtEd.shtm. An important component of the Texas Medication Algorithms Project (TMAP) is education about mental illness and medications. At this website you can access TMAP's consumer and family educational materials, including fact sheets about psychiatric disorders, medication benefits, symptom and side effect monitoring, and suggestions for coping with persistent symptoms and side effects. A session-by-session Peer Facilitators' Guide can also be downloaded, which includes drawings by consumers to illustrate key points and questions to guide discussion.

www.mentalhealth.com. Click on "Contents," then on "Medication," then click on the name of the medication that you wish to learn more about.

Possible Antipsychotic Medication
Side Effects Checklist

Instructions: Check possible side effects of antipsychotic medication your relative may have. This form can be completed in collaboration with your relative.

Side effect	Not present	Possibly present	Definitely present
Sedation, fatigue			
Muscular stiffness			
Headache			
Tremor			
Weight gain			
Blurred vision			
Dizziness			
Sexual difficulties			
Restlessness, feeling jumpy			
Sensitivity to sun			
Lack of facial expressiveness			
Nausea, vomiting			
Constipation			
Increased salivation (drooling)			
Tardive dyskinesia (see p. 149)			

The Pros and Cons of Taking Medication

Instructions: With your relative, brainstorm as many possible pros and cons of taking medication, with particular focus on what is important from your relative's perspective. When considering the pros, think about issues such as lower symptoms, staying out of the hospital, and pursuing goals in relationships, work, education, or recreation. When considering the cons, think about issues such as side effects, trouble remembering to take medication, being reminded that one has a disorder, and cost.

Pros of taking medication	Cons of taking medication

Medication Log

Instructions: Complete this worksheet for all medications your relative is currently prescribed. When a change is made, note the change, date, and reason for the change. When a prescription is stopped by the doctor, carefully draw a single line through the name of that medication. (*Note:* When photocopying this form, you may want to enlarge it to allow more room for writing.)

Medication name	Date	Dosage	Purpose	Date changed	Reason for change

CHAPTER 11

Managing Stress

The stress–vulnerability model of schizophrenia introduced in Chapter 1 suggests that the severity and course of symptoms are determined by four factors: biological vulnerability, stress, coping skills, and social support. This chapter explains how you can help your relative cope effectively with stress. Eliminating *all* stress is neither realistic nor desirable, but learning to *manage* stress is critical since stress is a natural part of working toward personal goals and taking on new challenges—what recovery is all about. As your relative becomes increasingly able to manage stress, he will be less vulnerable to symptom relapses and also able to enjoy life more fully.

Reducing the effects of stress is important for both your relative and you. It's difficult to enjoy yourself when you're constantly feeling tense and pressured. And stress tends to be passed on, so reducing your own stress can reduce it in the whole family.

Identifying Sources of Stress

Stress is a term used to describe a feeling of strain, pressure, or tension. People say they are "under stress" when forced to adjust their behavior to cope with a difficult circumstance or event. Stressful events can be thought of as threats or challenges from the environment. The environmental challenge is called a *stressor*. People differ markedly with regard to what they find stressful; what is stressful to one person may be exciting to another. Some people find activities like rock climbing, taking a trip, or going to a party enjoyable, whereas others find them stressful. Similarly, some people look forward to challenges as opportunities for change, whereas others see challenges as threats to their control and experience them as stressful.

To cope effectively with stress, you first need to be able to identify what is stressful in your life. Stressors can be divided into two broad categories: *life events* and *ongoing stressors*.

Life Events

Although each person is unique in how she perceives stress, there are certain types of experiences that most people find stressful—life events. *Life events* are major life occurrences, such as having a baby, starting a new job, moving, being ill, experiencing a death in the family, and getting a divorce. Even when life events are a source of happiness—for example, getting married—they can be stressful. Some stressors are more severe than others; for example, divorce is certainly more stressful than getting a traffic ticket. Regardless of the severity of stressors, recognizing that a life event is likely to be stressful for your relative will prepare you to help her cope.

The Stressful Life Events Checklist (Worksheet 11.1) at the end of the chapter can give you an idea of how much stress you and your relative have experienced over the past year. You or your relative might have experienced other stressors as well, but this checklist sums up the most common life events that cause stress.

Ongoing Stressors

In addition to stressful life events, most people are faced with ongoing stressors, from financial difficulties to crowded or noisy living conditions, minor medical problems, repeated arguments or conflicts, frequent criticism or intrusions, a long commute, or unpleasant household chores. Ongoing stressors can be quite severe, such as living in poverty in an unsafe neighborhood, poor-quality housing, or having a family member with a serious mental illness, substance abuse problem, or medical disorder. Discuss ongoing stressors with your relative. You may find it helpful to make lists of what each of you finds stressful on a regular basis. Your lists may overlap, or you may be surprised at the differences.

Recognizing Signs of Stress

Stress can have a wide range of effects on people, including changes in physiology, thinking, mood, and behavior. Just as people differ in what they find stressful, their responses to stress also differ. Some show only physical signs, such as headaches, indigestion, increased heart rate, or muscular tension. Others have difficulty with their thinking and concentration or their mood, becoming irritable, anxious, or depressed. Still others may show their stress through behaviors such as restlessness, nail biting, explosive outbursts, drinking, or using drugs.

Most people respond to stress with a combination of physical, thinking, mood, and behavior changes.

Talk with your relative about the way each of you responds to stress and make separate lists of individual signs of stress. Understanding how your relative responds to stress will help you recognize when he is under stress and offer assistance. Similarly, recognizing your own stress–response pattern will help you know when you are under stress so you can take action to reduce its effects.

Managing Stress

Many of us react to stress in ways that only make it worse, such as yelling, blaming ourselves, or withdrawing. Better options include eliminating the stressor or minimizing its negative effects, both of which are discussed below.

Reducing the Sources of Stress

When possible, try to reduce stress by addressing the cause.

• *Avoid or modify situations that caused stress in the past.* If a situation was stressful before, it's highly likely to cause problems again. A person who became tense and agitated during the last big family Thanksgiving celebration, for example, might consider abbreviating her visit or staying home this year. If you find it stressful to drive at rush hour, try scheduling your car trips at other times of the day when possible.

• *Set reasonable expectations.* It's important not to expect too much from ourselves or from others. Setting realistic goals can reduce stress. Encourage your relative to develop a meaningful but not overly demanding schedule, with expectations that he can comfortably meet. People with schizophrenia tend to benefit from moderate, but not excessive, structure.

Problems can result when the environment is either overstimulating or understimulating. Helping your relative find the right balance of stimulation and reasonable expectations will minimize stress. For example, one young man found volunteering twice a week to deliver meals to housebound seniors preferable to attending a day treatment program 3 days a week.

• *Schedule meaningful activities.* Having activities that you enjoy and find meaningful makes a significant difference in reducing stress. For some people, work is enjoyable. For others, volunteering, hobbies, music, sports, reading, or art provides meaning and enjoyment. It all depends on the individual.

• *Maintain good health habits.* Eating right and getting enough sleep can help buffer the effects of stress by fortifying you to deal with hassles and crises. Scheduling regular physical exercise can also help you decrease stress and increase your sense of well-being. Taking walks, riding a bicycle, swimming, bowling, tennis, and jogging are examples of exercise that people often enjoy. If possible, schedule some form of exercise two to three times per week.

• *Schedule regular leisure activities*. Most people find that taking a break from their normal routine is refreshing. For example, going to a movie, walking in the park, eating out, or shopping can all help to reduce stress. Having a hobby such as music, knitting, reading, or drawing can be an enjoyable way of spending leisure time. Planning leisure activities on a regular basis is especially helpful; this gives you something to look forward to and prevents stress from accumulating.

Because of the negative symptoms of schizophrenia, some people have difficulty thinking of enjoyable activities. Your relative may appreciate help in reviewing pastimes he enjoyed before the illness. Chapter 28 provides more suggestions for helping your relative identify leisure and recreation activities. For yourself, schedule leisure activities that you find relaxing and enjoyable; doing so will help you "recharge" your energy.

• *Avoid being hard on yourself.* People often increase their stress by being critical of themselves and belittling their accomplishments. Remember to give yourself and your relative credit for the many tasks you accomplish, even if they seem like small steps. One parent reported that he finds it useful to take time each day to note the positive things that happened. "I'm proud of how persistent my daughter has been in pursuing her art career in spite of the many difficulties she's encountered," he said. "We both have a lot to learn about coping with this illness, but we've also come a long way."

Coping with Stress

Some stressors are unavoidable, and some are part of pursuing important personal goals. Being able to cope effectively with stressful situations is therefore important.

• *Communicate directly about stress*. Talking about feelings can keep stress from building up once it occurs. Letting someone know how you're feeling often provides some immediate relief and also invites the other person to share ideas for dealing with a stressor that you haven't thought of. It's especially important for your relative to tell someone when she is feeling under stress, because these feelings can be an early warning sign of relapse. For yourself, talking to someone who understands the factors involved can help you feel under less pressure and better able to cope with a difficult situation.

• *Hold a family problem-solving discussion*. If just talking to someone doesn't help, consider meeting with family members (including your relative, when possible) to discuss the situation and explore possible solutions to the problem causing the stress. Openly discussing the problem with others and trying to resolve it can reduce stress. Chapter 15 describes effective ways that families can solve problems together.

- *Use relaxation techniques.* Certain methods of reducing the effects of stress require learning and practicing specific techniques. Some examples are breathing exercises, progressive muscle relaxation, imagery, meditation, and yoga. These methods can be learned from books, classes, or sessions with trained practitioners. At the end of this chapter is a list of books and tapes about relaxation and stress reduction, which may be useful to both you and your relative.

In the table on pages 183–184 you'll find step-by-step examples of three simple relaxation techniques: relaxed breathing, muscle relaxation, and peaceful imagery. Relaxation techniques are most effective when practiced regularly, such as once a day. When you're first learning a technique, you usually concentrate on doing the steps according to the instructions. As you become familiar with the steps, you'll be able to concentrate more on the relaxation you're experiencing.

- *Use positive self-talk.* The more negatively you view a particular situation, the more stress you experience from it. Many situations that people encounter are very tough, and self-defeating thoughts such as "This is awful," "I can't stand it," or "I'm a nervous wreck" are common. These self-defeating thoughts can be replaced with more positive self-talk that includes saying coping-oriented things to yourself, such as "This is a challenge, but I can handle it," "I'm going to do the best that I can do," and "It's too bad that this happened, but I can deal with it."

For example, instead of saying to yourself "I'm hopelessly disorganized," try saying "I'm organized in some ways but not in others." You can use this strategy in a variety of circumstances, and you can help your relative by suggesting different ways of thinking about a stressful situation. For example, when one man's daughter expressed feeling like a failure for needing a hospitalization, he said, "I'm sorry you had to go through that, but I'm proud of you for getting help when you needed it and for being so strong in dealing with this illness. You're a survivor." Further information about positive self-talk is provided in Chapter 21, under "Correcting Unhelpful Thinking."

- *Maintain your sense of humor.* The old saying "laughter is the best medicine" also applies to the management of stress. Granted, many times there seems to be nothing to laugh about. However, if you can manage to see the lighter side of a stressful situation, you may be able to keep from being totally overwhelmed by it. For example, an argument can sometimes be derailed by a humorous remark, particularly if you poke fun at yourself and not the other person. Many people with schizophrenia have a good sense of humor and respond well to a good-natured joke. You and your relative may also enjoy a humorous movie, video, or television show to take your mind off stress.

- *Use religion or other spiritual inspiration.* For thousands of years people have been comforted and guided by religious beliefs that give meaning to their lives. These beliefs can help people cope with stress arising from difficult circumstances. For some people, prayer or other religious activities (attending services at their church, synagogue, or mosque) may substantially reduce stress. For less religious people, communion with nature is a source of inspiration that can

Three Relaxation Exercises

I. Relaxed Breathing

The goal is to slow down your breathing, especially exhaling.

1. *Sit in a comfortable chair* with your back fully supported.
2. *Choose a relaxing word or phrase to say* as you practice inhaling and exhaling slowly. Examples include "peaceful," "relax," "slow down," and "stay calm."
3. *Slowly inhale* through your nose and exhale through your mouth. Take normal breaths, not deep ones. Be especially conscious of exhaling slowly and completely.
4. *While you breathe, say the relaxing word or phrase of your choice.* If there are two syllables or words, say one while you inhale and the other when you exhale. For example when you inhale, say *re* and when you exhale, say *lax*.
5. *Pause after exhaling* before taking your next breath. Try counting to 4 before inhaling each new breath.
6. *Concentrate on your breath* as it travels through the air passageways.
7. *Repeat the sequence 10 to 20 times.*
8. *Gradually return to breathing normally.* Sit quietly for a minute or two, focusing on your natural breathing.

II. Muscle Relaxation

The goal is to gently stretch your muscles to reduce stiffness and tension, starting at your head and working down to your feet. Do this exercise while sitting in a chair.

1. *Head.* Drop your head gently forward so that your chin is near your chest. Count to 5, then return to the neutral position. Tilt your head to the right so that your right ear is approximately over your right shoulder. Count to 5, then return to the neutral position. Let your head drop gently backward, with your chin pointing toward the ceiling. Count to 5, then return to the neutral position. Tilt your head to the left and count to 5, then return to the neutral position. Repeat this sequence three to five times.
2. *Shoulders.* Lift both shoulders as if shrugging. Try to touch your ears with your shoulders. Hold the position for a few seconds. Let your shoulders drop. Hold the position for a few seconds. Repeat three to five times.
3. *Arms.* Raise both arms straight above your head. Interlace your fingers, like you're making a basket, with your palms facing down toward the floor. Now stretch your arms toward the ceiling and hold this position for a few seconds. Then, keeping your fingers interlaced, rotate your palms to face upward, toward the ceiling. Stretch your arms toward the ceiling again and hold this position for a few seconds. Repeat this sequence three to five times. If doing this exercise with your arms overhead is uncomfortable, try it with your arms reaching out in front of you.
4. *Knees.* Reach down and take hold of your right knee with one or both hands. Pull your knee up toward your chest, as close as is comfortable. Hold your knee there for a few seconds before lowering it and returning your foot to the floor. Reach down and take hold of your left knee with one or both hands and bring it up toward your chest. Hold it there for a few seconds before lowering it. Repeat the sequence three to five times. If you're not comfortable doing this exercise by pulling up your knees, try raising your knees by lifting up just your heel from the floor. Hold this position for a few seconds, then return your heel to the floor. Repeat with each knee three to five times.

(cont.)

5. *Feet/ankles*. Lift your right foot from the floor and stretch your leg out straight in front of you. Rotate your foot at the ankle, keeping your leg stationary. Repeat three to five times in each direction. Then do the same rotating exercise with your left foot, repeating three to five times in each direction.

III. Peaceful Imagery

The goal is to "take yourself away" from stress by picturing yourself in a peaceful scene.

1. Think of a scene that you find peaceful, calm, and restful. If a scene does not come to mind, consider the following examples:
   - Walking in a park
   - Watching waves at the beach
   - Floating in a canoe or sailboat
   - Sitting on a park bench
   - Walking in the woods
   - Having a picnic in a meadow
   - Traveling on a train
   - Watching a waterfall
   - Watching the sunrise or sunset
   - Riding a bicycle
   - Visiting a farm
   - Hiking up a mountain
   - Looking out the window of a tall building at the city below
   - Petting a cat or dog
   - Watching logs burning in a fireplace

2. After selecting a scene that is peaceful to you, imagine as many details as possible, using all your senses.

3. What does the scene look like?
   - What are the colors?
   - Is it light or dark?
   - What shapes are in the scene?
   - If it's a nature scene, what kinds of trees or flowers do you see? What kinds of animals?
   - If it's a city scene, what kinds of buildings do you see? What kinds of landmarks?

4. What sounds do you hear?
   - Can you hear people?
   - Are there sounds from birds or animals?
   - Can you hear the breeze rustling or the sound of rain?
   - Are there sounds from water, such as waves lapping?

5. What do you feel with your sense of touch?
   - What are the textures?
   - Is it cool or warm?
   - Can you feel a breeze?

6. What are the fragrances?
   - Are there flowers to smell?
   - Can you smell the ocean?
   - Can you smell wood burning?
   - Can you smell food cooking?

7. As you continue to imagine your peaceful scene, disregard any stressful thoughts that come to mind. Keep your attention on the details of the peaceful scene and what it would be like to be there.

8. Allow at least 5 minutes for this relaxation technique.

lower stress. Religious organizations can also be a source of social support, which can reduce feelings of isolation and stress.

• *Exercise regularly.* Almost any type of physical exercise has a positive effect on reducing stress, lifting mood, and improving sleep patterns. Some people find it relaxing to take a walk, work in the garden, or take a leisurely bike ride. Others prefer running, swimming, aerobics, or lifting weights. The most important point is for you and your relative to choose a form of exercise you can both do regularly, at least three times per week. Some people find they enjoy exercising more with someone else. For example, your relative may enjoy taking a walk with a family member or friend rather than by himself.

• *Keep a journal.* Being able to express your thoughts and feelings is important to relieving stress; bottling up your feelings only makes things worse. Even if you have someone to talk to, it may be additionally beneficial to write in a journal. One family member told us she needed a place where she could just vent without worrying what someone else's response might be. Another said writing helped her to think things through and get a better perspective on her experiences. Your relative may also find it helpful to keep a journal. Many people with schizophrenia say that writing down what they experience, think, and feel is an important outlet. Some people also like to use their journals for their own drawings, poetry, or song lyrics.

• *Make or listen to music.* Many people find it relaxing to either play a musical instrument, such as piano, guitar, or recorder, or to sing. What matters is not how expertly you play or sing, but rather how much you enjoy it and how relaxed you feel afterward. There are several ways you or your relative can be involved in making music, ranging from playing or singing on your own, to taking lessons, to joining an amateur group. If you or your relative do not find it relaxing to make music, you may enjoy listening to musical recordings or live performances.

• *Create artwork or view art.* Drawing, painting, sculpting, pottery, and weaving are just a few of the types of artwork that people find relaxing. As in music, what matters is not whether you're creating professional-quality artwork, but rather how much you enjoy it and how relaxed or satisfied it makes you feel. You or your relative might enjoy doing artwork on your own or taking classes. Or you might enjoy going to look at art at a museum or gallery, which many people say helps take their mind off stress.

• *Play games or pursue a hobby.* Pastimes such as playing cards, checkers, chess, word games, and board games have been a source of relaxation for centuries. You or your relative may enjoy playing familiar games with family members or friends, or you may want to join a group of people with similar interests, such as a bridge club. Or you or your relative might enjoy taking up a hobby (such as knitting, collecting coins, or birdwatching) or reviving one that you used to enjoy.

• *Make a plan to increase your coping strategies.* Review the coping methods described in this chapter and discuss with your relative which ones each of you uses and which ones might be worth exploring. Then develop a plan for trying out one or two new coping methods. Think about the steps for implementing the method, materials you might need (e.g., an instructional videotape and a mat for doing yoga exercises), people who could help, and appropriate locations and times to practice the new method. Bear in mind that any method will take some time to be effective, so be sure to give an adequate trial period for whichever techniques you and your relative choose.

Reducing Stress Is a Family Affair

Stress can affect everyone's mental and physical health. This impact is especially true for people with schizophrenia, who are more sensitive to the effects of stress because it can trigger symptom relapses and rehospitalizations. Learning how to manage stress effectively can improve your relative's life by helping him deal with the ordinary challenges involved in pursuing personal goals. Of equal importance, having a relative with schizophrenia can contribute to stress in your life and other family members' lives. Decreasing your own experience of stress and that of other family members can be equally beneficial. Working with your relative to develop more effective ways of handling stress can be a rewarding way of sharing time and can strengthen your relationship by giving you something to work on together that will improve the quality of *both* your lives.

Resources

Books about Reducing Stress

Benson, H., & Klipper, M. Z. (2000). *The relaxation response* (reissue). New York: HarperTorch. Originally published in 1976, this classic describes how to relax and the benefits of relaxation.

Davis, M., Eshelman, E., & McKay, M. (2000). *The relaxation and stress reduction workbook* (5th ed.). Oakland, CA: New Harbinger. A comprehensive guide to recognizing, reducing, and managing stress.

Feuerstein, G., & Bodian, J. (1993). *Living yoga: A comprehensive guide for daily life*. New York: Tarcher. Easy-to-use guide to yoga.

Franklin, E. (2002). *Relax your neck, liberate your shoulders: The ultimate exercise program for tension relief*. Princeton, NJ: Princeton Book Company.

Harvey, J. (1998). *Total relaxation: Healing practices for body, mind and spirit*. New York: Kodansha America. Describes different methods for relaxing and includes a CD with step-by-step relaxation techniques.

Kabat-Zinn, J. (1990). *Full catastrophe living: Using the wisdom of your body and mind to face stress, pain, and illness*. New York: Delta. Principles of Zen Buddhism applied to everyday life.

McKay, M. (1997). *The daily relaxer*. Oakland, CA: New Harbinger. Simple tension-relieving exercises that can be learned and used quickly.

Miller, F. L. (2002). *How to calm down: Three deep breaths to peace of mind.* New York: Warner Books. This brief book describes different ways of calming down, including using one's senses, breathing, imagery, and thinking.

Wilson, P. (1999). *Instant calm: Over 100 easy-to-use techniques for relaxing mind and body.* New York: Plume Books. Helpful and creative strategies for relaxing.

Zeer, D. (2000). *Office yoga: Simple stretches for busy people.* Yoga stretches designed to be done anywhere, whether at home, in the office, or in bed.

Audiotapes for Reducing Stress

Fanning, P., & McKay, M. (1993). *Time out from stress: Lakeside and the path to Lookout Mountain.* Oakland, CA: New Harbinger. Two guided imagery exercises, one beside a lake, the other hiking up a mountain.

McKay, M., & Fanning, P. (1987). *Progressive relaxation and breathing.* Oakland, CA: New Harbinger. Includes deep muscle relaxation, brief "pick-me-ups," and yoga alternative breathing.

Meyerson, M. (2001). *Drifting off to sleep.* Oakland, CA: New Harbinger. Contains soothing sounds of music and nature.

Sanders, H. (1993). *Body relaxed–Mind at ease.* Oakland, CA: New Harbinger. Learn to breathe calmly, using images of calming lights and colors.

Videotapes and DVDs for Reducing Stress

Cappy, P. (2001). *Yoga for the rest of us: A step-by-step yoga workout* (VHS). Boston: WGBH. Yoga for people who may be inflexible or out of shape.

Ivanhoe, S. (2001). *Basic yoga workout for dummies: An easy-to-follow yoga practice.* (DVD). Troy, MI: Anchor Bay Entertainment. Yoga and breathing techniques.

Stressful Life Events Checklist

Instructions: Check each life event that you or your relative has experienced over the past year. Use two checkmarks for any event that you or your relative found especially stressful. Count up the total number of checkmarks to find out how much stress you and your relative have experienced in the last year.

0–3 = mild stress   4–6 = moderate stress   7 or more = high stress

Event	Experienced by your relative	Experienced by you
1. Moving		
2. Family vacation		
3. New baby		
4. Marriage		
5. Family holiday at your house		
6. Family member moves out		
7. Family member moves in		
8. Financial problems		
9. Buying a house		
10. Inheriting or winning money		
11. Physical illness		
12. Physical injury		
13. Caring for an ill relative		
14. Hospitalization		
15. Hospitalization of a relative		
16. Death of someone close		
17. Victim of a crime		
18. Retirement		
19. New job (paid or volunteer)		
20. Loss of job		
21. Reduction in income		
22. Conflict at work		
23. Separation/divorce		
24. Change in time spent with friends		
25. New boy/girlfriend		
26. Reduction in leisure activities		
27. Starting a diet		
28. Stopping smoking		
29. Legal problems		
30. Car accident		

CHAPTER 12

Developing a Relapse Prevention Plan

*T*he course of schizophrenia is usually episodic, with symptoms varying in severity over time. Significant worsening of symptoms or reappearance of old symptoms is usually referred to as an *episode of the illness* or a *relapse*. Some severe relapses require hospitalization to protect the person or others; hospitalization can be disruptive to everyone involved. After receiving treatment for a relapse, some people feel better right away, but many people take weeks or even months to regain their prior level of functioning. Therefore, preventing relapses or minimizing their severity and disruption is an important treatment goal.

You can play a critical role in preventing relapses in your relative. You can monitor the illness over time and take steps to prevent a relapse when it begins to happen. You and your relative can work together to prevent relapses by developing an awareness of the *early warning signs* that occur in the days and weeks before a major relapse and hospitalization. By carefully monitoring early warning signs, you, your relative, and his treatment providers can work together as a relapse-prevention team, helping to improve the course of the illness and minimizing setbacks.

Recognizing the Early Warning Signs of a Relapse

Even when people with schizophrenia are doing well, their symptoms may flare up. Some relapses may occur over short periods of time, such as a few days, with little or no warning. However, most relapses develop gradually over longer periods of time, such as several weeks. The early changes in behavior, mood, and thought processes tend to be rather minor and may seem unimportant. When people look back after a relapse, however, they often realize that these early changes were signs that they were starting to have a relapse. Recognizing and responding to these subtle changes can prevent relapses and hospitalizations.

People with schizophrenia are often not aware when they are experiencing an early warning sign of relapse. For example, one person reported that she did not realize she was feeling unusually irritable before a relapse. Instead, it seemed to her that everyone around her was being especially annoying. If you have regular contact with your relative, you're in a good position to detect when she is experiencing early warning signs of relapse. Family members, friends, coworkers, treatment providers, fellow participants in peer support programs, and others who have regular contact with your relative may also notice when she is behaving in an unusual way or responding to things differently. With your relative's permission, these individuals can be her "extra eyes and ears" for detecting early warning signs. It may be helpful to involve willing participants in developing a relapse prevention plan, as described later in this chapter.

Common Early Warning Signs

Certain early warning signs of relapse are experienced by many people with schizophrenia—among them, increased social withdrawal, irritability, sleep problems, and depression—but everyone is unique. It's therefore important for you and your relative to become aware of his personal early warning signs.

Tension and Nervousness

Many people feel tense, anxious, or worried before a relapse.

Jacob reported feeling so nervous the week before he had a relapse that he couldn't spend time with his 5-year-old nephew, an activity he usually enjoyed. He said his nephew's movements seemed too quick and his voice was too loud, and that he couldn't relax around him.

Linda reported feeling so tense that she was unable to sit still, and she kept pacing back and forth during the day.

Sleep Disturbance

Sometimes you'll become aware of your relative's increased difficulty in sleeping by noticing changes in the person's nighttime behavior, such as pacing in the middle of the night, playing the stereo loudly late at night, or tossing and turning in bed.

Several days before Tom had a relapse, his family noticed that his bed had not been slept in. When they asked him about this, he said he had been having trouble sleeping, and had been spending his nights watching television or looking out the window.

Janell had the problem of sleeping too much before she had a relapse. Although usually an early riser, she couldn't get up in the morning. She stayed in bed until her mother woke her up for lunch.

Depression

Many people feel sad, discouraged, and hopeless in the weeks before a relapse. They may appear "down" or uninterested in their usual pastimes. Some may have a feeling that life is not worth living and may contemplate, or attempt, suicide.

Two weeks before relapsing, Elise said she had had difficulty facing the day and felt like crying much of the time.

William wondered out loud, "What's the point in living?"

Jennifer managed to perform her daily activities but got no pleasure from them.

Before having a relapse, Samuel would become preoccupied with thoughts of killing himself; he had been hospitalized after attempting suicide in the past.

Social Withdrawal

Some people may pull back from social situations before they relapse. This social withdrawal may occur because an individual feels less comfortable around others, or it may be in response to small increases in psychotic symptoms, such as hearing voices or believing that people are against him. In the most extreme example, the person might refuse to leave his room even to eat.

Rachel lived with her parents and usually enjoyed eating dinner with them. Two weeks before she relapsed, she started taking a tray of food up to her room at dinner.

Dan lived in his own apartment and usually went out for coffee and donuts with a friend twice a week. One month prior to relapsing, he found he did not want to spend time with anyone and made excuses for not going out for coffee.

Concentration Problems

Before some people have a relapse, they have more difficulties paying attention. They may take longer to do tasks or have trouble finishing them. They may have difficulty following a conversation or focusing on a topic.

Grace said she would find herself staring for 20 minutes at a familiar bus schedule, unable to locate the bus she wanted to take.

José found he could not keep up with conversations with his friends. "When there was more than one person," he said, "I kept losing track of who was talking and what they were saying. I felt lost in all the words."

Irritability

Some people describe feeling touchy, impatient, or on edge in the weeks before a relapse.

A few weeks prior to Michelle's relapse, her husband noticed that she would "fly off the handle" at things that would not ordinarily bother her. For example, she got angry if he rattled the dishes while loading the dishwasher, and she slammed the door if he asked where she was going when she left the apartment.

Ted usually enjoyed listening to the radio, but when he started to relapse, he found that he "couldn't stand the noise" of music.

Decreasing or Stopping Medications or Other Treatment

When some people are about to experience a relapse, they stop complying with treatment recommendations. They may stop taking their medications, refuse to see the doctor, or skip their vocational program.

One of Eleanor's early warning signs was throwing away her bottles of medicine.

Jerry stopped going to his support group 3 weeks before he had a relapse.

Eating Less or Eating More

Change in appetite is an early warning sign of relapse.

One family noticed that 3 weeks before Annie's relapse, she stopped eating breakfast and lunch. She ate only a very small amount at dinner and reported having no appetite. She lost over 10 pounds before she was admitted to the hospital for treatment.

Bob found himself eating constantly and gaining weight in the month before he had a relapse.

Early Warning Signs in People Who Have Persistent Symptoms

Your relative may continue to have symptoms even when taking optimal doses of medication. For example, some people hear voices all the time. Often they can learn to ignore the voices and accomplish tasks in spite of them. Other people have delusions, such as believing that people are plotting against them. For these individuals, a relapse is defined as a dramatic increase in symptoms or a decrease in their ability to control their behavior in response to the symptoms.

Steven was generally suspicious of people around him, but a week before his relapse he became more paranoid. He believed that neighbors were talking about him and plotting to kidnap him.

Alyssa always heard voices but was usually able to ignore them. Prior to her relapse she began to obey commands that her voices made of her, for instance, following a stranger home from the video store.

Unique Early Warning Signs of Relapse

Some people have unique, rather than common, early warning signs of relapse. You and your relative are in the best position to recognize these signs. Examples of unique early warning signs include dressing all in black, buying lots of lottery tickets, collecting weapons, whistling constantly, not answering the phone, or suddenly getting a close-cropped haircut.

To determine which unique early warning signs your relative with schizophrenia might have, ask yourself the following questions:

- Did any unusual changes in your relative's behavior occur in the weeks before her last relapse?
- Did she do things that seemed "out of character" before a relapse?
- Have the same behaviors preceded other relapses in the past?

The Early Signs Checklist

Several researchers have studied the early warning signs that people experience before a relapse. Marvin Herz, MD, used the results of his research to develop the Early Signs Checklist, which is included as a checklist in Worksheet 12.1 at the end of the chapter. You and your relative may find it helpful to review the questionnaire together to check off any early warning signs that he experienced before the most recent relapse. The questionnaire includes blank spaces at the end to record unique warning signs.

Responding to Early Warning Signs

The primary goal of monitoring early warning signs is to be able to act quickly to prevent relapses. The earlier you take preventive steps, the more likely that a relapse can be averted. Even if a relapse does occur, early intervention can decrease the severity of the episode and avoid hospitalization. Even if hospitalization is necessary, recognizing and responding quickly to the early warning signs of relapse usually results in a briefer stay.

When Bernice started to spend more time alone in her room, which was one of her early warning signs, her parents talked to her about their concern, and she agreed to see her psychiatrist that week. At that meeting, she agreed to increase her medication for a few weeks or a month. After a few days of taking the increased dosage, she began to leave the house and spend more time with other people. Both Bernice and her family felt that a relapse had been averted.

Christopher's early warning signs included feeling depressed and suicidal, and he had been hospitalized because of suicide attempts. After he and his wife identified his early warning signs, they were able to prevent several relapses by alerting his treatment providers when he showed the first signs of feeling sad or depressed. On one occasion when Christopher felt suicidal, he was hospitalized for 4 days, which was much shorter than his previous hospital stays. Most important, actual suicide attempts were avoided by Christopher and his wife's awareness of his early warning signs.

Most relapses in schizophrenia occur when the person stops taking medication, experiences more stress, or abuses alcohol or drugs. When early warning signs are noted, the major strategies you can take to avoid a relapse are:

1. Meet as a family to discuss concerns.
2. Evaluate whether the person is taking medication as prescribed.
3. Determine whether she is abusing alcohol or drugs.
4. Lower the level of stress.
5. Assess the need for an increase in medication.
6. Monitor the early warning signs until the situation is resolved.

These critical steps of responding to early warning signs are described in detail below.

1. *Meet as a family to discuss concerns about early warning signs as soon as possible.* Either you or your relative can call a meeting to discuss concerns about early warning signs. Whenever possible, all meetings should include your relative as well as any other family members involved. Create an open, nonjudgmental atmosphere for this discussion. The more your relative is involved and the more people can communicate openly, the easier it will be to determine whether a relapse is likely and how it can be prevented.

In the family meeting, explain to your relative why you're concerned. Describe the specific changes you've observed in his behavior, how long you've noticed these changes, and how the behavior is different from his usual pattern. Explain your concern that these changes preceded relapses in the past and consider whether there are alternative explanations for your relative's behavior. For example, although Rodrigo was spending more time in his room, his behavior did not reflect social isolation, which was one of his early warning signs of relapse, because he was enjoying listening to some new CDs. On the other hand, Alan was sleeping most of the morning, not coming down to meals, not participating in family activities, and not able to explain why. He agreed with his family that his behavior was probably an early warning sign of relapse.

By the end of the family meeting, try to reach a consensus with everyone about whether or not early warning signs of a relapse have appeared. If you conclude that no early signs are present, you can assure your relative that you will check periodically to make sure the problem has not worsened. If you decide that your relative has shown early warning signs of a relapse, proceed to the next step.

2. *Evaluate whether your relative has been taking medication regularly.* Early warning signs and relapses often follow soon after a person with schizophrenia has stopped taking medication. If you do not already monitor your relative's adherence to medication, try to evaluate her medication routine as soon as early warning signs appear. Start by asking your relative directly whether she has been taking medication or by checking how much medication is left in the bottle or pill box. If you confirm that medication has not been taken regularly, discuss how to improve this situation with your relative and other family members. Increased monitoring, reminders, encouragement, and addressing issues related to side effects are all possible paths toward improvement (see Chapter 10). If taking medication regularly is not the problem, proceed to the next step.

3. *Determine whether your relative has been abusing alcohol, street drugs, or over-the-counter drugs.* Substance abuse can worsen the symptoms of schizophrenia and increase a person's vulnerability to relapse. You can determine whether your relative is abusing alcohol or drugs by asking him directly and/or by your own observations. For example, you may have smelled alcohol on your relative's breath or noticed that he had episodes of poor balance, slurred speech, and difficulty completing ordinary tasks. Or you may have noticed the odor of marijuana or crack cocaine smoke or seen drug paraphernalia such as rolling papers, cut plastic tubes, empty vials, or small plastic baggies. If substance abuse is confirmed, first remind your relative how it contributes to relapse, then talk about ways that he can reduce or stop using substances to avert a relapse. For example, your relative may benefit from (a) the removal of liquor and/or drugs from the house, (b) identifying other activities he can engage in, (c) contacting his treatment team, or (d) talking with a substance abuse counselor. You will find more suggestions for responding to substance abuse in Chapter 22.

4. *Evaluate your relative's stress level and plan how to lower it* Stress is an especially important factor for people with schizophrenia because it can lead to symptom relapses. In addition, people with schizophrenia tend to be highly sensitive to the effects of stressful situations such as arguments, criticism, and sudden increased responsibilities.

When Ellie's brother moved back home, he was very critical of her, making frequent negative comments about her weight and lack of friends. He often argued with her about money, household chores, and tastes in music. After a few months, Ellie's auditory hallucinations had worsened and she experienced more difficulty concentrating–her early warning signs of relapses in the past.

In evaluating whether your relative might have had a recent increase in stress, you can ask yourself some of the following questions:

- "Has my relative experienced a recent life event, such as the loss of a job, illness, reduced income, or death of someone close?"
- "Has there been a significant change in my relative's routine over the past 2 weeks? Was there a change in the treatment program, school, or living situation?"
- "Have there been arguments, conflicts, or strong disagreements between my relative and other family members or friends or coworkers?"
- "Did my relative experience a change in an important relationship? Break up with a boyfriend or a girlfriend? Start a new relationship? See a different therapist, psychiatrist, or case manager?"
- "Has my relative experienced a sudden increase in responsibilities, such as working several more hours a week?"
- "Did my relative stop participating in some leisure activities she usually enjoyed and found relaxing?"

These questions point to common areas of stress for people with schizophrenia. Remember, however, that what is stressful for one person is not necessarily stressful to another. It's important, therefore, to ask your relative whether something was experienced as stressful before assuming it's a problem. Evaluating stress can be especially difficult because people are often not aware when they're under stress and they may deny that it is a problem. In addition, bear in mind that not all relapses are precipitated by stress.

Once you and your relative have identified sources of stress that might be contributing to early warning signs, your next step is to put your heads together to figure out how to deal with that stress. There are two basic ways of responding to stress: You can try to reduce the source of the stress itself, or you can help your relative cope better with the stress that exists. Reducing stress involves such steps as cutting back on responsibilities, looking for new leisure activities, getting a temporary loan to reduce financial distress, or resolving a pressing conflict. Coping with stress involves strategies such as using relaxation techniques, talking to a counselor, or engaging in recreational activities. Other strategies for reducing stress are noted in Chapter 11.

5. *Consult the doctor or nurse to evaluate the need for a change in medication.* Sometimes your relative's usual dose of medication is not enough to keep his

symptoms under control, even when efforts are made to reduce stress. Your relative's psychiatrist will need to meet with him to evaluate whether temporarily increasing the dose of medication is needed to prevent a relapse. If early warning signs clearly indicate an impending relapse, it may be necessary to arrange a special appointment for your relative before the next one scheduled. Providing additional medication during the first few days or weeks after early warning signs have been detected is a powerful strategy for preventing relapses and hospitalizations.

6. *Monitor the early warning signs until the situation is resolved.* Once you and your relative have detected early warning signs and have taken steps to address the problem, it's important for both of you to monitor those signs until you see clear improvement. Monitoring will provide important information about whether a relapse has been averted. Useful questions for you and your relative to ask include:

- "Is the sign (or symptom) still the same?"
- "Has it gotten worse?"
- "Has it improved?"

While you're monitoring early warning signs, it's best that your relative not feel spied on or that other family members are "walking on eggshells" around her. Try to keep your family routines normal and include relaxing activities each day. Plan to follow up with a family meeting every week (or more often) until the problem is resolved.

Developing a Relapse Prevention Plan

Formulating a specific plan for how you, your relative, and other family members will respond to early warning signs allows your family to take advantage of its own unique combination of resources to prevent relapses. Being *proactive* rather than *reactive* will prepare you and your relative to respond to early warning signs quickly and effectively.

Decide How to Conduct a Family Meeting for Preventing Relapses

Determine in advance who will be present at the family meeting, where it will be held, and how people will be contacted when early warning signs are first suspected. In addition, some families find it useful to have a "chairperson" for the meeting who guides the process. You can list the people that should be included in a family meeting on step 1 of the Relapse Prevention Plan (Worksheet 12.2) at the end of the chapter.

Discuss Past Relapses

To develop a relapse prevention plan, first talk with your relative and other family members about past relapses. It may be easiest to focus mainly on the last relapse or the last two relapses. Ask questions such as:

- "What early warning signs of relapse were observable?"
- "What were the very *earliest* clues that a relapse was about to occur?"

As noted, the Early Signs Checklist (Worksheet 12.1) is a standard form for assessing common early warning signs of relapse as well as listing signs that are unique to your relative. If you have not already done so, complete this questionnaire with the help of your relative and other family members who are in close contact with her. Put a star next to the early warning signs that were the most troublesome. Only these signs (and not the entire list) need to be monitored on a regular basis. As an aid to remembering which of your relative's signs are most important to track, complete step 2 of the Relapse Prevention Plan by listing three to five of the early warning signs that you and your relative need to monitor. (Do not write down more than five signs, because it will be too difficult to monitor them all.)

Discuss Past Stressful Experiences

You also need to talk about which types of situations have been stressful for your relative in the past and what has helped him reduce stress. Ask other family members what they noticed about their relative's symptoms in relation to a particular event or problem. There is no right or wrong answer to the question of what is stressful, so it's important to listen to everyone's point of view. You can record the situations your relative identified as stressful on step 7 of the Relapse Prevention Plan.

Put Together a Relapse Prevention Plan

After you, your relative, and other family members have identified the pattern of early warning signs, discussed strategies for dealing with stress, and resolved logistical questions about family meetings, you're prepared to put together a Relapse Prevention Plan. Many families have found it important to include the following steps in their plan:

- Meet to discuss the concern about your relative's early warning signs.
- Evaluate whether medication is being taken regularly and, if necessary, plan how to deal with any nonadherence.

- Evaluate whether your relative is abusing alcohol or drugs and, if necessary, plan how to deal with it.
- Evaluate stress and, if necessary, plan how to alleviate it in some way.
- If the early warning signs are still a concern, contact the treatment providers.
- Monitor the early warning signs until the problem is resolved.

Worksheet 12.2 provides a form on which you can assemble all the important information in your relative's Relapse Prevention Plan. This form can be used to record your relative's early warning signs and previous stressful situations as well as to list the steps of the plan for preventing her early warning signs from developing into a full-blown relapse.

The following is an example of how one family developed a Relapse Prevention Plan and used it to respond to early warning signs.

During a period when Ed's symptoms were under control, he and his family held a meeting to develop a Relapse Prevention Plan. The meeting was attended by Ed, his mother, father, brother, sister, and brother-in-law. First they discussed Ed's last relapse and the early warning signs that preceded it. Then Ed completed the Early Signs Checklist (Worksheet 12.1) with input from family members. Ed said that before his last relapse, he had felt more tense (item 23) and had difficulty sleeping (item 20). His parents and brother also noted that Ed had become very preoccupied with talking about a girlfriend he'd had in high school more than 10 years ago. This unique early warning sign, along with the two signs from the questionnaire, were recorded on step 2 of the Relapse Prevention Plan.

Next the family reviewed what had been most stressful for Ed in the past. Ed noted that he found it stressful to be around crowds of people and that deep breathing usually helped him relax in a crowded situation. His sister said she had noticed that Ed sometimes "flew off the handle" when he became involved in an argument or disagreement. Ed agreed that arguments were upsetting. He said taking a break when there was an argument helped him cool off, and talking to either his dad or brother about the argument and how he felt helped too. The stressful situations were recorded on step 7 of the Relapse Prevention Plan.

In discussing how to hold a family meeting when early warning signs were detected, the family decided Ed's mother would call a meeting at their home. Ed asked to include his uncle Bud, because he felt close to him. The individuals to be included in a family meeting were recorded on step 1 of the Relapse Prevention Plan.

Six months later Ed's mother heard him pacing back and forth in the hall in the middle of the night on three occasions. When she asked Ed about this, he said he was getting only about 2 or 3 hours of sleep each night. Because sleeping difficulties had been identified as an early warning sign, Ed and his mother decided to call a family meeting the next day. At the meeting, when asked about the two other early warning signs (irritability

*and preoccupation with his past girlfriend), Ed said that he wasn't feeling tense or irrita-
ble but had been thinking of his high school girlfriend frequently in the past few weeks.*

*Ed was taking his medication as prescribed, and he was not abusing alcohol or
drugs. When the family asked about stressful situations he might be experiencing, Ed said
he was enjoying taking a new computer course but was feeling stressed by the crowded bus
ride to the community college. When various strategies for dealing with the bus ride were
suggested, including getting rides from Uncle Bud, Ed said he preferred the independence
of taking the bus and would like to try taking an earlier, less crowded bus and using deep
breathing to help himself relax. He also wanted to try his sister's suggestion of listening to
music on headphones to help him stay calm on the bus. The plans for reducing stress were
noted on step 8 of the Relapse Prevention Plan.*

*One week after the meeting was held and the suggestions for reducing stress were
enacted, another family meeting was held. Ed said he was feeling better and no longer
thinking about his high school girlfriend. He had been listening to music and practicing
deep breathing on the bus and was feeling significantly less stressed out by the ride. However, he was still having difficulty falling asleep at night. After the family meeting, he
called his doctor and described his early warning signs. The doctor set up an appointment for him to come in the next day. At the appointment the doctor suggested that he take
an extra dosage of medication a few hours before going to bed at night. The following week
another family meeting was held. Ed reported his sleep had returned to normal. One more
follow-up meeting was held a week later, and Ed said the sleep problem was still resolved.*

*Both Ed and his family agreed no more family meetings were needed at this time. Ed
continued to take an extra dosage of medication for 1 month, after which his doctor
reduced his medication to its previous level. By addressing early warning signs promptly
and holding follow-up meetings, Ed and his family were able to prevent a relapse.*

If You Live Alone with Your Relative

If you live alone with your relative, planning how to prevent relapses can be more
difficult. For example, if your relative is uncomfortable talking about past
relapses and early warning signs, the pressure is on you to identify the core components of your Relapse Prevention Plan. However, there are a number of steps
you can take ahead of time to make it easier to head off a relapse when one
threatens.

First, find someone who can support you in your efforts to cope with your
relative's schizophrenia—someone you can "bounce ideas off of." Relatives who
are not living at home, friends, clergy, and counselors can all be helpful people
to talk with in times of need. Even if the supportive person lives far away, talking
to him on the phone can give you perspective on your observations and help you
arrive at a decision about what to do next. When you've identified someone who
can fulfill this role, ask him to help you to develop a Relapse Prevention Plan.

Second, develop stronger relationships with your relative's treatment team members. When you think your relative may be facing an impending relapse, you can contact a team member and discuss your observations with her. Explore in advance which team members would be accessible and willing to discuss your concerns. The most likely possibilities are your relative's psychiatrist, social worker, case manager, or counselor.

Third, join a self-help advocacy association such as the National Alliance on Mental Illness (NAMI). Having the support of other families who have gone through similar experiences can help you make plans to prevent relapses in your relative.

Putting Your Relapse Prevention Plan into Place

You now know how to set up a Relapse Prevention Plan. However, this plan will work only if you actually put it into place. Make sure everyone involved knows the steps of the plan, has his own copy of it, and is confident about his role in carrying it out. Review the plan together at least every 6 months to ensure that everyone is still familiar and comfortable with the plan, making revisions as indicated. We strongly encourage you to take the steps necessary to implement this powerful technique. You, your relative, and your family will reap the benefits of a Relapse Prevention Plan by avoiding (or minimizing) the disruptive effects of relapses and rehospitalizations on everyone's lives and enjoying the rewards that come from long-term stabilization and the ability to focus on both personal and shared goals.

Resources

Herz, M. I., & Mueser, K. T. (2002). *Coping skills training program*. Wilmington, DE: AstraZeneca Pharmaceuticals. Written and videotaped materials for teaching consumers and their families about the relationship between symptoms and life stresses, recognizing early warning signs, and developing coping strategies.

Symptom Self-Management. A social skills training program aimed at teaching people how to cope effectively with symptoms and prevent relapses. Available through *www.psychrehab.com*: click on the "Modules" part of the home page.

Instructions: Below is a list of early warning signs that people with schizophrenia and their family members have observed the week before a relapse. With your relative, talk over each sign and try to agree whether it was noticeable in the week prior to his/her most recent relapse. There are blank spaces at the end of the checklist to add any unique early warning signs. After checking off the early signs that your relative experienced, put a star next to the ones that were most troublesome.

Early warning sign	Experienced
1. Mood shifted back and forth.	
2. Energy level was high.	
3. Energy level was low.	
4. Lost interest in doing things.	
5. Lost interest in the way I looked or dressed.	
6. Felt discouraged about the future.	
7. Had trouble concentrating or thinking straight.	
8. Thoughts were too fast to keep up with.	
9. Afraid of going crazy.	
10. Puzzled or confused about what was going on.	
11. Felt distant from family and friends.	
12. Had the feeling of not fitting in.	
13. Religion became more meaningful than before.	
14. Felt afraid that something bad was about to happen.	
15. Felt that others had difficulty understanding what I was saying.	
16. Felt lonely.	
17. Felt bothered by thoughts that I couldn't get rid of.	
18. Felt overwhelmed by demands or that too much was being required.	

19. Felt bored.	
20. Had trouble sleeping.	
21. Felt bad for no reason.	
22. Worried about physical problems.	
23. Felt tense and nervous.	
24. Got angry at little things.	
25. Had trouble sitting still; had to keep moving or pace up and down.	
26. Felt depressed and worthless.	
27. Had trouble remembering things.	
28. Ate less than usual.	
29. Heard voices or saw things that others didn't hear or see.	
30. Thought that people were staring at me or talking about me.	

Relapse Prevention Plan (p. 1 of 2)

Instructions: Hold a family meeting when your relative is feeling well to develop a plan for preventing relapses in the future. Review all the steps and complete in advance steps 1, 2, 7, and 9. Refer to the form when you or your relative becomes concerned that he/she may be experiencing early warning signs of relapse.

Step 1. Who should participate in a family meeting if early warning signs are a concern? List below:

Step 2. What are your relative's early warning signs? Talk about past relapses, use the Early Signs Checklist (pp. 202–203), and list 2–5 early warning signs of relapse:

Step 3. If your relative is experiencing early warning signs, evaluate whether he/she is taking his/her medication regularly:

Step 4. If your relative is not taking medication regularly, make a plan for helping him/her to resume doing so:

Step 5. Evaluate whether your relative is abusing alcohol or drugs:

Step 6. If your relative is abusing alcohol or drugs, make a plan for helping him/her to reduce or discontinue the substance abuse:

Step 7. What situations have triggered relapses in the past or does your relative find stressful? Note these situations below:

Step 8. If your relative is experiencing stress or is in a situation that has triggered relapses in the past, make a plan to reduce the stress or deal with the situation:

Step 9. List treatment providers (and other supportive people or agencies) to contact if early warning signs persist for more than a few days. Names and phone numbers:

1. Psychiatrist:

2. Nurse:

3. Case manager:

4. Social worker:

5. Therapist or counselor:

6. Other:

Step 10. Set date for a family meeting to follow up: _____. At the follow-up meeting, evaluate whether the early warning signs are still a problem. Make a new plan and set a date for additional follow-up, as necessary.

CHAPTER 13

Responding to Crises

M any serious illnesses require loved ones to respond to crises. Severe diabetes and asthma, for example, can lead to frightening symptoms, midnight visits to emergency rooms, and hospitalizations. Schizophrenia can also lead to crisis situations in which immediate action must be taken. In this chapter we focus on the most serious kinds of crises related to schizophrenia: situations in which someone's safety is threatened. Violent/destructive behavior, suicide attempts, and threats of hurting oneself or others are all crises that require immediate attention. We distinguish crises from other situations that need attention but allow you more time to respond, such as when your relative stops taking her medication but threatens no one's safety.

Most crises in schizophrenia involve a worsening of symptoms that may include psychotic experiences (hallucinations, delusions) and suicidal behavior. It's also possible for people with schizophrenia to have crises that are not related directly to a symptom relapse; for example, disinhibition due to drinking or using drugs, medical crises, severe financial problems, and housing crises. The general principles of responding to crises, however, are similar regardless of their origin. Therefore, although not all crises in schizophrenia are related directly to symptoms, we focus on those that are, recognizing that you can apply the general principles to other types of crises that may occur in your relative's life. Procedures for seeking involuntary psychiatric evaluations and treatment for people with psychiatric illnesses are also reviewed in this chapter.

Like other families, you may have painful memories of dealing with a crisis involving your relative and find that you don't even want to think about it—much less make plans for how to deal with it, should it happen again. These feelings are understandable. However, reviewing your previous experiences and making plans for the future may be your best bet for preventing such crises from recurring. Even if you haven't experienced a crisis with your relative, it pays to learn strategies for dealing with common crises related to schizophrenia. By being well informed, you may be able to keep a problem situation from developing into a full-blown crisis.

Experiencing Crises

Several characteristics of schizophrenia can lead to crises:

- The symptoms of the illness fluctuate. Even when your relative is taking medication, he may be vulnerable to relapse. This vulnerability is increased if medication is not taken.
- The nature of the symptoms themselves can contribute to crisis. For example, when people with schizophrenia have strong paranoid delusions, they may react aggressively to defend themselves.
- People with schizophrenia are prone to depression and suicidal thoughts and may try to hurt themselves.

Malik was 19 and lived with his mother and teenage sister Shayna. He spent most of his day alone and was not involved in any work, school, or treatment activities. After being diagnosed with schizophrenia, he had taken medication for a year when he began to have problems sleeping at night. After several weeks of disrupted sleep, he got into the habit of being awake all night and sleeping all day, which resulted in getting off schedule with his medications. He often did not take his "morning" dose because he was sleeping until mid-afternoon, and he frequently lost track of when his "evening" dose should be taken. Malik spent a great deal of time alone in his room, and his mother and sister saw him for only a few hours every day, finding him very quiet and withdrawn. He denied any problems, saying "I'm fine. I just don't like being around too many people."

At 3 A.M. one morning, Malik's mother and sister heard noises in the living room and went to investigate. They found Malik dragging the couch to block the front door; books had been thrown from the shelves and empty bookcases were shoved up against the windows. The television was turned to the wall. Malik was dressed in all black and was very agitated. When he saw his mother and Shayna, he yelled, "Get down, quick, before they see you!" When they asked him who he was talking about and what was happening, he rushed over and pulled them down behind the couch. "The silver soldiers have surrounded our house! We don't want them to find us here."

When Malik's mother peered out the window, she couldn't see or hear anyone outside. He said the "silver soldiers" were part of a secret army that had targeted their house, and that they had been talking to each other through the family television. Malik's mother tried to persuade him that there was no danger, but he was convinced that they were being attacked by a secret army. He wouldn't let his mother or Shayna leave the living room for nearly an hour. Eventually he agreed to let his mother crawl into the kitchen (so as not to be seen from the windows) to use the phone to call the police for a "military consultation." When the police arrived, Malik's mother managed to call them aside to tell them about his psychiatric disorder. Malik was finally convinced to let the police drive him to the emergency room of the local hospital. His mother met them there and stayed with Malik in the waiting room. She accompanied him to the examination room, where he talked to the attending psychiatrist.

Guidelines for Dealing with Crises

Despite everyone's best efforts, you and your relative may not be able to prevent a return of symptoms such as Malik experienced. Schizophrenia can be an unpredictable illness. Therefore, we advise you to be prepared to respond to a crisis, should one occur—especially if your relative has had a crisis in the past.

• *Evaluate the urgency of the situation.* Many situations are upsetting but do not constitute a crisis. For example, you may be disturbed if your relative refuses to bathe for a week, but body odor does not constitute an emergency. Asking the following questions will help you determine if a situation is a crisis and requires immediate attention:

— Has anyone been hurt? Is your relative or someone else in danger of harm?

— Has property been damaged? Does it appear likely that it will be?

— Does the current behavior indicate that a serious relapse has occurred?

If the answer to any of these questions is "yes," the situation is a crisis and *you need to take immediate action.*

• *Use crisis services when necessary.* Learn about services that can help you in a crisis and make a list of their phone numbers *before* a crisis erupts. This list should include your relative's treatment team, a crisis hotline, a mobile crisis team, a suicide hotline, the nearest emergency room, the police, and any other services you think might be helpful.

• *Behave calmly.* Your primary task is to help your relative regain control. One of the best ways to do this is to show that you're in control of yourself. Speak slowly and clearly, in a firm tone of voice. Keep communication brief. Avoid panicking or acting hysterical, which will upset her even more. For example, shouting, hurrying around, or attempting to physically restrain your relative (unless there is no other recourse) can worsen the situation.

• *Determine how much time you have to respond.* If your relative reports feeling irritable because of increased voices, scheduling an evaluation at the clinic the next day is probably sufficient. If your relative reports hearing voices that tell him to hurt himself and he feels that he may do so, however, an immediate evaluation needs to be conducted by either his psychiatrist or an emergency room physician. Some situations may be so urgent that you need to call 911 to get help in maintaining safety. For example, if your relative is beginning to *obey* voices that tell him to defend himself forcefully or to hurt other people, you must act *immediately*.

• *Get help in handling the situation*. It's hard to stay calm and organized when you have the full responsibility for managing a crisis. When possible, enlist another family member, someone from the treatment team, or a neighbor or friend to help you deal with the situation. Working with another person to resolve a crisis will lighten your burden and may help you respond more effectively.

• *Make a specific plan to manage the crisis*. Decide exactly what should be done about the crisis and determine the first step, second step, and so forth. Keep your plan simple and realistic. Determine what you need to carry out your plan, such as specific information, phone numbers, and additional people. Take action as soon as possible to keep the situation from worsening.

For example, if your relative were to experience severe paranoid delusions that family members were trying to hurt her, your plan might include the following steps:

— Call a treatment team member to alert the team to the situation.
— Arrange an immediate evaluation at the clinic.
— Contact a relative or friend to drive you both to the clinic.
— Help your relative remain calm while waiting for the appointment by sitting with her and listening to her favorite music.

• *Keep safety in mind at all times*. Although most people with schizophrenia are not aggressive or violent, there is an increased chance of such behavior during a crisis. Even people who ordinarily would never act aggressively may do so in response to severe symptoms. Being aware of the importance of safety, therefore, can prevent someone from getting hurt. For example, during a crisis it's best to avoid blocking your own or your relative's way out of a room or other setting, in case your relative feels threatened. We discuss the issue of potential violence in more detail later in this chapter.

Developing a Crisis Prevention and Response Plan

After a crisis has been resolved but is still fresh in your mind, review what happened and plan how to prevent a similar crisis from developing in the future. First, review the crisis with everyone involved: family members, friends, professionals, and (when possible) your relative. You may do this individually or in a group. In either case, during your meeting(s), try to take a positive, constructive approach and avoid blaming or finding fault. The Crisis Prevention and Response Plan (see Worksheet 13.1 at the end of the chapter) contains questions that will help you consider your relative's most recent crisis by identifying which actions were effective in the crisis and developing a plan of action for coping more effectively, should a similar situation occur again. Even if it has been some time since your relative's last crisis, the information-gathering and planning process may prove invaluable in the long run.

Advance Psychiatric Directives

Advance psychiatric directives provide an opportunity for people with mental illness to plan ahead for the treatment they would like to receive if they have a crisis that renders them unable to make decisions about treatment. In most cases, people use advance psychiatric directives to clearly state their preferences for the following:

- A health care agent to make decisions on their behalf.
- Hospitals and other treatment facilities.
- Physician(s).
- Psychiatric medication(s).
- Electroconvulsive therapy (ECT).
- Emergency interventions (such as seclusion, restraints, specific medications).
- Persons to be notified about an admission to a psychiatric facility.
- Care and temporary custody of children.

Because advance psychiatric directives are relatively new, several legal issues are still in contention, especially in crises that involve safety issues. Nonetheless, when your relative is feeling well and able to make sound decisions, it may be beneficial for him to complete an advance directive to designate a health care agent and to make his other preferences known. At the very least, you will feel more confident that you know the kinds of choices your relative would prefer if a crisis situation were to arise in which he is not competent to make decisions.

An Example of a Crisis Prevention and Response Plan

At the beginning of this chapter you read the example of Malik, who experienced a crisis involving delusions that his house was being attacked by a secret army.

After the crisis was resolved, Malik's mother spoke individually with him, his sister Shayna, and members of the treatment team, using the questions on the Crisis Prevention and Response Plan (Worksheet 13.1) as a guide. Then she met with Malik and Shayna, and they used the information she had gathered to come up with a specific plan that they could follow in the future. The completed worksheet follows.

1. Briefly describe the crisis.

   — Malik had a relapse of symptoms and was paranoid about being attacked by a secret army. He wouldn't let Mom and Shayna leave the living room for an hour. Mom had to call the police.

2. What was happening in your relative's life before the crisis occurred?

   — Bored, problems sleeping, stopped taking medication regularly.

3. What were the early signs that a crisis was building up?

   — Sleeping all day and awake all night; incomplete taking of medications (some pills left in bottle at end of the month); quiet and withdrawn; lots of time in room.

4. What actions were taken to resolve the crisis? Put a star next to actions that were most effective.

   — Listening to Malik when he tried to explain what was happening.
   — Calling the police.
   — Seeing a psychiatrist at the emergency room.
   — Following up with the regular doctor the next day.

5. What could have been done to improve how the crisis was resolved?

   — Take it more seriously when Malik reverses night and day and is extra quiet; call the mobile crisis team instead of the police.

6. What is the plan of action for preventing a similar crisis in the future?

   — Be aware of early signs that a crisis was building up (see #3).
   — Help Malik find some regular structured activity during the day.
   — Improve communication so Malik can tell Mom or Shayna if he starts to experience any of the signs in #3 or if he hears voices.
   — Help Malik set up appointment with treatment team if signs in #3 show up.
   — Have dinner together three times a week so family can touch base.
   — Set up system to help Malik take medications regularly, such as weekly pill box.
   — Have clear understanding about hours when everyone in house will be awake.

7. What is the plan of action for responding to a similar crisis if it occurs in the future?

   — Mom and Shayna will avoid going into any barricaded room with Malik, so that their access to a phone will not be blocked.
   — Call the treatment team if the crisis is during working hours (XXX-999-2222).
   — Call the mobile crisis team if the crisis is on the weekend or after hours (XXX-777-3333).
   — Call the police if safety is threatened.

Example of a Completed Crisis Prevention and Response Plan.

Guidelines for Involuntary Commitment

If your relative presents a serious danger to others or herself during a crisis, she needs to be evaluated for admission to a psychiatric hospital. This evaluation can be arranged relatively easily if your relative agrees that a psychiatric evaluation is in her best interests. However, your relative may disagree, and it may be difficult to convince her to get an evaluation. For example, if your relative has delusions that people are conspiring to harm her through hospitalization, she would be likely to refuse. If your relative will not agree to an evaluation, your next step is to seek an involuntary evaluation. (If you're convinced that your relative, or someone else, is in imminent danger of being harmed, however, don't wait to seek the involuntary evaluation; call the police immediately by dialing 911 to ensure safety for all concerned.)

Each state has its own laws governing involuntary commitment, but there are also many similarities. In most states, a concerned person, such as a family member or treatment provider, must file a petition for a warrant to require the person to submit to a psychiatric evaluation. These petitions are granted based on a combination of two factors that must have existed within the past 30 days: (1) evidence of serious danger to the person or to others and (2) evidence of severe mental illness. The petitioner must have *directly observed* the person behave in a way that presents an immediate threat of injury to himself or others. In some states being unable to care for himself to the point where he might die if left alone is also grounds for involuntary psychiatric evaluation.

To file a petition, the family member or professional must usually go to the nearest psychiatric emergency center—often a community mental health center or hospital emergency room. Once the petition is completed, the staff contacts the local branch of the state office of mental health (or a similar legal authority) for approval to obtain a warrant for involuntary psychiatric evaluation. If the petition is approved and a warrant is obtained, the police are called, and they bring the person to the nearest emergency facility for an evaluation.

If the examining psychiatrist determines that the person meets the criteria for involuntary commitment to a hospital, she is committed for treatment for a specific time period (usually around 3–7 days) at the nearest appropriate psychiatric facility with an available bed. Prior to the end of the commitment period, the petitioner must appear at a court hearing and testify to the dangerous behavior that he witnessed. The person has the right to attend the hearing and can be represented by an attorney. The judge (or other designated legal representative of the state) considers all testimony and makes a ruling as to whether the person will be discharged or remain in involuntary treatment (usually for around 2–3 weeks).

Commitment laws can be very complicated. It's best to become knowledgeable about the specific laws and procedures for involuntary commitment in your state *before* a crisis arises. Contact your treatment team, local psychiatric emergency room, community mental health center, or chapter of NAMI to find out the necessary details.

Guidelines for Responding to Violent or Destructive Behavior

When a person with schizophrenia threatens others or acts in a violent manner, he may be having a symptom relapse. For example, if a person hears voices saying someone is trying to hurt him, he may strike out in self-defense. Although only a small percentage of people with schizophrenia become violent, effective strategies are needed to minimize the risk these individuals may pose to others and themselves. For example, it's important to be aware that problems with anger often presage violent behavior and that helping your relative with his angry feelings may reduce the risk of violent behavior. Chapter 23 focuses on strategies for dealing with anger.

Research has shown that the people who are most likely to become violent have been violent in the past. Also, when violence occurs in people with schizophrenia, relatives are the most likely victims, mainly because they spend the most time with the person. Other factors sometimes associated with violence in schizophrenia include high levels of tension, active hallucinations or delusions, and drug or alcohol abuse. However, these factors are less important than a past history of violence.

Responding to Violent Behavior

Here we provide some suggestions for responding to threats of violence or violent behavior. These suggestions can be used in addition to the general guidelines described earlier for dealing with crises.

- *Step 1: Evaluate the potential for actual violence*. If your relative threatens to hurt someone or break things, the best indication of whether she will act on these threats is past behavior. If your relative has been violent in the past few hours or days, threats of violence must be taken very seriously, because she is likely to be violent again. Similarly, if your relative has made threats and acted on them in the past, there is a good chance she will act on the current threat. We emphasize, however, that even if your relative has never made threats in the past and does not have a history of violent behavior, it's best not to ignore any threat of violence toward people or property.
- *Step 2: Take action to minimize the chance that someone will get hurt*. Try to avoid handling any situation with a significant threat of violence by yourself.

Don't be embarrassed to ask for help from professionals, other family members, or even the police. Also, don't be embarrassed to leave your house if you fear harm to yourself.

Keep in mind that people who make violent threats often feel threatened themselves. This sense of threat can lead to violence when they feel cornered or under pressure to defend themselves. If you're in the same room, allow enough physical space so that your relative does not feel crowded and avoid blocking his "escape route" from the room. Stand at least 3 feet away from your relative. Avoid approaching your relative suddenly, and carefully evaluate whether touching him might be perceived as threatening.

Speak in a firm but nonthreatening and nonchallenging manner. Acknowledge that your relative feels upset and try not to judge her feelings. Remember that even though your relative's perceptions may not be based in reality, to her the dangers are very real. For example, you could say, "I can understand that you're upset. I'd like to help you with this problem." Avoid attempting to interpret why your relative is upset; instead, focus on making the situation as safe as possible.

Remove any weapons or objects that could be used as weapons from your relative's access. If there are other people in the house, alert them to the situation, because if they are not aware of what is happening, they may inadvertently provoke your relative. They may also be able to help you cope with the situation. Remember, if at any time you believe you are in imminent danger, leave the area as soon as possible and call 911. Avoid making sudden moves or being overly dramatic in your departure.

• *Step 3: Resolve the immediate crisis.* Once safety has been ensured, you can focus your attention on rectifying the situation and helping your relative get his symptoms under control. The usual first step is to contact your relative's treatment team to arrange for an immediate evaluation. If the treatment team cannot arrange an evaluation, take your relative to the nearest emergency room or crisis center. In some areas, local community mental health centers have emergency services and mobile crisis teams to help families in crisis. If your relative refuses to be evaluated, you will need to seek an involuntary evaluation, as described in the preceding section.

• *Step 4: Develop strategies to prevent future violence.* After the immediate crisis is over, get together with family members (including your relative, if possible) to review what happened and develop a plan for preventing a repetition of the situation. Use the Crisis Prevention and Response Plan (Worksheet 13.1) to record your plans for preventing the same kind of crisis and for responding more effectively if it does occur.

In the process of discussing the event, it is important for your relative to acknowledge if someone was injured or if property was damaged by her behavior. Making this point explicit can help your relative remember why a similar crisis needs to be prevented in the future. In addition, other family members may feel less angry and more understanding toward her if your relative expresses concern over harm done and offers to pay for any costs incurred.

Because some violent episodes seem to come "out of the blue," you may not be able to see a pattern that would have helped predict or prevent the crisis. When there is little or no predictability, or when a past episode contained a very high risk of actual harm (or someone was seriously hurt), we recommend that you seek alternative living arrangements for your relative where he can receive more supervision. You can still maintain your relationship with your relative without exposing yourself to risk if he lives elsewhere, such as in a supervised residence in the community.

Guidelines for Responding
to Suicidal Thoughts or Attempts

It is very upsetting when someone you love has thoughts about hurting herself or committing suicide. This is a particular concern for relatives of people with schizophrenia, because individuals with this disorder have a higher risk of having suicidal thoughts or trying to hurt themselves than people in the general population. Depression is common among people with schizophrenia, and when it is severe, they may think of taking their own lives.

The most important predictor of whether your relative will attempt suicide is a past history of attempts. Other important predictors are thinking about suicide, being preoccupied with death, or feeling very depressed. Individuals who are younger, have feelings of hopelessness, and abuse alcohol or drugs are also at higher risk for suicide.

Common Myths about Suicide

There are several common myths about suicide that are important to dispel.

* *Myth 1: Talking about suicide with your relative may give him the idea to try it.* Talking about suicide does not cause people to start thinking about it. Most people who have been thinking about suicide experience some relief when asked about it. People who have not had such thoughts usually simply dismiss the question. By asking questions about how your relative feels, you show that you're concerned about his welfare.
* *Myth 2: People who talk about suicide don't act on it.* Talk about suicide should not be ignored. Most people who commit suicide talk about it before they make an attempt. Even statements made jokingly, such as "I guess I'll just jump off a bridge," may indicate serious intent. Only by knowing your relative well and by asking questions will you be able to evaluate the seriousness of what she says.
* *Myth 3: If someone really wants to commit suicide, no one can prevent it.* Most

people who talk about suicide have mixed feelings about ending their life. Often, they want to live but find living very painful. Sometimes a person's desire to end his life is a temporary urge that is difficult to resist; it may seem at the time like the only solution. Timely intervention can help the person get past this urge and begin to address the problems in his life.

Suicide Prevention Guidelines

• *Step 1: Be alert to warning signs of suicidal intent.* Symptoms of severe depression, including pervasive feelings of worthlessness, excessive guilt, and hopelessness about the future, are an important warning sign. Other signs include preoccupation with thoughts of death, the presence of voices telling the person to hurt herself, and increased risky behavior, such as walking into traffic or heavy use of alcohol or drugs.

Pay close attention if your relative begins to verbalize suicidal thoughts. Statements such as "I wish I were dead," "I would be better off dead," "I'm not afraid to die," and "I have nothing to live for" are reasons for concern. Your relative may also refer to a specific plan for hurting himself or to methods other people have used to commit suicide. This kind of talk can be a warning of serious suicidal intent.

Increases in symptoms, such as auditory hallucinations or delusions, often accompany suicidal thoughts in people with schizophrenia. Relapses that involve hearing extremely critical voices or voices that command the person to hurt herself are especially related to suicide attempts.

• *Step 2: Behave in a supportive manner.* If your relative is suicidal, it will probably help to express your concern and affection for him. Refusing to acknowledge your relative's suicidal thoughts or trying to gloss over these feelings by making dismissive remarks such as "You don't really feel that way" only make matters worse. Speak calmly and try not to respond to your relative in a judgmental way; talking with him openly keeps a vital channel of communication open, which may provide a ray of hope.

• *Step 3: Evaluate the risk for self-harm.* Any discussion of suicide should be taken seriously. It's impossible to predict perfectly when someone will follow through on suicidal thoughts or plans. Evaluating suicidal intent is a complicated and difficult matter and is usually best done by a professional. However, situations may arise at a time when the person's treatment team cannot be reached immediately, and it falls to family members to evaluate whether there is an immediate danger of self-harm.

If your relative has already tried to harm herself, you must take emergency action and get help immediately. If no actual self-harming behavior has taken place in the past, ask specific questions to evaluate the immediate danger. The following questions will elicit the kind of information that you need to know:

"Have you been feeling sad or unhappy?"

"Does it ever seem like things will never get better?"

"Have you felt so bad that you thought about hurting yourself?"

"Do you have any thoughts of ending your life?"

"Have you had thoughts of how you might kill yourself?"

"Have you made any plans to do so?"

"What are your plans? What do you intend to do? When do you plan to do it?"

"Is there anything that might hold you back, such as people you care about, religious beliefs, responsibilities to others, or something you still want to do or see?"

As you go down the list, the questions indicate progressively more danger of a suicide attempt. Thus, the danger is very high if the person feels hopeless about the future, has made a plan for carrying out his intentions, has already taken steps toward this plan, and feels there is nothing to hold him back. If your relative expresses such conviction, he should be evaluated immediately by professionals, and steps should be taken to prevent him from carrying out the plan (see step 4). Even when the danger is not immediate, the situation should be monitored closely and a professional consultation sought. *Do not try to handle the situation alone*; the circumstances can be very intense and demanding.

On rare occasions, people may develop a habit of talking about suicide when they do not sincerely feel suicidal. If your relative has a history of this behavior, talk it over with the treatment team and formulate a plan about how to respond. Bear in mind, however, that no talk of suicide can be ignored.

• *Step 4: Take steps to protect the person in the immediate situation.* If your relative appears to pose a grave danger to herself, remove any potentially lethal instruments from the home (including guns, knives, sharp scissors, medicines, alcohol, and car keys) and do not let your relative out of your sight. Keep communication open. Your relative may experience some relief as a result of expressing her feelings, and family members can keep abreast of any changes in the seriousness of the threat. Although you need to give your relative space, keep a careful watch and stay close enough that you could reach her quickly, if needed.

Talking with staff members at a suicide or crisis hotline can be helpful to both you and your relative. Keep the phone numbers of such hotlines, as well as other emergency numbers, in a convenient spot (see Worksheet 13.1).

• *Step 5: After the situation has been resolved, develop strategies to prevent suicide attempts in the future.* Complete the Crisis Prevention and Response Plan (Worksheet 13.1) and pay special attention to developing strategies for maintaining good communication with your relative. If he can learn to discuss his suicidal thoughts with others before making an attempt, you can intervene early enough to help him before the urge becomes overwhelming. To encourage open communication, be receptive and listen to your relative when he expresses feelings, even if they are frightening or hard to comprehend.

Because many people who attempt suicide suffer from feelings of depression, it's also essential to monitor the symptoms of depression (see Chapter 21). Furthermore, staying alert to various life stresses, which can contribute to feelings of depression, may help you identify times when your relative is at greater risk for a suicide attempt.

Talking about Crises

A crisis is a frightening event that creates unpleasant memories that everyone would prefer to avoid. However, the best way to prevent a crisis is to prepare for it in advance. Keep in mind the saying "Those who forget the past are condemned to repeat it." Talking about past upsetting events or crises can lay the groundwork for preventing future ones—which is what everybody wants.

Resources

The Bazelon Center for Mental Health Law is an excellent source of information about advance psychiatric directives and other legal issues pertaining to mental illness. Their website is *www.bazelon.org*; the page *www.bazelon.org/issues/advancedirectives/ FAQ/index.htm* is particularly relevant.

Crisis Prevention and Response Plan

Instructions: After gathering information from your relative and everyone else involved in his/her most recent crisis, summarize what you have learned by completing this worksheet.

1. Briefly describe the crisis.

2. What was happening in your relative's life before the crisis occurred?

3. What were the early signs that a crisis was building up?

4. What actions were taken to resolve the crisis? Put a star next to actions that were most effective.

5. What could have been done to improve how the crisis was resolved?

6. What is the plan of action for preventing a similar crisis in the future?

7. What is the plan of action for responding to a similar crisis if it occurs in the future?

8. Whom can we contact for help? On the back of this page, write down phone numbers for the treatment team, mobile crisis team, crisis hotline, emergency room, and police.

PART IV

Creating a Supportive Environment

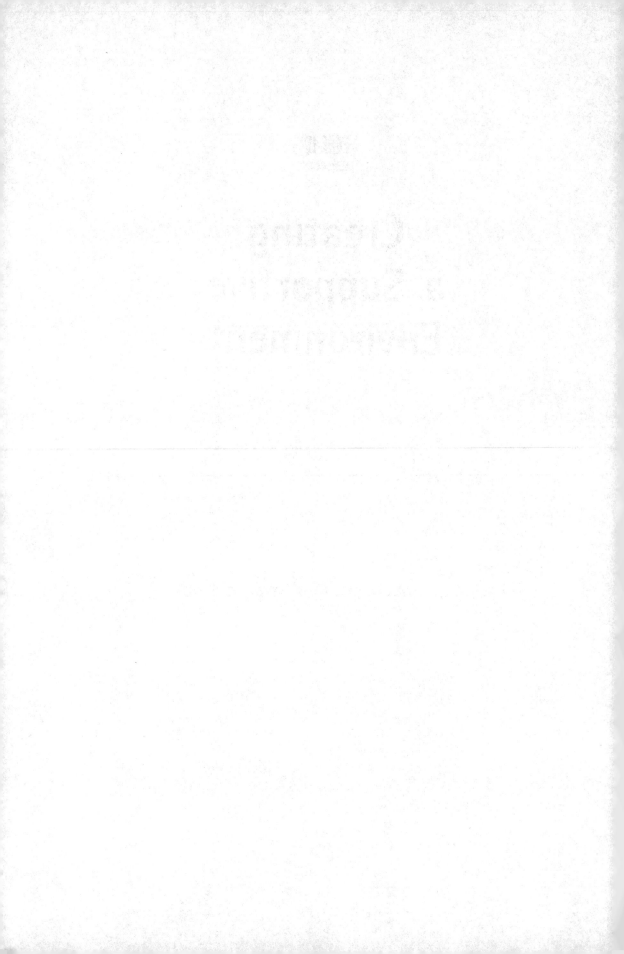

CHAPTER 14

Communicating Effectively

All families have communication problems from time to time, but these problems are particularly common when one member has schizophrenia. Symptoms can make it difficult for your relative to communicate with you and cause high levels of stress that may lead to frequent arguments, family members not talking to each other, and hurtful misunderstandings. Schizophrenia heightens the importance of effective communication because family members must often work closely together to manage the disorder. Direct and clear communication can go a long way toward preventing conflicts and preserving positive relationships when you're trying to help a loved one get his needs met. We hope the suggestions in this chapter will help you interact more productively with your relative.

Why Communication Is Often a Problem

Symptoms of the Illness

Many of the communication problems you experience with your relative may be linked directly to her symptoms of schizophrenia. Being able to recognize when your relative's symptoms are causing difficulty in communicating will help you be more understanding and more effective in your responses.

Cognitive (thinking) problems are a common source of difficulty for people with schizophrenia. These problems may lead to reduced ability to concentrate, difficulties reaching conclusions (deductive reasoning), and memory problems. In addition, people with schizophrenia may need more time to process what others say and to formulate a response.

Walter often finds it very difficult to stay focused on the topic of a conversation. He becomes distracted by irrelevant stimuli and finds it hard to follow the other person's line of reasoning. He often takes such a long time to respond that the other person gives up. To others, it seems that Walter is just not trying to concentrate or is uninterested in what they are saying–even though this is not true.

Delusions and hallucinations can be distracting and make it difficult for your relative to know what's real and what's not. They can also interfere with trusting other people and feeling safe in expressing feelings.

Jasmine hears voices much of the time and finds it hard to ignore her hallucinations when talking with someone. Sometimes her voices actually tell her not to listen to the real person.

Alexis feels distracted when she hears auditory hallucinations while she is trying to converse with someone. She describes the experience as like "too many tennis balls coming over the net at once–I don't know which one to hit."

Gerardo has delusions that FBI agents are recording his conversations, which makes him reluctant to express his feelings to anyone for fear that they will be used as evidence against him.

The negative symptoms of schizophrenia pose a special set of problems when it comes to communication. Negative symptoms include *blunted affect* (the person's face does not indicate the emotion felt), *poverty of speech* (not having much to say), *anhedonia* (not being able to experience pleasure), and *apathy* (not caring about what happens). These symptoms can make it difficult to get an accurate "reading" of how your relative is feeling. Not knowing how the other person feels can make conversations more difficult.

Jared's father feels frustrated when trying to communicate with him. He says, "I don't know where Jared stands on so many things. Sometimes he says one thing, but then his facial expression suggests something different. At other times he hardly wants to talk at all. I want to help him, but I don't know what he wants."

You may have also found it difficult to communicate with your relative because she is demoralized and appears to have given up. It may seem like nothing you say to your relative makes a difference.

Kate's mother describes feeling discouraged because her daughter will not engage in conversations aimed at helping her identify activities she might enjoy doing. Whenever her mother tries to talk with her, Kate puts her off by saying "It's hopeless anyway–what's the point of talking about it?" Kate's unwillingness to talk about making changes affects her mother, who is beginning to feel that the situation actually is hopeless.

Stress of Coping with a Psychiatric Illness

Difficulties interacting with a relative who has schizophrenia can also arise from the stress you may be under from coping with your relative's illness. When people live under a strain, regardless of the source of the stress (financial, medical, legal, emotional), communication often breaks down. Coping with schizophrenia can be a major strain on everyone, especially when the majority of care falls on the family. Sometimes family members feel additional stress because they blame themselves for problems in communicating, even though it's not their fault.

The stress you may have experienced can be worsened if your relative doesn't express appreciation to you for your efforts. Jasmine's sister says, "Jasmine's a nice person, but it's so hard to talk to her, and I don't know if she even notices what I do for her. I don't expect a lot of thanks, but a little would be nice once in a while."

You may have also found it frustrating to try to distinguish between communication problems that are caused by your relative's illness and those that are not. Jared's father says, "When he doesn't want to talk to me, I don't know if it's because of his symptoms or because he's mad at me."

How Improving Communication Can Help

The stress–vulnerability model of schizophrenia (Chapter 1) indicates that stress puts a strain on the person's biological vulnerability and can lead to increases in symptoms and relapses. Better communication can lower the amount of conflict and stress in the family, thus decreasing your relative's biological vulnerability and improving her long-term outcome. Improving your skills at communicating with your relative may therefore reduce her risk of relapse and improve symptoms.

In addition, improving communication among family members can affect the overall quality of family life. Effective communication can lead to an expression of more positive feelings, an improvement in relationships, a reduction in conflicts, and resolution of disagreements with a minimum of stress. Also, reducing stress through improved communication skills benefits all family members given that stress is related to many health problems such as high blood pressure and heart disease.

Skills for Communicating Effectively with Your Relative

The communication skills discussed in this chapter may enhance your interactions with people in many different contexts. However, these skills are especially important to use when communicating with your relative, so that you can compensate for problems related to the symptoms of schizophrenia.

• *Get to the point.* People with schizophrenia often have difficulty following conversations, so it's helpful to be brief and stick to one topic at a time. Keep communications simple and direct and avoid complex language and roundabout introductions to a topic. Getting to the point quickly will result in fewer misunderstandings between you and your relative. Instead of "I was at the post office today after lunch. Remember we had ham sandwiches but we ran out of mustard, so I was going to pick up some mustard at the market, too. Anyway, guess who I ran into? It was Lee Thompson, that boy in your high school class who got in trouble for the senior prank. He has a new haircut, very sharp looking. It might look good on you. And I asked what he's doing now and he said something about computer school, but I didn't catch it. Didn't you like computers in high school? Anyway, he said to say, 'Hi' to you. I went to the market after that but they didn't have the kind of mustard we like, so then I . . ." Say something like "I saw Lee Thompson today. He asked me to say 'Hello' to you."

• *Express your feelings directly.* People with schizophrenia often have difficulty recognizing others' feelings. They may miss subtle cues about others' emotions, such as changes in facial expression or tone of voice. Verbally expressing your feelings, including both positive and negative ones, will reduce the amount of guessing your relative must do to discern your feelings. Using direct verbal feeling statements will result in less confusion and less tension, even when you're upset about something.

One way of being clear about your feelings is to use "I" statements such as "I was really pleased when you set the table tonight" or "I'm upset that you haven't taken medication for 2 days." Using "I" statements lets your relative know directly how you feel. Taking responsibility for your own thoughts and feelings is more effective than referring to someone else (e.g., "Uncle John thinks you're doing better") or generalizing (e.g., "Some people should do more chores around the house").

• *Give lots of positive feedback.* People with schizophrenia often feel demoralized and think they can't do anything well. It will help your relative to know when he has done something that pleased you or when you are proud of something he did. By praising your relative for specific behaviors, you encourage him to do more of the things that foster the pursuit of personal recovery goals. Praise can also encourage your relative to follow through with treatment recommendations and increase his independent behavior.

Your relative may be painfully aware of her own limitations. Giving positive feedback will help her become more aware of her strengths. People with schizophrenia tend to make progress in small steps. Recognizing and encouraging your relative when she achieves each small accomplishment can help her see that progress is possible and that effort is rewarded.

- *Make positive requests.* Making requests of each other is an everyday event in most families. Requests perceived as demanding or nagging, however, usually arouse resentment and hurt feelings and discourage the other person from complying with the request. This is especially true for people with schizophrenia, who are highly sensitive to criticism and stress. Making requests of your relative in a nondemanding, positive manner can minimize stress and make it more likely that he will try to carry out your request. It helps to be brief and specific about what you would like him to do and to use a calm, pleasant voice. It may also help to start your request with phrases such as "I would like you to . . ." or "I would appreciate it if you would. . . ."

- *Express upset feelings constructively.* We all get upset with one another from time to time, feeling anger, annoyance, sadness, anxiety, or worry. When expressing these kinds of feelings to your relative, it helps to focus on her specific behavior rather than her attitude, character, or personality traits, which are more difficult to change. It also helps to suggest to your relative how she might correct the situation or prevent it from happening again in the future. When speaking, avoid using a harsh or critical tone of voice: "You're wasting your life away by doing nothing all the time." While it's important to express upset feelings, doing it in the least stressful way is likely to be more effective. "I'm concerned that you're home alone all day. I'd like to set aside some time this week when we could sit down together and talk about some activities that you might enjoy doing with other people." Also remember to use verbal statements to express your feelings, because people with schizophrenia often have difficulty distinguishing between different negative feelings (such as anger, anxiety, and depression) based on facial expression and voice tone.

- *Check out what the other person thinks or feels.* If your relative has blunted affect (not much facial expression) or poverty of speech (not talking much), you may often have to guess at what he thinks or feels, and you're often likely to be wrong, which can cause misunderstandings and frustration. Rather than guessing, listen carefully to what your relative says, ask questions when you don't understand, and check out what you've heard to make sure you understood correctly. Rather than "You must be angry at me," say "You haven't spoken to me today. I'd appreciate it if you could tell me what's on your mind." One way of verifying your perception is to paraphrase what you heard and to ask your relative if that was what he meant.

- *Suggest taking a break from stressful situations.* In spite of using these effective communication skills, at times you may find yourself in a stressful or emotionally charged situation with your relative. Taking a break can often help both people calm down so that they are better able to communicate and solve problems later. Avoid staying in a stressful or emotionally charged situation. Instead, try saying something like "I'm feeling stressed out by our conversation right now. I'd like to take a break and go for a walk. I think I'll feel calmer and better able to solve this problem when I return."

Managing Conflict

When any group of people live together or spend significant time together, conflicts are inevitable, but when one family member has schizophrenia, conflict is even more likely.

Your relative's cognitive problems may make it difficult for her to anticipate problem situations or recognize the negative repercussions of her behavior. Helena didn't think ahead about the consequences of leaving leftover food in her room (ants). Your relative may also have difficulty coming up with possible solutions to problems or may find it hard to express her point of view.

Communication problems are compounded by the fact that your relative is especially vulnerable to the negative effects of conflicts. Frequent or intense conflicts can increase the stress on your relative, resulting in a worsening of symptoms. Therefore, rapidly resolving conflicts through good communication can have beneficial effects for both of you.

Strategies for Managing Conflict

In general, it's best to address a conflict as soon as it's recognized. Don't be reluctant to take the initiative and address the conflict in a conversation with your relative. Conflicts involving your relative's behavior are usually easier to resolve *before* the situation has resulted in negative consequences or the behavior has become entrenched. When discussing a disagreement or concern, stay calm and in control of your temper, express yourself clearly, and listen to your relative's perspective. Approach conflicts with an open mind. Rather than trying to convince your relative that he is wrong, express your views and listen to what he has to say. Then think of solutions that take into account both your concerns and your relative's.

When Lisa stopped taking her medications, her mother raised the problem with her as soon as possible, before the lack of medication led to a worsening of symptoms and a reduction in Lisa's ability to respond to logical reasons for resuming medication. Lisa's mother spoke to her in a calm manner, which made her more receptive to listening and talking about the issue. Lisa's mother was also willing to listen when Lisa told her about the sedating side effects of the medication, which she found distressing. Together they came up with the solution of setting up a special doctor's appointment for Lisa to explain her concerns about the medication side effects. At the appointment, the doctor suggested taking the medication at night, before she went to sleep, so that the sedating effects would be less intrusive. Lisa agreed to try this schedule, and after a week she noticed a decrease in daytime sleepiness. Lisa has been taking her medication regularly, using the new regimen, since then. By attending to Lisa's concerns about side effects, her mother avoided a potentially volatile conflict and addressed the medications problems in a collaborative manner that led to an effective solution.

Resolving conflicts requires the same communication skills described earlier in this chapter. The following strategies may also help:

• *Avoid blaming.* People often feel criticized or guilty when blamed for something. Rather than blaming your relative, describe the problem, explain how you feel, and focus on finding solutions. "It's a problem for me that you've asked me for several loans since December but haven't paid me back," Terrence told his older brother with schizophrenia. "I feel frustrated because I run short of money at the end of the month. I'd like to talk about this and see what we can do to solve this problem." By focusing on solutions instead of placing blame, he was able to have a more constructive dialogue with his brother.

• *Speak in a calm voice.* People tend to be more receptive to a calm tone of voice than one that is harsh, loud, sarcastic, or angry. Some people with schizophrenia are particularly sensitive to harsh, critical tones. A negative tone of voice or shouting can put your relative on the defensive, making it difficult for her to hear what you say and making it less likely that you two will come up with a solution to the situation.

• *Use short, clear statements to highlight the main points.* When discussing a point of conflict, it's vital that you help your relative focus on the major topic. Short, clear, and specific statements are easier to understand and respond to than lengthy statements. Avoid talking about things that don't relate to the problem at hand and pause frequently to review what has already been said. One father, concerned that his daughter would lose her subsidized housing because of the fire hazard of numerous piles of newspapers and magazines, got lost in digressions about how she used to keep old magazines when she was a teenager, her housekeeping habits in general, and the possibility of replacing her furniture with some new upholstered chairs that her cousin was giving away. His daughter didn't understand her father's point and didn't know how to respond.

• *Elicit your relative's point of view.* One-sided discussions of conflicts don't lead to lasting resolutions. Because your relative may have trouble expressing himself, you may need to actively ask for your relative's opinion. Try saying "I'm interested in your perspective"; "How would you describe this situation from your point of view?"; "What do you think?"; "What's your opinion?"; or "What do you think might be some possible solutions?" Be sure to allow enough time for him to answer. If you solicit his point of view, chances are good that he'll have some ideas for resolving the problem. If you don't seek his opinion, he may feel frustrated and less invested in resolving the problem.

• *Focus on the present situation and on specific behaviors.* Personality, attitudes, and feelings can be very difficult to change. In contrast, people often find it easier to change their behavior. People with schizophrenia are easily discouraged by criticism. For example, comments about being lazy or irresponsible can be upsetting and may distract your relative from attending to the problem at hand. One husband found it more constructive to concentrate on how they could follow a budget for the coming month and avoid referring to past financial problems or describing his wife as "extravagant."

- *Be open to compromise.* If you and your relative disagree about a solution to a particular conflict, a compromise may be the best solution. In working out a compromise, each person generally gets some of what she wants but also has to give up something. The goal is to reach a solution that is acceptable to both you and your relative. If, for example, you're uncomfortable with your relative's sleeping until noon or later every day, could you two agree on his sleeping until 10 A.M. on weekdays and as late as he wanted to on weekends?

An Example of Resolving a Conflict

The following example of resolving a conflict has two parts. In the first part, the family attempts to address a conflict but, in the heat of the moment, does not use good communication skills. In the second part, after the family has a chance to cool off, they approach the conflict again, this time using more effective communication skills.

Dylan has schizophrenia and lives at home with his mother and two sisters, Rose and Amy. Each person in the household is expected to do some housework. Dylan's task is to set the table for dinner. At first he did this on a regular basis. As the weeks went on, however, he stayed in his room more and two or three times a week neglected to set the table. At first his mother did not want to talk to Dylan about this, hoping the lapse would be temporary. The problem persisted, however, until Dylan ceased setting the table altogether. One evening, Dylan's mother and Rose were talking about how much they resented the fact that he wasn't helping out anymore. When Dylan came down for dinner, Rose yelled at him, "You're making Mom upset. You never do anything around this house. You're lazy!" When Dylan didn't answer, his mother said in an angry tone, "Maybe your sister is right; you should do more to help." Dylan looked confused and retreated to his room, saying "I'm not hungry." Tension continued to mount in the family as the conflict remained unresolved.

Perhaps this conflict could have been resolved if better communication skills had been used. First, it would have been helpful for Dylan to hear right away that he had forgotten to set the table. At that point a gentle reminder could have been given. By the time Dylan heard about his mother's and sister's concerns, their feelings had already intensified and the conflict simply erupted. Even at that point, however, it would have been easier for Dylan to listen to his mother and sister if they had not yelled at him. Their communication would have been more effective if they had spoken to him calmly, been specific about which behaviors they wanted changed, and made clear statements about how they felt. Although Dylan probably recognized that his mother and sister were angry with him, they did not explain the exact reason for their anger. Referring specifically to Dylan's failure to set the table could have helped him understand the basis of their concern.

Even when conflicts develop into misunderstandings and arguments, all is not lost. You can always take some time to cool off and address the disagreement again, as Dylan's mother and sisters did.

Dylan's mother and his sister Rose later regretted having spoken harshly to him and asked him and his sister Amy to participate in a family meeting over dessert one night. His mother began the discussion, saying "I'm very sorry that I yelled at you last week about not doing enough around the house. I didn't mean to hurt your feelings." Rose added, "Me, too. I wish that I hadn't said those things to you. I was out of line." Dylan said, "I didn't know what you were talking about." His mother continued in a calm voice, "I think it would be a good idea to start our conversation over. Would that be okay with you?" Dylan agreed. "Your sisters and I have noticed that you haven't been setting the table like you used to. We were wondering if there was a reason for that." After a pause, Dylan said, "A few times I lost track of what time it was, and when I came downstairs someone else had already set the table. I thought that maybe you didn't like the way I was doing it or something. So it seemed better for me not to set the table." Rose said, "I'm sorry there was a misunderstanding about that. I really like the way you set the table. And I appreciate your help." Dylan's mother said, "I appreciate your help, too, Dylan. I can understand that it's easy to lose track of the time. What could we do to help you with that?" Dylan said that he would like it if someone would knock on his door to say that it was time to set the table. Amy volunteered to do this. They agreed to try the plan for a week to see if it was working. Dylan's mother ended the discussion by making sure Dylan was comfortable with the plan and then thanked everyone for working together on the problem.

Common Pitfalls in Effective Communication

So far we've focused on communication skills that we recommend you use. There are also some common problems that we advise you to *avoid*. These pitfalls in effective communication are summarized in the following table. It's not always easy to avoid these common problems, but as you become aware of them, you'll be rewarded by fewer arguments and a calmer atmosphere at home.

Although good communication can resolve many conflicts and can often prevent problems from occurring in the first place, some disagreements between people living together or in frequent contact are inevitable. Chapters 15 and 16 focus on additional strategies that will help you resolve conflicts and prevent others from happening.

Common Pitfalls in Effective Communication

Communication problem	Example of problematic statement	Alternative statement
Coercive statements ("shoulds" and "musts")	"You should know when to put out the trash."	"I would appreciate it if you would take out the trash every night after dinner."
Mixing positive and negative statements	"You look nice today, but why did you wear those shoes?"	"I really like the dress you're wearing today."
Speaking for others ("we" statements)	"We are concerned that you have been sleeping a lot lately."	"I am concerned that you have been sleeping a lot lately."
Mind reading	"You're angry at me for forgetting our movie date."	"You look angry. Are you feeling that way?"
Criticism	"You're so inconsiderate."	"I feel upset when I see your clothes in the living room. I would appreciate it if you would take them to your room."
Dwelling on the past	"You're not coming home for Thanksgiving, just like you didn't come home for Dad's birthday, Christmas, or your brother's wedding."	"I'm disappointed that you don't plan to join us for Thanksgiving dinner this year. Is there anything we can do that would help you reconsider?"
Overgeneralizations	"You never eat with the family."	"I missed you joining us for dinner the past two nights."
Arguing about delusions	"There is no reason whatsoever to be afraid of the police."	"I'm sorry you're feeling afraid. I'd like to help you with that."
Bringing up multiple problems	"You stay in bed until noon, don't keep track of your medications, and haven't called your brother in weeks."	"I'm worried that you haven't taken your medications in the past 2 days."
Giving inconsistent verbal and nonverbal signals	"It's okay with me if you want to move to Arizona" (while sighing and rolling eyes).	"I don't feel good about your moving to Arizona."

Good Communication

Communication is an essential and rewarding aspect of all human relationships, especially among family members. When a loved one has schizophrenia, communication can suffer due to a combination of factors: the symptoms, thinking and mood disturbances related to the illness, and the stress and frustration experienced by everyone in the family. However, these difficulties can be overcome, and conflict reduced, by understanding how schizophrenia can interfere with communication and attending to a few simple rules. Good communication skills will enable you to enjoy your relative's company, minimize unnecessary tension, and strengthen your appreciation of each other.

Resources

Hoffman, D., & Chamberlin, K. (1999). *Find something nice to say: The power of compliments.* Hopkinton, NH: Two Friends Publishing. A wonderful book—the title speaks for itself!

McKay, M., Davis, M., & Fanning, P. (1995). *Messages: The communication skills book.* (2nd ed.). Oakland, CA: New Harbinger. Provides practical suggestions for how to communicate more effectively with your children, partners, coworkers, and friends.

CHAPTER 15

Solving Problems

*E*very day we confront any number of challenges, from the mundane to the profoundly life-changing. Having a relative with schizophrenia can add to the challenge. Given all the possible problems you might encounter in coping with your relative's illness, it would be impossible to tell you how to solve each one specifically. The goal of this chapter is to provide you with a practical method for solving a variety of problems effectively. This method has been found to be helpful by many other families with a relative who has a mental illness. By developing your problem-solving skills, you will be better able to solve both current problems and those that arise in the future.

The Active Style of Problem Solving

We all have our own way of solving problems, but the most effective methods generally are characterized as having an *active style*. People with this style of solving problems have the attitude "If there is a problem, there must be a solution." Usually these problem-solvers recognize problems quickly, get others involved as much as possible, and take steps toward putting plans into action. The active style is particularly effective when combined with a strong desire to develop consensus about the nature of the problem and how to deal with it.

The active style has also been called the *problem-solving coping style* by Thomas J. D'Zurilla, PhD, an expert on problem solving at Stony Brook University. According to D'Zurilla, people who develop the problem solving coping style are better able to adapt to stresses and are less vulnerable to negative feelings such as depression and anxiety. Their positive attitudes toward problems are summarized in the table on page 235. If you think that you don't currently use the active style, you can begin to foster a positive, coping-oriented frame of mind by reviewing the attitudes in this list before tackling a problem.

> ## Attitudes of People with an Active Style of Solving Problems
>
> "Problems are inevitable. I don't blame myself for having problems."
>
> "A problem is a challenge to be confronted, not a threat to be avoided."
>
> "It is better to try to solve a problem and fail than never to try to solve the problem at all."
>
> "There is a solution to every problem, or at least every problem situation can be improved on. If I set my mind to it, I can find a solution and carry it out."
>
> "Solving most problems takes time and effort, but it's worth it."

A Step-by-Step Method of Solving Problems

Some people find a structured approach to solving problems helps them stay focused and come up with more effective solutions. Here we describe a six-step method for solving problems that has been found to be helpful in families with a member who has a mental illness. We refer to this method as *step-by-step problem solving*. Remember that regardless of which method of problem solving you use, it's best to start with a positive frame of mind, as summarized in the preceding table.

The step-by-step method can be used by individuals or groups. We recommend you keep records of your problem-solving efforts to keep you on track when working on a problem. These records can also be referred to later if the initial plan does not solve the problem. The Problem-Solving Worksheet (Worksheet 15.1 at the end of the chapter), which you may photocopy, lists the six steps of problem solving and provides spaces for recording important points. If you're tackling problems as a family, it's helpful to have a chairperson who guides everyone systematically through the steps. The chairperson can also complete the Problem-Solving Worksheet during the family meeting, or a different member may act as secretary. The primary role of the chairperson is to keep family members focused on the task, to remind them of the steps of problem solving, to get all family members involved in the discussion, and to prevent the discussion from deteriorating into arguments. The six steps of the method are described below.

Step 1: Define the Problem

This step is perhaps the most important of all. Defining a problem as specifically as possible sets the stage for the most effective problem solving. If you're meeting together as a family, it's crucial to talk about how the situation is a problem for each person. Once each person has expressed his point of view, the chairperson helps the group arrive at a common definition of the problem. It's essential that each person agree with the definition to ensure that everyone will be invested in solving the problem. This may require family members to compromise with one another when defining the problem. Reframing the problem as a goal to be accomplished or a situation that needs improvement sometimes helps family members agree on a definition. If you're solving the problem on your own, you'll still need to begin by defining the problem; you may find it helpful to consider how others (mainly your relative with schizophrenia) perceive the problem.

The Gordon family often had disagreements about how much time Tyler spent sleeping while other family members were working or going to school. Usually when they talked about the problem, each had a different point of view that led to misunderstandings and heated exchanges. Working on the first step of problem solving by defining the problem, Tyler's mother said she thought the problem was that "Tyler needs to set his alarm." In contrast, his father said, "He should get a job." Tyler said he was bored but not ready to go back to work. His brother thought the problem was that Tyler lacked friends to do things with. After much discussion, some compromising, and reframing the problem as a goal, they came up with a definition that all felt comfortable with: "Tyler would like to participate in an activity during the day where he could meet other people." Instead of arguing, they all became invested in finding solutions.

Step 2: Generate Possible Solutions

The goal of this step is to brainstorm as many solutions as possible. If you're working as a family, each family member should try to offer at least one idea, but the more possible solutions generated the better. If you're solving the problem alone, think of as many solutions as you can. Don't evaluate or criticize the solutions at this point—be as creative as possible. Even outlandish solutions are welcome. These solutions can help loosen people up and may even lead to a creative idea that actually solves the problem.

When the Alvarez family first tried to think of possible solutions to the problem of being able to meet everyone's transportation needs with only one family car, they fell into an old habit of evaluating the solutions as they were suggested, by saying "That's definitely the best one—let's just go with that" or "That would never work." This made it difficult for ideas to flow freely and to get beyond the solutions they had already tried. The father, who was the chairperson, realized they were getting bogged down and said, "Remember, this is the part where we brainstorm. At this point we just write down everyone's ideas and don't decide which solutions are good or bad. We want to get creative here. Carmen, we haven't heard your idea yet." By brainstorming, they eventually came up with a new and more effective plan, which included making a weekly transportation schedule at a regular Sunday night family meeting (with dessert) and Carmen teaching her mother how to take the bus to the library.

Step 3: Evaluate the Advantages and Disadvantages of Each Solution

After you've come up with five or six possible solutions, it's time to discuss the advantages and disadvantages of each. This can be done briefly by highlighting the main strengths and weaknesses of each solution. It may be helpful to put one to three stars next to the solutions that seem especially promising.

Step 4: Choose the Best Solution

When choosing a solution, consider its practicality, its probable impact on the defined problem, and the resources needed to implement it. Sometimes after evaluating the solutions, one solution clearly stands out as the best. Other times two or more solutions have merit. Solutions can be modified or combined to arrive at a "best" one.

When solving problems as a family, you all need to agree on a solution. Sometimes this means agreeing on a compromise between two or three solutions. If it's extremely hard to agree, however, select one option to try first, with the understanding that another idea will be tried if the first doesn't work.

Step 5: Plan How to Carry Out the Best Solution

Selecting a solution is an important achievement, but now you need to come up with an explicit plan for implementing it. The best plans break down a solution into several specific steps and assign someone to carry out each step. If you're solving problems as a family, individual members can divide up the tasks based on ability and available time. It's also helpful to specify when each task will be completed and to set a date to follow up on the plan. Many people find it useful to post the completed Problem-Solving Worksheet on the refrigerator or somewhere else in the house where everyone involved is likely to see it.

The Goldman family had engaged in several family discussions about wanting to do something together as a family. Using problem solving, they came to an agreement on attending one of the summer outdoor concerts in their community. However, they stopped short of making a concrete plan about how to carry out this solution. Two weeks later they realized they had not made any progress toward going on a family outing and decided to meet again to make a step-by-step plan to follow up on their solution. When they made a plan that assigned specific steps to individuals (Emily: find out the date and time of the next concert; Quentin and Emily: prepare picnic supper; Mom: locate blankets and chairs; Dad: do the driving, etc.), they succeeded in attending the concert. This was the first time they had done something together as a family in over a year.

Step 6: Evaluate Whether the Solution Was Implemented and the Problem Solved

Set a date to evaluate your progress. If you're meeting as a family, discuss the steps accomplished and praise all efforts. If you're on your own, give yourself credit for what you have accomplished. The evaluation process involves determining which steps of the plan were carried out, how effective each step was, and whether the overall problem has been solved. Sometimes plans are carried out only partially. When this happens, further plans are made to complete the steps. Other times the steps are carried out but the problem remains, in which case alternate solutions must be considered. The Problem-Solving Worksheet completed during the first attempt can help remind you of other solutions considered.

The more you practice the step-by-step approach to problem solving, the more efficient you will become and the less time the process will take. Often a problem can be discussed, solutions generated and selected, and a plan of action agreed on in just 10–15 minutes. This method can be used for new problems or for reviewing old problems. It can also be used to set goals and make plans for achieving them. Many families report that using this approach helps them make decisions about a variety of problems, from crisis situations to long-term planning issues.

Twenty-six-year-old Brandon lived at home with his parents and younger sister, Sophia. Although Brandon usually got along with his sister, he began getting into frequent arguments with her. Sophia was very upset by this behavior and started spending more and more time away from home. Brandon's parents became aware of the situation and called the family together to discuss it. Although Brandon was initially reluctant to participate, saying "People will only pick on me," his parents reassured him that they would not allow that to happen. They arranged to meet after dinner one evening when everyone was feeling relatively calm and in a good mood.

Brandon's parents started the discussion by saying they had noticed more arguments recently and would like to hear everyone's point of view. They avoided blaming Brandon or Sophia, and they maintained a positive tone in the discussion, focusing on how to improve the situation. In the process of getting each person's point of view, Brandon revealed that he had been hearing more voices recently. After being questioned gently, Brandon said the voices were warning him that Sophia was stealing his possessions and wanted to hurt him. He said he was very troubled by the increase in voices.

Family members brainstormed with Brandon and came up with several ideas for what he could do in response to the voices:

- *Ignore them.*
- *Play music on his headphones to drown out the voices.*
- *Avoid contact with Sophia.*
- *Consult his doctor about a medication adjustment.*

Although the rest of the family wanted Brandon to call the doctor immediately, he was opposed to this idea because he thought the doctor would automatically increase his medication, which would worsen his side effects. After more discussion, everyone agreed to a compromise. Brandon would try playing music to see if he could distract himself from the voices when they became intrusive. If this didn't work, Brandon would call his doctor.

The family made a plan to implement the solution as follows:

1. *Brandon will play music to distract himself from the voices for 3 days.*
2. *Brandon will post a sign in his room reminding himself to listen to music when the voices bother him.*
3. *If, after the 3 days, he is still troubled by the voices, Brandon will call the doctor on the morning of the fourth day.*
4. *Brandon's father will give him a ride to the doctor for the appointment.*
5. *The family will meet again in 1 week to evaluate how the plan worked.*

General Guidelines for Problem Solving

Whether you like the step-by-step method or prefer to use only a few of the steps or to have less formal discussions, the following guidelines will help you come up with effective solutions together:

- Develop a positive, optimistic attitude toward dealing with the problem.
- Respect everyone's point of view.
- Avoid blaming and faultfinding.
- Identify as many solutions as possible.
- Be willing to compromise.
- Formulate a plan of action, including a follow-up step.

Solving Problems with or without Other Family Members

In general, problem solving is most effective when everyone involved in the problem situation is included. Some people's symptoms are well controlled, and they are excellent problem solvers. However, not all people with schizophrenia are able to participate actively in solving problems with others. Those who have persistent auditory hallucinations or delusions, impaired attention, poor concentration, or chronic apathy may find participating in problem-solving meetings stressful and nonproductive.

If your relative has persistent symptoms but can be reoriented easily and guided to focus on the problem, it's important to try to include her. Some people with the illness may prefer to participate in some of the steps of problem solving, but not others. However, it is sometimes more effective for family members to solve problems alone.

The following example describes how one parent, working alone, used the guidelines to solve a problem involving her daughter, who refused to participate in problem solving.

Thirty-year-old Almira lived in a community residence. She had phone contact several times a week with her mother, who was a single parent with no other children. Her mother also tried to visit her at least once a week. Almira looked forward to these visits.

Although Almira's mother cared deeply about her, she often felt uncomfortable spending time with her because of her poor grooming and hygiene. She felt especially embarrassed by Almira's appearance when they went out into the neighborhood together. Previous attempts to get Almira to take better care of her appearance had failed, and she now refused to discuss the situation with her mother, insisting "I look fine."

Because Almira did not want to participate in solving the problem, Almira's mother decided she would have to do it by herself—although she would try to take Almira's point of view into consideration. After consulting with the staff at the community residence, Almira's mother made a list of strategies for dealing with the problem, including:

- *Try not to care about Almira's appearance.*
- *Suspend visits until staff members report that Almira is well groomed.*
- *Point out Almira's shortcomings in grooming at every visit.*
- *Reward Almira for good grooming by spending more time with her when she is clean and neat.*

Her mother decided that rewarding Almira for good grooming was the best solution. She formulated a specific plan, which she shared with Almira and the staff members at the residence. If Almira was appropriately groomed when her mother arrived, she would praise her for this and then take her out to the local coffee shop. If Almira was not appropriately groomed, she would comment on this, spend about 15 minutes visiting with her, and leave. Almira's mother explained to her that "appropriate grooming" means a clean body, unsoiled clothes, and combed hair. Her mother decided to evaluate whether this solution was working after 6 weeks.

At first Almira did not take her mother's plan seriously and expected that she would be taken out regardless of her appearance. Her mother was clear and firm about following through, however, and Almira began to spend more time on her hygiene before her mother arrived. At the end of 6 weeks Almira had been neat and clean for three of her mother's visits. Her mother was very pleased and praised Almira for the improvement. She planned to keep her plan in place for the next 6 months.

Wrap-Up on Problem Solving

There is no magic formula for solving problems and achieving goals. Each family must discover which strategies work best for them. However, with teamwork and determination it's possible to find solutions that will improve many of the situations that family members face when a loved one has schizophrenia.

Resources

Gause, D. C., & Weinberg, G. M. (1990). *Are your lights on? How to figure out what the problem really is.* New York: Dorset House.

Jones, M. D. (1998). *The thinker's toolkit: 14 powerful techniques for problem solving* (rev. ed.). New York: Three Rivers Press.

Straker, D. (1997). *Rapid problem solving with Post-It notes.* New York: Da Capo Press.

Problem–Solving Worksheet

Step 1: What is the problem or what do you want to achieve?

Talk about the problem or goal, listen carefully, ask questions, get everybody's opinion. Then write down *exactly* what the problem or goal is.

_____

Step 2: List all possible solutions.

Write down *all* ideas, even bad ones. Encourage everybody to come up with at least one possible solution. List the solutions *without discussion* at this stage.

1. _____

2. _____

3. _____

4. _____

5. _____

6. _____

Step 3: Discuss each possible solution.

Quickly go down the list of possible solutions and discuss the *main* advantages and disadvantages of each one. Put one to three stars (∗s) next to the best solutions.

Step 4: Choose the best solution.

Choose the solution that can be carried out most easily to solve the problem.

Step 5: Plan how to carry out the best solution.

List the resources needed and major obstacles to overcome. Assign tasks and set time table.

Step 1: _____

Step 2: _____

Step 3: _____

Step 4: _____

Step 6: Set a date to review implementation and praise all efforts.

First focus on what you have accomplished, then review whether the plan was successful and revise it, as necessary.

CHAPTER 16

Establishing Household Rules and Sharing Responsibilities

Creating and enjoying a harmonious living environment with others is part of what makes life worthwhile. Often the rules that family members live by have an important bearing on how they get along and on their feelings of mutual support and well-being. Many families function quite well with implicit (unstated) rules. When one member has schizophrenia, however, more explicit household rules are often necessary to maintain a peaceful and comfortable environment. This chapter will be of special interest to you if you share your home with a relative who has schizophrenia. In addition, if you feel unsafe, tense, or uncomfortable at home or have come to feel resentful or taken advantage of by the behavior of a relative with schizophrenia, you'll find the suggestions in this chapter helpful. Having explicit rules as a point of reference can help you assert your right to live in a positive, supportive home.

The Value of Explicit Rules

Relying on unspoken rules often leads to problems and misunderstandings because schizophrenia impairs (1) understanding of common social norms and (2) following of implicit rules.

Schizophrenia Impairs Understanding of Common Social Norms

People with schizophrenia often lack an understanding of the many unwritten rules that govern social behavior, including how to live and get along with others.

They may also find it difficult to judge other people's feelings by their tone of voice and facial expression. The result of these impairments is that many people with schizophrenia are isolated from the world around them and have difficulty taking into consideration the needs and feelings of others, including their own family members. A common example is staying up late at night and making noise that keeps other family members awake. Spelling out explicit household rules can help compensate for your relative's lack of social judgment by making it clear what is expected and what is not allowed.

Symptoms Interfere with Following Implicit Rules

Many of the symptoms of schizophrenia can interfere with your relative's ability to follow conventional rules for living with others. People with schizophrenia often suffer from low energy and have little motivation (negative symptoms), resulting in a lack of initiative for activities, including doing household chores. Furthermore, psychotic symptoms such as paranoid delusions or auditory hallucinations can decrease your relative's ability to understand what is expected or make him suspicious of ordinary requests. If your relative experiences persistent symptoms, he may have difficulty following conventional implicit expectations.

Clear Household Rules Reduce Stress for Everyone

The unpredictable behavior of your relative, coupled with her lack of awareness of the needs of others, may result in your doing extra work. Naturally, this extra work can cause you to experience stress as well as anxiety, annoyance, and frustration. Many family members deal with these feelings either by openly criticizing their relative or by simply bearing the added responsibilities silently but resentfully. Neither of these responses is likely to lead to positive changes, and the discomfort of living with someone who doesn't follow the basic rules of communal living can pervade the family atmosphere, increasing the stress on your ill relative as well.

Clear Household Rules Can Improve Your Relative's Quality of Life

When expectations are clear and realistic, your relative is more likely to contribute to the household, and doing so will improve his self-esteem and confidence. If your relative is able to follow through with tasks independently without being reminded or nagged by other members of the household, he will feel less stressed and proud of pulling his own weight.

Who Should Establish Household Rules?

Ideally, household rules should be established in a collaborative spirit, with all members agreeing on what is important to maintaining a safe, clean, and pleasant household. Rules are usually not well received (or followed) when imposed on people who have had no say in developing them. The more input your relative has into the discussion of household rules, the more invested she will be in carrying them out.

Although it's important to take a collaborative approach to developing household rules, anyone with primary responsibility for maintaining the home—the owners or renters, those persons who pay the majority of expenses, and those who coordinate cooking, cleaning, and shopping, for example—have the right to take the lead. If you have a child, sibling, niece, nephew, or grandchild with schizophrenia who lives at home, you should take the lead in establishing the household rules. If you're the partner or spouse of someone with schizophrenia, however, it's more effective to work together to establish clear expectations of what each will contribute to the household, as described later in this chapter.

Common Household Rules or Expectations

You and your family must decide what household rules work best for all concerned. (You may prefer to use terms such as *guidelines* and *expectations* rather than *rules*.) The following rules are common in most families, regardless of whether one member has schizophrenia:

- No violence to people or property.
- Respectful communication with one another.
- Assistance with meals and chores.
- Regular bathing or showering.
- No activities that put the household in danger (e.g., no smoking in bed, no leaving doors unlocked).

Household Rules Related to Schizophrenia

In addition to these common household rules, others may be necessary to address specific difficulties related to schizophrenia. Three problems are especially common for people who have schizophrenia: (1) not taking medication regularly, (2) engaging in disruptive behavior, and (3) failing to do household chores. You can establish specific household rules to deal with each of these problems.

- *Make a rule about taking medication regularly.* As Chapter 10 discussed, people with schizophrenia may stop taking their medication regularly for a variety of reasons. But if they have agreed to this course of treatment to begin with, the relatives they are living with have the right to insist that they take medication on a regular basis and see their doctor regularly. You can, in fact, establish medication adherence as a condition of your relative's continuing to live at home. Specific strategies for monitoring and improving medication adherence are described in Chapter 10, but your first step is to establish medication adherence as a clear rule for your relative. Your second step is to follow up to make sure the rule is followed.

• *Set limits on disruptive behavior.* The symptoms of schizophrenia can lead people to behave in ways that are upsetting, annoying, or anxiety provoking. Some upsetting behaviors may be beyond your relative's control. However, many behaviors can be managed by establishing clear household rules. Remember that your goal in setting rules is to limit the disturbing effect your relative's behavior has on you and your family, not to actually change the symptoms that cause the behavior. Therefore it's reasonable and realistic to establish the rule "There will be no shouting in the home" but not a rule that states "You will not hear auditory hallucinations." The following table lists examples of upsetting behaviors that are common in people with schizophrenia. For each behavior we suggest a household rule that may help you deal with it.

• *Identify household chores.* Lack of initiative and low energy can make doing chores challenging for people with schizophrenia, yet it's still reasonable for you to expect your relative to do something useful around the house. Even if your rel-

Examples of Household Rules to Manage Disruptive Behaviors	
Common disruptive behaviors	Suggested household rules
Staying in bed most of the day	Get out of bed by 10 A.M. on weekdays and noon on weekends.
Shouting	No raised voices.
Offensive language	No swearing or insulting people.
Watching TV most of the day and evening	No more than 3 hours of TV watching per day.
Poor personal hygiene	Bathe or shower twice weekly.
Constant smoking	Smoke outside the house (or in a designated room).
Lack of involvement in constructive activity	Must participate 3 days a week in one of the following: classes, work (paid or volunteer), parenting tasks, treatment program, vocational program, support group, housework.
Not taking medication regularly	Take medication as prescribed by the doctor (same dosage and frequency).

ative can only do one or two minor chores, you will probably both feel better knowing she is trying to contribute.

Make a list of the regular chores and additional jobs you need performed routinely in your household. To get you started, here is a list of some of the most common household chores:

- Shopping for groceries
- Preparing meals
- Setting the table
- Clearing the table
- Washing dishes
- Taking out the trash
- Doing laundry
- General cleaning
- Cleaning the bathroom

With your relative, select one or two chores that match her interests and abilities for her to do on a regular basis. These chores will be incorporated into the household rules. You can discover your relative's interests by asking her directly or by observing which chores she is naturally drawn to; for example, you may have noticed that your relative seems to enjoy helping with meal preparation or that she is meticulous about folding laundry.

You and your relative can also evaluate potential new chores by breaking them down into small steps and then determining what she feels comfortable doing. (See Chapter 27 for examples of the steps involved in several common household tasks.) Your relative may feel confident in doing some, but not all, of the steps involved in certain chores. For example, she may like cooking dinner but find it difficult to plan menus in advance.

When you're first establishing household rules regarding chores, err on the side of too few, rather than too many. If you start out with fewer rules, your relative is more likely to experience success and pride in doing a job well. After your relative has shown some consistency in doing the chores agreed on, you can gradually add more responsibilities over time. This approach will build up your relative's confidence that she can play an important role in maintaining the home.

The Process of Establishing Household Rules

Here are several steps you can use to effectively establish your own family rules.

- *Step 1: Meet as a "committee."* Arrange a meeting of the family members who have primary responsibility for running the household. Often it's the parents, but it may also be siblings or other family members, including your relative.

At this meeting, find out what each person thinks is important to maintaining an orderly and low-stress household. Hold the meeting at a time when there is a minimum of tension. Rules made in the heat of an argument tend to be overly rigid and punitive. Setting rules before tension builds, on the other hand, can help prevent arguments and stress.

• *Step 2: Briefly discuss the basic rules.* You can use Worksheet 16.1 at the end of the chapter, which contains a list of common household rules, to facilitate the discussion. If you agree on these basic rules, briefly define them so that everyone knows what is meant, for example, by "helping with meals and household chores."

• *Step 3: Develop additional household rules to address selected problems.* If there are problems related to the running of the household, select a few of the most important ones and agree on a tentative rule for each one. Rules should be realistic, based on a clear rationale, and described in terms of specific behavior (e.g., rather than the vague rule "keep your room neat," use specific indicators such as "make your bed and hang up our clothes"). Add no more than five household rules and give priority to problems that most upset your family's equilibrium. For example, your relative's not taking medication regularly and disrupting the household would be more urgent than her occasionally forgetting to dry the dishes after dinner.

While you're setting household rules, think through whether there are some situations or behaviors that you're no longer willing to tolerate. For example, you may decide that hitting other people is intolerable to you and that you're ready to put your foot down. Rules about intolerable behavior should be nonnegotiable.

• *Step 4: Set consequences.* When everyone knows there are concrete consequences for violating household rules, the rules are much more likely to be taken seriously and followed. When determining the penalties for breaking a rule, we recommend that you consider two factors. First, breaking more serious rules should result in more severe consequences. For example, smoking in bed and destroying property are more serious infractions and should have greater penalties attached than forgetting to take out the garbage. Second, you must be willing (and able!) to enforce any consequences you establish. Don't, for example, establish moving out of your home as a consequence unless you're truly willing to follow through on it. Unenforced rules will rapidly lose their meaning and undermine the purpose of establishing the rules to begin with.

Determining the appropriate consequences for violating household rules is an individual matter that you and your family must decide on your own. The most natural consequences available to you may include limiting privileges over which you have control, such as use of the family car or spending money for cigarettes, special foods, movie rentals, and so on. In most families, the people who carry the major household responsibilities (e.g., those who pay the rent or the mortgage) ultimately have the right to insist that a person who does not follow the basic household rules cannot continue to live at home. Although you may not choose this possible consequence, it's important to keep in mind that if you are financially and legally responsible for running your household, you do have the right to set rules and to expect others to follow them if they want to live with you.

The table on page 249 contains examples of household rules and possible consequences for breaking them.

• *Step 5: Meet with the entire family.* Meet with everyone in the family, including your relative, to discuss household rules. Be clear and firm about the nonnegotiable rules, but encourage discussion of the other ones and be open to suggestions and compromises. Just be sure not to agree to a compromise you will feel uncomfortable with. For example, a smoking rule could be modified to include a more acceptable smoking area, but it would be unwise to change it to allow smoking in bed.

• *Step 6: Record your decisions.* Using Worksheet 16.1, write down the rules and consequences agreed on. As you record the rules, make sure they are realistic, based on a clear rationale, and about specific behavior. Also check to make sure consequences are clear and you are willing and able to enforce them. Then read the list aloud, making sure each family member agrees to follow the rules as listed. Give a copy of the completed worksheet to each member of the household and post one copy in a prominent location, such as on your refrigerator.

• *Step 7: Plan follow-up.* It is critical to schedule a time for following up on whether the household rules are being obeyed. Otherwise they will become just scribbles on a piece of paper on the refrigerator. When you are first establishing household rules, we recommend having weekly meetings for the family to talk about how the new system is working.

Following Through on Household Rules

Once household rules have been established and plans have been made to follow up on them, it's important to recognize everyone's efforts and to troubleshoot any problems encountered.

Providing Positive Feedback and Encouragement

The most powerful tool for helping a family member follow household rules is *praise*. Regular positive feedback for following the rules acknowledges effort and helps build a cooperative spirit. For example, a mother might tell her son, "I'm really pleased to see you did your laundry today without my reminding you."

One way to get your regular family meetings off to a good start is to begin each meeting by pointing out what is going well. For example, a brother might tell his sister, "I like the way you've been turning off your stereo at 11:00 P.M. I can go to sleep a lot more easily." As you discuss the rules, you may need to make some modifications, such as making a rule more specific or lowering the task or

Household Rules and Consequences Defined by Different Families

Rule	Possible consequences for violating the rule
1. No violence to people or property, defined as no hitting or using weapons and no breaking objects.	• Violence to others will receive one warning; if it happens again, the person may no longer live at home. • Damaged property must be replaced.
2. Respectful communication, defined as no shouting, offensive language, or insults.	• The person must apologize. • The person must spend an hour away from the rest of the family.
3. Help with meals and chores, defined as setting the table each day by 5:30 P.M. and taking out the garbage each day by 9:00 P.M.	• If the person does not set the table, he/she will be asked to clear the table. • If the person does not take out garbage, he/she will be asked to sweep the kitchen.
4. Bathe or shower regularly, defined as twice weekly.	• The person's spending money will be reduced each week that showers or baths cannot be confirmed.
5. No activities that put the household in danger, defined as no smoking in bed.	• Cigarettes will be managed by someone else. • No cigarettes will be given out after 9:00 P.M.
6. Medication must be taken as prescribed, defined as taking the prescribed dose each day. Person will set up a medication box every week and Dad will monitor daily.	• No use of the family car for 24 hours each time that a dose of medication is not taken.
7. Everyone will get up by 10:00 A.M. on weekdays and noon on weekends.	• The person who does not get up by the specified time must do an extra load of laundry.
8. The stereo cannot be played after 11:00 P.M. each night.	• If the person plays the stereo after 11:00 P.M., he/she will be asked to stop playing the stereo at 7:00 P.M. the next day.
9. Three days a week the person must participate in one of the following: class, volunteer work, paid employment, or peer support program.	• On the specified day, if the person does not participate in an activity, he/she will be asked to do an errand, such as mailing letters, taking clothes to the cleaners, going to the bank, or picking up groceries.

requirement to something more realistic. When one family had decided to rotate the chore of cleaning the bathroom, they found that each family member had a different idea of what that chore required, so they worked together on a common definition: clean the toilet, scrub the sink and tub, wash the floor. Another family found their expectation that each person would take full responsibility for cooking one dinner a week was unrealistic, so they changed the rule to "each person will help Mom once a week by getting out the ingredients, making the salad, cutting up vegetables and/or meat, putting the ingredients away as they're used, putting in the dishwasher the dishes used in preparing dinner, and wiping off the counters." Another family found that the household rule requiring the person with schizophrenia to set up his medication box independently was unrealistic, so they decided he should assist his father in this task by bringing out the medication bottles and helping to count the pills.

People with schizophrenia often lack motivation because of the negative symptoms of the illness. One way to provide additional motivation is to celebrate rule following. For example, you might plan to go out to eat or to a movie if the rules are followed successfully for 2 weeks. Another way to increase your relative's motivation is to give him the opportunity to earn special privileges (such as using the family car) or something else that he wants (such as a music CD). Keep in mind that *rewarding* your relative for following household rules is not the same as *bribing*. A reward is a positive reinforcement that is given to the person *after* he has performed a desirable behavior, whereas a bribe is an incentive given *beforehand*.

What to Do When Rules Are Not Followed

Don't panic if your new rules aren't immediately successful. It will take time for your family to learn the rules and get used to following them daily. Your relative or another family member may need to find out whether you're serious by testing the rules. Testing new rules is natural, and you can best respond to these challenges by remaining calm but firm.

A good first response to a rule violation is to remind the person of the rule that he has broken. Your relative may have forgotten the rule or perhaps did not fully understand it or its rationale. After being reminded, he may respond by following through with the behavior described by the rule. Let your relative know that you appreciate this shift and you would like him to follow the rule in the future. If your relative still does not follow the rule, you may have to impose the consequences established.

If your relative does not follow the rule despite experiencing the consequences, review the rule itself. Ask yourself the following questions:

- Is the rule defined in terms of specific behavior?
- Is your relative capable of following the rule?
- Is the reason for the rule clear?

You may need to modify the rule based on how you answer these questions. If you do modify it, call a family meeting to review the change and alter your list of rules accordingly.

When Your Relative Doesn't Live at Home

Household rules can also be established for your relative if she does not live at home but visits regularly. In such instances, the basic rules apply during visits, and you can develop additional rules to address specific problems that arise surrounding these visits. For example, special rules can be made concerning phone calls home, surprise visits, smoking at home, requests for money, and helping out around meals.

A Portrait of Effective Household Rules

Daniel is 35 years old and lives with his parents, who are retired. His sister, Chloe, is 28 and lives at home to save money while attending graduate school. Daniel spends most of his day watching television in the living room, especially game shows and sports. Daniel frequently hears voices that criticize him and say that other people want to harm him. He often shouts back at the voices, which makes his parents feel tense and on edge. They also resent the fact that neither Daniel nor Chloe helps with meal preparation or household chores. After talking it over, they decided to work on these problems by developing some household rules.

Their first step was to set aside time to meet privately to discuss household rules with each other. They reviewed the list of common household rules (Worksheet 16.1) and agreed that they were good basic rules for their own home. Four of the rules were already being followed without difficulty: no violence, respectful communication, bathing regularly, and no dangerous activities in the house. They agreed, however, that they needed to establish a rule about each person contributing something to the running of the household. They made a list of chores that needed to be done regularly and checked off four tasks they wanted help with.

Daniel's parents then discussed the problem areas that would require special rules in addition to the common ones. They decided to focus on the problem of Daniel's shouting back at voices, which was disturbing to everyone, especially to Chloe when she was studying. After much discussion, they decided they could no longer tolerate shouting in the house and a rule should be made to prohibit this behavior.

Next they discussed possible consequences for not following the rules. After brainstorming several different options, they decided that the consequence for not doing chores would be losing the privilege of using the family car for a day. The consequence for shouting in the house would be losing 30 minutes of television time for each incident. They recognized that Daniel could not control the voices he heard and that it would be important to help him develop other ways of responding to them.

When Daniel's parents felt confident about the rules and consequences they wanted to propose, they asked Daniel and Chloe to set aside time after dinner the next night to meet as a family. They introduced the topic by saying that although there were many things about living together that pleased them, there were also some things that could be improved and that might reduce stress on everyone in the household. They then introduced the idea of household rules, saying it would be helpful to be more direct about what was expected of everyone. They briefly reviewed and discussed the common household rules, starting with the ones that were already being followed. Then they said they would like to talk more about the household rule of everyone helping with meals and chores.

Chloe and Daniel initially protested, saying they were too busy or too stressed to do specific chores around the house. Their parents remained calm but stated firmly that living in their household involved sharing some of the chores involved in maintaining it. They said they didn't expect Daniel and Chloe to do an unreasonable amount of work and they would particularly like assistance with certain chores, bringing out the list they had prepared. They asked Chloe and Daniel to choose two chores each. After some discussion, Chloe chose grocery shopping and clearing the table, and Daniel selected setting the table and vacuuming.

Next Daniel's parents said they wanted a rule about not shouting in the house. Daniel looked startled and said, "But I can't help it!" His parents were sympathetic, acknowledging that his hearing of voices was beyond his control. They were firm, however, that he needed to learn to respond to these voices in other ways. They said they recognized it would take time and practice to develop other strategies and that they would help him in any way possible. However, they said it was very important to their peace of mind to live in a household where people don't shout. They briefly talked about other options for dealing with the voices (which they had learned from Chapter 17), such as distracting himself (listening to music or reading the newspaper), using positive self-talk (saying to himself "I'm not going to listen to these voices"), humming to himself, or engaging in a physical activity (walking around the block). Daniel said he was most interested in trying humming to himself to see if that would drown out the voices.

Finally, Daniel's parents talked about the consequences of not following the household rules (i.e., losing television time or the privilege of using the family car). At the end of the family meeting, Daniel's parents asked Chloe, who was skilled at the computer, to type up the new household rules and make copies to post on the refrigerator and to give to each family member. They also set up family meetings for the next several Wednesdays to talk about how the rules were working.

The Rights of Caregivers

You and other family members have the right to live in a peaceful home and to expect everyone to behave in an acceptable manner. In some families, in spite of vigorous attempts to establish basic rules for the person with schizophrenia living at home, the stress and burden on the family members become too great. If you're feeling this way, you may decide it's best for your relative to live elsewhere, such as in a community residence, boarding home, shared apartment, or independent apartment. A variety of housing resources are available to help people with mental illness live as independently as possible, as described in Chapter 5.

It is not a failure on anyone's part if the decision is made for your relative to live elsewhere. You can still maintain regular contact with him and continue to be an important person in his life. For many people with a psychiatric illness, leaving their home of origin is an important *positive* step toward more independent living. If such a transition can be made smoothly and with the support of you and other family members, the result can be a reduction of stress for everyone. An additional consideration is that your relative's capacity for independent living may increase when he moves into a different living situation supervised by a non-family-member. Changing living arrangements is not something that is done lightly, but there are a number of positive consequences for both you and your relative that can follow such a transition.

When Your Partner Has Schizophrenia

If your spouse or partner has schizophrenia, it's helpful to agree on rules or expectations for living together. The process is similar to the one just described but differs in that you need to come up with the rules *together* and be willing to negotiate and compromise to make sure you're both satisfied with the agreement. Some partners prefer the term *mutual expectations* to *rules* to reflect the joint development of guidelines. Regardless of the term used, you first need to identify for yourself which problem areas are most critical and then formulate tentative rules or expectations for each area. When you have an idea of the expectations you would like to establish, meet with your partner and explain that you would feel more comfortable if the two of you could agree on what each of you expects from the other when sharing a home. Discuss the expectations you've identified. Be open to establishing expectations concerning your own behavior so that your partner can address some of her specific concerns. The process of negotiating expectations with your partner can improve the overall quality of your relationship.

Maria is 27 and has schizophrenia. Five years ago she married Anthony, age 29, and they now have two children, ages 2 and 4. Anthony works full-time as an X-ray technician at a hospital, and Maria is a part-time file clerk at a real estate office, working Monday, Wednesday, and Friday mornings. When both parents are at work, the children are in daycare. In the past, Anthony and Maria informally took turns with the tasks related to running the household and caring for the children, often figuring out what each of them would do at the last minute. This arrangement often led to confusion and stress because of a lack of routine. Anthony decided that it would be a good idea to talk to Maria about trying to reduce stress in the household. Before meeting with Maria, he reviewed the common household rules in Worksheet 16.1 and noted that, in most areas, they were doing well. However, he thought they had problems in routinely dividing household chores and childcare. Anthony considered some possible solutions for these problems but held off making any decisions until he talked with his wife. Anthony then approached Maria, saying "I'd like to talk to you about how we share some of the jobs around the house. I think some things are going really well, but we're a little disorganized about some other things. If it's all right with you, I'd like to put aside time to talk after the kids go to bed tonight." Maria agreed but said that she was very tired and would prefer to go to bed early and talk the following night.

The next night Anthony started the conversation by praising Maria's parenting and saying how much he appreciated the income she contributed to the family. He then said he would like to talk about how they divided some of the household chores and childcare duties and that he also wanted to know if Maria had any concerns. Maria said she would like to go out as a couple more often, like they used to, instead of either working or taking care of the children all the time. Anthony and Maria then discussed what needed to be done on a regular basis regarding the household, such as grocery shopping, preparing meals, and cleaning. Maria said she found it difficult to think of menus and prepare meals every night, and although she was willing to do the grocery shopping, it was stressful for her because she usually took the children with her.

After some discussion and compromise, Anthony and Maria worked out a schedule whereby each of them would cook a simple dinner three times a week and order a take-out meal once a week. When one person cooked, the other would clean up. Maria liked Anthony's suggestion of taking care of the children while she did the grocery shopping on the weekend so she could be less distracted while she shopped. They agreed to split the weekly housecleaning tasks, such as vacuuming, on the weekend. Finally they talked about Maria's desire to go out more often as a couple. Anthony said he would like this too and offered to talk to his parents, who lived nearby, about babysitting for a few hours each weekend so they could have more time alone together.

At the end of their meeting Maria and Anthony wrote down the schedule they had agreed on and planned to follow up every Saturday for several weeks to evaluate how it was working.

Everyone Benefits from Clear Expectations

Establishing household rules or agreeing on expectations for living together can help reduce stress for everyone in your home. Your relative with schizophrenia will feel more secure knowing what he is expected to do and will gain skills and self-esteem by contributing to the running of the household. You will benefit because you'll get more help and spend less of your time reminding others about what they need to do (and resenting them for it). When expectations are equitable, clear, spelled out in advance, and followed up, your household will be calmer and more peaceful.

Household Rules Worksheet

Household rule	Consequence for not following rule
1. No violence to people or property, defined as:	
2. Civil communication, defined as:	
3. Helping with meals and household chores, defined as:	
4. Bathe and shower regularly, defined as:	
5. No activities that put the household in danger, defined as:	
6.	
7.	
8.	
9.	

Coping
with Specific Problems

CHAPTER 17

Psychotic Symptoms

A ntipsychotic medication makes it possible for most people with schizophrenia to live in the community with only occasional hospitalizations to manage symptom relapses. However, many people continue to experience psychotic symptoms such as hallucinations, delusions, and strange or bizarre behavior. Fortunately, there are many strategies that you and your relative can use to cope with and overcome the effects of these troubling symptoms on all areas of her life: in her relationships (including with you), at work or school, in self-care tasks, and in overall enjoyment of life.

Persistent Psychotic Symptoms

Virtually everyone with schizophrenia has had psychotic symptoms at some time during the illness. If your relative experiences psychotic symptoms only during a relapse, your need to cope with them is limited to monitoring and recognizing their reemergence so you can take immediate action to prevent a major relapse, as described in Chapter 12. But about half of the people with schizophrenia have psychotic symptoms most or all of the time. If your relative experiences persistent psychotic symptoms, they probably cause some distress, and when they lead to strange or threatening behaviors, they can have a negative effect on you as well. Coping effectively with psychotic symptoms, therefore, reduces stress on both you and your relative.

Your relative may have mild symptoms between episodes, such as occasionally hearing voices or believing others are talking about him. Or the symptoms may be more severe, such as relentless auditory hallucinations, delusions that others can read her mind, or stable paranoid (harm-related) delusions. Before considering how to help your relative cope more effectively, it's important to be aware of the factors that can contribute to the severity of these symptoms.

Factors That Can Influence Psychotic Symptoms

As mentioned earlier, the stress–vulnerability model of schizophrenia points to three factors that could contribute to more severe, persistent psychotic symptoms: inadequate medication treatment, substance abuse, and high levels of stress. Is your relative receiving optimal doses of medication? This is not an easy question to answer. One indication that your relative is receiving the right medications is that he has tried different antipsychotics at different dosages to find the right one. Also, research has shown that clozapine (brand name Clozaril) is more effective than other antipsychotics at treating persistent psychotic symptoms, so it should be considered if your relative has not tried this medication.

As discussed in Chapter 22, drug and alcohol use can undermine the effects of medication and worsen psychotic symptoms. If substance abuse is a problem for your relative, you'll need to address it to reduce his psychotic symptoms. When alcohol or drug abuse occurs as an attempt to cope with, or *self-medicate*, persistent psychotic symptoms, you can combine the strategies described in this chapter with those in Chapter 22 for dealing with it.

High levels of stress can also worsen psychotic symptoms, but stress is usually not the major reason for persistent symptoms. If stress is playing a role in your relative's psychotic symptoms, it may be due to *chronic* stressors, such as living in an extremely demanding or unsupportive environment (e.g., with people who are tense or hostile). Making the environment more supportive by establishing realistic expectations, encouraging small steps forward, and communicating in a more positive and constructive manner may improve your relative's psychotic symptoms (see Part IV for more on creating a supportive environment).

Although it's important to evaluate the contribution of these factors to your relative's psychotic symptoms, the fact remains that many people have persistent symptoms even when their medication is well managed, they don't use substances, and their families and friends are supportive. The coping strategies described here can help. First, however, to understand your relative's needs and to consider possible coping strategies with her, you need to be able to talk to her in a sensitive and caring manner.

Having a Dialogue with Your Relative about Delusions and Hallucinations

The key to helping your relative deal with persistent psychotic symptoms is being able to communicate with him about those symptoms and being able to listen empathically. The guidelines for empathic listening differ somewhat for delusions and hallucinations.

Delusions

When talking with your relative, avoid trying to convince her that her delusional beliefs are not true. Most people with delusions are incapable of logically debating the accuracy of their beliefs, except in the rare instances when they themselves question their beliefs and ask others for feedback. In fact, confronting or attempting to persuade your relative that her beliefs are inaccurate can actually backfire. Research has shown that when people with delusions are confronted by others about their beliefs, they may show an initial decrease in their convictions, but this is followed by a rebound in which the conviction actually increases. The nature of delusions is that people cling to them in spite of overwhelming evidence against them. For this reason, you're not likely to succeed in talking your relative out of a delusion, and you may inadvertently increase tension between the two of you.

As an alternative, listen carefully and show your concern. To your relative the delusion seems totally real, and if it causes anxiety or frustration, those feelings are also quite real. You can validate your relative's feelings about delusional beliefs without reinforcing the actual beliefs. To show your relative you understand his feelings, use empathic listening skills such as paraphrasing and asking clarifying questions to reflect back what you've heard. By focusing on *feelings* rather than *beliefs*, you avoid unnecessarily challenging your relative, as illustrated in the following example with Mabel (a woman with schizophrenia) and her mother, Rita.

MABEL: I can't go to my job.

RITA: What seems to be the problem? [clarifying question]

MABEL: Everybody can read my mind there—and they talk about me.

RITA: Does that make you feel uncomfortable? [clarifying question]

MABEL: Sure it does! I feel scared.

RITA: It sounds like when you're at your job, you feel scared when you think other people can read your thoughts or are talking about you. [paraphrasing]

MABEL: Yes—it makes me want to hide.

RITA: I can understand that; those feelings must be difficult for you. [empathic validation]

MABEL: They are.

RITA: I can see how worried you are. Maybe we could see if there are some ways of helping you deal with this situation of feeling frightened that others can read your thoughts. [paraphrasing]

By reflecting back your relative's feelings, you communicate that you're on her side and want to help. If your relative is willing to talk about these feelings, the discussion can turn to strategies for dealing with them and the delusional beliefs associated with them.

Hallucinations

Unlike delusions, which people lack insight into, hallucinations are sometimes recognized as unreal. However, emphasizing to your relative that the hallucinations are not real is likely to serve little purpose, because real or not, they cause distress. Talking about the *feelings* associated with the hallucinations is more productive and can convey your concern more effectively. It can also be a starting point for working with your relative to improve his ability to cope with the hallucinations.

Some people with schizophrenia are reluctant to talk about their hallucinations and how they affect them. Your relative may be suspicious of you due to past experiences with others who reacted negatively when she talked about her hallucinations. Your relative may have a strong sense of privacy that makes her reluctant to talk about these symptoms. If your relative does not want to talk about these symptoms, respect her wishes. You may still be able to address some of the feelings associated with hallucinations without talking about the symptoms themselves.

Specific Coping Strategies

Even if your relative is willing to talk about symptoms, he might not be interested in developing strategies to deal with them more effectively. Some people don't mind their psychotic symptoms, and without distress, they have little motivation to work on coping with them. For example, some people hear voices that are kind, encouraging, or interesting. If psychotic symptoms cause distress but your relative does not want to talk about them, you can still work together on developing strategies for managing the depression or anxiety that results from the symptoms (see Chapters 20 and 21).

If your relative is interested in coping more directly with psychotic symptoms and their associated feelings, you can work together to identify strategies, plan how to try them out, and follow up to evaluate their success. *Coping strategies* are specific methods that can be used to reduce symptoms, the negative feelings related to them, or both. A wide range of different strategies can be used. In general, these strategies involve changes in physiological arousal level (heart rate, breathing rate), behavior, or thinking (cognition). Specific strategies are summarized in the table on the following page.

Strategies for Coping with Persistent Psychotic Symptoms	
Strategies	Examples
Arousal level	
Decreasing arousal	Relaxation exercises (such as deep breathing), blocking ears, closing eyes
Increasing arousal	Getting physical exercise, listening to loud, stimulating music
Behavior	
Increasing nonsocial activity	Walking, doing puzzles, reading, pursuing hobby
Increasing interpersonal contact	Initiating conversation, playing a game with someone else
Reality testing	Seeking opinions from others
Cognition	
Shifting attention	Thinking about something pleasant, listening to the radio
Fighting back	Telling voices to stop
Positive self-talk	Telling oneself "Take it easy" or "I can handle it"
Problem solving	Asking oneself, "What is the problem?" or "What else can I do about it?"
Ignoring the symptom	Paying as little attention to the symptom as possible
Acceptance	Accepting that the symptom is not going to go away and deciding to get on with other goals
Prayer	Asking for help from a higher power

Changes in Physiological Arousal Level

Increasing or decreasing inner or outer sources of stimulation can reduce psychotic symptoms. Physical exercise or listening to loud, stimulating music can increase arousal; relaxation exercises, deep breathing, imagery, closing eyes, or blocking ears (e.g., using earplugs) can decrease arousal.

Behavioral Strategies

Participating in more activities can lower psychotic symptoms, probably because it involves a shift in attention away from the psychotic symptoms to the activity. Taking a walk, doing a puzzle, reading, playing a musical instrument, having a conversation, and playing a game with someone can all reduce the disruptive effects of these symptoms. Some people with persistent auditory hallucinations experience relief when they hum or sing to themselves. People with frequent ideas of reference (such as thoughts that others are talking about them) can benefit from reality-testing strategies; that is, checking out with another person whether their thoughts seem realistic. When selecting behavioral coping strategies, focus on those behaviors that your relative can most easily do.

Cognitive Strategies

A variety of different strategies related to thinking patterns can be useful for coping with psychotic symptoms. *Shifting attention* involves engaging in some mental activity that competes with the psychotic symptom by drawing attention away from it (e.g., working on a crossword puzzle to counter auditory hallucinations). Thinking about something pleasant is one strategy for shifting attention, although most people find this difficult to do when feeling stressed or upset. Passive diversions such as watching TV or listening to music can be helpful. Sometimes people with chronic auditory hallucinations find music a particularly useful diversion, especially listening with earphones.

In contrast to shifting the focus of attention, *fighting back* involves responding directly to these symptoms. For example, a person who hears voices yelling at her might *think* back at the voices, "Stop! I'm not listening to you! I don't care what you say!" Sometimes people fight back by talking out loud to voices—which may have positive effects for them but can also be socially disruptive and lead others to avoid them.

Positive self-talk involves focusing on one's own strengths. You may be able to help your relative identify a few positive things to say to himself to cope with hallucinations or delusions. For example, a person with many paranoid feelings may say to himself, "I'm afraid, but I can handle it. I'll be all right." A person with frequent hallucinations can say "Take it easy, I'm not going to let these voices get to me. Stay cool."

Problem solving involves exploring ways of overcoming the difficulties associated with the symptom. Asking questions such as "What's the problem?" "How can I help you with it?" "What else can I do?" and "How could you and I try out this idea?" can promote a positive approach to the problem. More information on problem solving is provided in Chapter 15.

Ignoring the symptom by paying as little attention to it as possible is a useful strategy for some individuals. This can be combined with positive self-talk, such as saying to oneself "I'm not going to let these voices keep me from doing things."

Prayer can provide hope, understanding, and acceptance of difficult situations, including psychotic symptoms.

Acceptance involves accepting the hard fact that the voices (or delusions) are here to stay but that the person doesn't have to let them run her life. Acceptance is different from ignoring the symptom because it involves acknowledging its presence. Sometimes the person can "just notice" the symptom by accepting it but not giving it undue attention. Developing acceptance helps people get on with their lives without having to try to change their delusions or hallucinations.

Juan had prominent delusions in which he believed others were talking about him on the bus, in stores, and at work. He was eventually able to accept and expect these delusional experiences even as he pursued his goals. This approach enabled him to make more progress toward his goal of working part-time. It also helped him realize that the best type of job for him was one that did not involve very much contact with other people.

Emma had a delusion that she had designed a building for which she never received credit. After years of frustration with trying to get compensation for her "stolen" idea, she began to accept the fact that she would never get the recognition she "deserved." Although she continued to believe she had designed the building, she no longer devoted efforts to proving this and started to pursue other, more realistic goals.

Geoff heard voices almost continuously. After years of trying to make the voices go away, protesting them, or trying to ignore them, he eventually learned to accept that they were not going to go away. When his voices became especially loud, he would "thank his brain" for its spontaneous contributions and go on with what he was doing.

When Sam heard frequent voices, he would say to himself, "More comments from the peanut gallery," and continue with whatever he was doing.

Research conducted by Steven Hayes, PhD, at the University of Nevada in Reno on an approach to psychotherapy called *acceptance and commitment therapy* has shown that helping people accept unwanted or unpleasant thoughts and feelings, including those related to psychotic symptoms, is more effective at reducing distress and improving functioning than attempting to suppress those thoughts and feelings.

Helping Your Relative Develop Coping Strategies

Because most coping strategies take time to learn and become comfortable using, a team approach to working with your relative is best. *Coping strategy enhancement* was developed by Nicholas Tarrier, PhD, at the University of Manchester in England and provides the following guidelines by which you can help your relative develop better coping skills:

• *Step 1: Choose one psychotic symptom to work on.* Choosing a single symptom to work on at a time increases the chances of finding effective coping strategies that really make a difference. The more specific the symptom you want to address, the more rapid change will be. Examples of specific symptoms include

auditory hallucinations, delusions that others are talking about you, and paranoid thinking (that others are trying to harm you).

• *Step 2: Gather information about the symptom.* Determine what the symptom
is, how it affects your relative, how often it occurs, under what circumstances and
at what time, and how long it lasts. Find out how your relative currently deals
with the symptom, including what things he does that seem to help and what
makes it worse. Explore whether there are any consequences that might "reinforce" the psychotic symptom, such as the "reward" of avoiding responsibilities.
Learning as much as possible about the symptom and how your relative manages
it will help when it comes to planning specific coping strategies. Worksheet 17.1
at the end of the chapter is provided to help you do this.

*Anna Marie was troubled by persistent auditory hallucinations. These hallucina-
tions usually involved a male voice telling her she was "a no-good slut" and she had "no
reason to keep on living." Sometimes she heard more than one voice. The hallucinations
made her feel anxious and depressed. She heard the voices almost all the time. However,
they were worst in the late afternoon, when she was sitting around the house after her program. She sometimes responded to the voices by retreating to her room and relaxing, but it
didn't seem to help much. She noticed that when she got out of the house in the late afternoon, the voices were less intense. When the voices bothered her, Anna Marie would sometimes skip her evening chore of setting the dinner table.*

• *Step 3: Modify potentially reinforcing consequences of the symptom. Reinforcement*
refers to anything positive that happens as a result of a behavior, such as getting
a reward (*positive reinforcement*) or escaping something unpleasant (*negative reinforcement*), which can then increase the chances of the behavior's happening
again. Sometimes when people are distressed by symptoms they respond in ways
that inadvertently reinforce symptoms. For example, Anna Marie did not especially like setting the table, so when her voices bothered her, she would sometimes skip it. This doesn't mean that Anna Marie was *trying* to hear voices to get
special treatment or that she was using her symptoms to "manipulate" others.
Nevertheless, avoiding responsibilities can be an unintended consequence of
responding to symptoms in ways that can actually increase these symptoms. It's
important to be sensitive to your relative's feelings about experiencing and dealing with psychotic symptoms while working together to reduce any possible
rewards she may get due to those symptoms.

*Anna Marie's mother decided to encourage her to set the table even when her voices
bothered her. Her mother empathized with Anna Marie about the voices she heard but also
stressed the importance of her meeting her responsibility of setting the table. Anna Marie
agreed to try to be more consistent about doing this chore.*

• *Step 4: Select a coping strategy to work on.* In helping your relative select a coping strategy to work on, start with what has worked in the past or is working now
and try to help your relative use this strategy more often. Or, select a new strat-

egy from the list in the table on page 263 or by identifying other strategies that you or your relative have heard about. Together, talk over which strategy seems most promising. If your relative already uses one strategy and wants to try another, consider a different type.

André found that listening to music (a cognitive strategy) distracted him from his auditory hallucinations and decided to try another coping strategy for this symptom, engaging his wife in a conversation (a behavioral strategy) when the voices became worse.

Your relative may not be convinced that any particular strategy will be helpful. Encourage her to try a strategy by saying that if one doesn't work, another can always be tried ("Nothing ventured, nothing gained"). Acknowledge that it's hard to try to cope with symptoms, but affirm your belief that working together on reducing the distress of the symptoms will benefit your relative.

Anna Marie selected going out for a walk in the afternoon as the first coping strategy to use for dealing with her hallucinations. She had used this strategy in the past, but only very infrequently.

• *Step 5: Practice the coping strategy.* Helping your relative practice the coping strategy is critical to his being able to use the strategy in real-life situations. The best way to help your relative practice the strategy is for you to observe while he practices it. If your relative is not hearing voices at the time, he can practice the strategy by pretending the symptom is present or you can play the role of the voices, verbalizing what they say while your relative practices the coping strategy. If the selected coping strategy involves a social activity, a third person can be enlisted so that one person plays the role of the voices and the other is involved in the social interaction with your relative.

The easiest way for your relative to practice coping strategies in the cognitive category is for her to first verbalize the thoughts out loud. Select a specific adaptive thought (e.g., "I can handle it") and practice it. Because many people aren't used to employing thinking strategies to cope with symptoms, it may be helpful for you to demonstrate the strategy first, by "thinking out loud," followed by your relative trying the strategy, also out loud. As your relative becomes more familiar with the strategy, she can practice it silently. You may find that your relative needs to practice the strategy many times on different occasions before it feels natural.

Anna Marie did not need much practice with her coping strategy of going out for a walk. Nevertheless, she and her mother did a few rehearsals in which Anna Marie prepared to head out the door for her walk while her mother played the role of her voices.

• *Step 6: Make a plan to implement the coping strategy.* Once your relative has practiced the coping strategy, you can plan together how to put it into effect in daily life, incorporating the information gathered about when and where the symptom is worst. Rather than trying the coping strategy every time the symptom occurs, focus initially on one or two of the situations in which it occurs most often. This plan will make it easier to ascertain whether the strategy is helpful.

When planning, consider how your relative will remember to use the strategy in the situation. You may be able to prompt your relative, or she can use written reminders or other cues. Rating how helpful the coping strategy was for dealing with her symptom can also be useful to your relative. Make up a record sheet that includes the date, time, and effectiveness of the coping strategy (with ratings such as 1 = not helpful, 2 = somewhat helpful, 3 = very helpful). This record sheet can be tailored to the specific plan that you and your relative develop and modified as the plan is changed. Worksheet 17.2 at the end of the chapter provides an example of a record sheet for evaluating the effectiveness of a coping strategy.

We all benefit from rewarding ourselves for working hard or making progress on a difficult goal. Many people promise themselves a new outfit if they succeed in losing weight, for example. Sometimes it can be useful to help your relative plan a reward for himself for implementing a coping strategy in a real-life situation. Your relative may prefer something that he provides himself, such as listening to music, or you may be able to do something special together, such as cooking a favorite meal.

Anna Marie and her mother agreed that Anna Marie would take a 15-minute walk each afternoon at 4:00 P.M., a time when her voices were often more intense. To help her remember, they posted a reminder sign in the living room, above the TV, where Anna Marie spent much of her time in the afternoon. Each day after the walk Anna Marie agreed to record her experience on a sheet that she and her mother devised, including a rating of how helpful the walk was. Her mother agreed to remind Anna Marie to complete the sheet if she forgot. She and her mother also reached an agreement that if Anna Marie succeeded in going out for a walk 6 of the next 7 days, her mother would buy her a new pair of walking shoes.

- *Step 7: Evaluate the success of the plan.* A strategy often needs to be used for several days or weeks before effectively reducing the symptom. Therefore, your first concern when following up on a plan is whether the strategy is being implemented, not how effective it is. You may need to encourage and support your relative to keep trying if she is following through on the plan but not experiencing any relief. Try to meet with your relative regularly (at least weekly) to see whether the plan is helping and, when success is apparent, to apply the coping strategy to other situations. Be positive about even small improvements and encourage your relative's continued use of strategies that seem to produce any benefit.

Anna Marie and her mother agreed to meet every Friday to discuss how the plan was working. After 1 week there was some success, which became more apparent after 2 weeks. At this time, Anna Marie and her mother agreed that an even longer walk might be helpful, so they arrived at a plan in which Anna Marie slowly worked up to 30 minutes a day, by increasing her daily walk by 5 minutes each week.

- *Step 8: Develop additional coping strategies.* If little or no improvement occurs after a few weeks, consider alternative strategies. Even if your relative has experienced success with the new coping strategy, you should help him develop at least one more strategy. Surveys conducted of people with schizophrenia have found that those who cope most effectively with their symptoms tend to use many different strategies.

Despite Anna Marie's improved ability to cope with her auditory hallucinations, they continued to disturb her. Because Anna Marie already used a behavioral coping strategy, she and her mother decided to explore a strategy that involved changes in thinking. Anna Marie was particularly interested in developing more positive self-talk, which she thought might also help with her tendency to become depressed. Therefore, she and her mother began to work on developing this strategy, practicing it, planning its implementation, and following it up. Eventually, Anna Marie developed several other strategies for coping with her hallucinations, which resulted in lowering her distress.

Tailoring Coping Strategies to Your Relative

The method described above is one general approach to helping a relative develop coping strategies for persistent psychotic symptoms, but it's certainly not the only way to help your relative. You may find a more informal approach easier to manage, such as suggesting different strategies to your relative, posting a list of strategies somewhere your relative will see it, or talking with her about ways of dealing with troubling symptoms.

Our most fundamental message is that, if your relative is willing to talk about his persistent psychotic symptoms, and if he experiences some distress due to them, you can help him cope more effectively with them.

Dealing with the Effects of Psychotic Symptoms on You

Your relative's persistent psychotic symptoms can have negative effects on you, especially if she lacks insight into these symptoms. People sometimes "talk crazy," are difficult to understand, or falsely accuse others of plotting against them or stealing their thoughts. These symptoms can lead your relative to engage in verbal or physical aggression or to act on the delusions by, for example, unplugging the refrigerator because she believes it is "bugged," staying up late at night and talking out loud to voices, or acting inappropriately in public. These types of behaviors can be disruptive to you and your family, leading to tension, anxiety, and frustration. In the following material, we describe strategies for handling disruptive behaviors caused by persistent psychotic symptoms.

- *Set realistic expectations*. High levels of tension are inevitable if your expectations for your relative's behavior differ radically from his actual behavior. Setting realistic expectations involves deciding what your relative is *capable* of, after taking into consideration his symptoms and problems related to schizophrenia. Your relative's past behavior is one indication of what he is likely to do in the future. Although improvements in behavior are possible, they tend to occur slowly, over long periods of time, and with much family support and encouragement. For your current expectations of your relative to be realistic, they should not involve major changes. For example, if for years your relative has responded to auditory hallucinations by loudly talking back, expecting him to simply stop talking back is probably not realistic. A more realistic expectation or goal for him might be (1) not to *shout* back at the voices, (2) to confine his talking back to a particular room, or (3) to whisper to the voices after 11:00 P.M.

- *Enforce household rules.* In the previous chapter we stressed the importance of developing household rules if your relative lives at home. Developing such rules helps structure your relative's time at home, builds self-esteem for contributing to the household, sets limits on disruptive or dangerous behavior, and reduces everyone's anxiety over unpredictable behavior. Although you can't create a rule that your relative will not have a particular symptom (such as hearing voices), you can establish rules regarding disruptive behaviors that are a response to the symptom (such as shouting back at the voices).

- *Use communication and problem-solving skills*. As reviewed in Chapters 14 and 15, using good communication skills and taking a problem-solving approach to problem behaviors in your relative can be very helpful. Communicating clearly with your relative about her behaviors can be achieved by (1) being brief and to the point, (2) making good eye contact, (3) being specific about the behaviors you would like changed, and (4) avoiding harsh and overly critical statements. Often a simple request can be quite effective, such as "It distracts me when you talk to yourself in the living room. I would appreciate it if you would go to your room when you want to talk to yourself."

Using problem-solving approaches can help generate a variety of solutions to problem behaviors. For example, family members may find it disruptive when the person talks about a particular delusion (e.g., believing that certain individuals are in league with "the devil") and may get together to plan how to handle the situation. Possible solutions that the family might consider include (1) ignoring such talk, (2) asking the person to stop, (3) listening sympathetically, (4) switching the topic, and (5) refocusing the person on another activity.

- *Provide structure.* There is strong evidence that the more structured the activity, the less severe the psychotic symptoms and the less likely disruptive or bizarre behavior will occur. Structured activities seem to divert the individual's attention away from hallucinations or delusional beliefs and toward the outside world of people, tasks, and activities. What this means for you is that increasing the structure of your relative's day can reduce her psychotic symptoms. Structure can be increased by helping her develop a routine around the house as well as elsewhere, such as working at a part-time or volunteer job or participating in a peer support program, organized sports, church, or community organizations.

Cognitive–Behavioral Therapy for Psychotic Symptoms

In recent years research has shown cognitive-behavioral therapy to be an effective treatment for persistent psychotic symptoms in people with schizophrenia. This approach involves helping people explore the basis of their psychotic symptoms and the evidence supporting these symptoms in a gentle, collaborative, understanding, and nonconfrontational manner. A variety of different cognitive-behavioral techniques are used to address psychotic symptoms, including the development of coping skills (described earlier in this chapter) and *cognitive restructuring*. Cognitive restructuring is a strategy in which people are coached to evaluate the evidence supporting (and not supporting) beliefs that lead to unpleasant feelings. Cognitive restructuring can help people deal with many negative feelings, including depression and anxiety, even when these feelings are related to delusions or hallucinations.

If your relative has persistent psychotic symptoms, you may consider trying to find someone with expertise in the cognitive-behavioral treatment of these symptoms. One such organization is the Association for Behavioral and Cognitive Therapies (formerly called the Association for Advancement of Behavior Therapy), whose website address is *www.aabt.org*. Although strong scientific evidence supports the effectiveness of cognitive-behavioral treatment for persistent symptoms, research in this area is relatively new—most of it has been conducted since 1995. Therefore, it may be difficult to find someone who has experience administering cognitive-behavioral therapy for psychotic symptoms. If you have trouble finding a cognitive-behavioral therapist, you may still be able to help your relative by applying some of the concepts of this approach in your day-to-day interactions with your loved one.

• *Focus on psychotic symptoms related to negative moods.* Most psychotic symptoms contribute to feelings of anxiety, depression, or anger, but some don't. For example, people with grandiose delusions (such as believing that one is a great inventor) often feel very good about themselves. Psychotic symptoms related to bad feelings are easier to explore because your relative will be more motivated to deal with them. Bad feelings can be related to grandiose delusions, however, because of the frustrations people experience when they don't achieve their unrealistic ambitions or aren't compensated for accomplishments they believe are theirs. Such negative feelings can serve as a basis for exploring the symptoms together.

• *Normalize your relative's psychotic symptoms.* The *normalization principle* is based on the fact that psychotic experiences lie on a continuum and that they are not qualitatively (or distinctively) different in people with schizophrenia than in others. In other words, lots of people with no mental illness have beliefs that aren't shared by others or are not supported by evidence, such as beliefs about aliens and UFOs, extrasensory perception (ESP), Elvis sightings, communication with people who have died, and past-life experiences. Furthermore, hallucinations are relatively common in the general population, and people from different ethnic or racial groups may differ in how often they have such experiences. For example, in one study Johns and colleagues asked "Over the past year have there been times when you heard or saw things that other people couldn't" and 4% of whites said yes, compared to about 10% of people from Caribbean backgrounds and about 2% of people from South Asian backgrounds. In another study of 13,057 people in the general population, Ohayon found that 38.7% reported having experienced hallucinations during their lives. Letting your relative know that having beliefs that aren't shared by others or hearing voices is part of the normal range of human experiences may make him feel less defensive when exploring these symptoms.

• *Explore evidence supporting delusional beliefs.* You may be able to help your relative reconsider her delusional beliefs by exploring together the evidence supporting them. First you might want to talk about the difference between strong and weak evidence, explaining that *strong evidence* is like *facts*, whereas *weak evidence* is like *guesses.* You can begin to help your relative practice distinguishing between facts and guesses by looking at pictures together and talking about what are the facts (Is the man wearing a hat? How many people are in the picture?) and what are guesses about those pictures (What is the man's relationship to the woman? Does the man *really* like the soda he's drinking?). You can then explore the kinds of questions he might have to ask to find out whether a guess about a particular picture is accurate and what kind of strong evidence would support the guess.

When helping your relative explore evidence related to a delusional belief, avoid directly confronting her with contradictory evidence; rather, encourage her to consider the evidence by asking questions and adopting a nonjudgmental, collaborative style in pulling the facts together. If your relative says things that seem contradictory to her delusions or she behaves in ways that seem inconsistent with those delusions, you can inquire about the contradictions in a genuinely curious fashion rather than directly pointing them out. When evaluating delusional beliefs that arise in a particular situation, help your relative consider factors related to that situation rather than herself. Asking questions and giving hints may be helpful. For example, if your relative believes that two people were talking about her when she got on the bus because they looked up at her and then started talking when she boarded, you could ask questions such as "What usually happens with the passengers on a bus when someone new gets on?" "Do people typically look up when someone gets on a bus?" "Let's think of some of the different things those people might have been talking about." This approach can help you both understand your relative's reasoning and may help her think about different ways of looking at the situation. After exploring the evidence with you and giving greatest weight to the strongest evidence, your relative may decide that a different explanation is more accurate or at least possible.

Jonathan, who had schizophrenia, and Julia, his wife, lived in a suburb where crime was not a problem. One day Jonathan saw some adolescents and young men near the bus stop who were dressed in the latest fashion, and this sparked a delusional belief that he was being pursued by inner-city gangs, in part because he had actually witnessed a crime many years ago while living in a different city. Jonathan refused to ride the bus to his job and started talking with Julia about the need for them to move, now that he had been "found out." Julia listened sympathetically and suggested they tackle this problem together. She got out a paper and pencil and made a list of all the evidence supporting and opposing the belief that these young people were gang members who were out to get Jonathan. In support of the belief, Jonathan pointed out that gang members often dress in the latest fashion, that he had in fact witnessed a crime committed by gang members, and that when these young men looked at him they had glared at him in a menacing way. With further exploration and questioning by Julia, Jonathan also acknowledged that he didn't recognize any of the gang members, no one had tried to chase or hurt him, sometimes young people dress fashionably even if they aren't in a gang, and the original gang members didn't know where he lived. After considering the evidence, Jonathan concluded that the young men he had seen probably weren't gang members, which allayed his concerns greatly.

• *Consider alternative explanations.* People with psychotic symptoms often jump to conclusions and don't consider alternative explanations for what happens around them. Encourage your relative to consider different explanations, not so much to find the single "true" explanation for an event but to see that multiple interpretations are always possible and more than one explanation may be accurate.

The best way to help your relative consider alternative explanations is by asking questions rather than providing other explanations yourself. This is called the *Socratic method* (named after Socrates' teaching style, as exemplified in Plato's writings such as *The Republic*), and it's often very effective because people are more likely to believe answers and conclusions that they come up with themselves than those provided by other people. You might ask your relative the following questions:

"What would you say to a friend who told you this?"
"Are there any other explanations for what happened?"
"Is there another way of looking at this?"

Encouraging your relative to consider more than one possible explanation helps increase the flexibility of his thinking—which, in turn, can *decrease* his conviction in specific delusional interpretations.

• *Conduct behavioral experiments.* Sometimes your relative may need more information about a particular belief to evaluate it, and the only way to get that information is by doing a real-life "experiment." *Behavioral experiments* involve actually doing something to get more information about the accuracy of a particular belief. Your relative must feel comfortable and safe to participate in a behavioral experiment, and you need to agree together on how the information gained may bear on the accuracy of the belief.

Hannah thought others could read her mind, and that made her very uncomfortable in public. After talking about some of these concerns with her adult children, they devised a behavioral experiment in which she would attempt to communicate to people through her thoughts. When she was in the waiting room to see her doctor, she would think the thought "Look at me, I have the head of a giraffe!" Hannah agreed that if she was able to communicate with people through her thoughts, most people would look at her to see her remarkable giraffe head. On the other hand, if people took no special notice of her, despite this thought, it probably meant she was not able to communicate with people through her thoughts. Hannah agreed to count the number of people in the waiting room who looked at her within a minute of thinking this thought. She agreed that if fewer than half the people in the room looked at her, it would mean her belief that others could read her thoughts was not supported by evidence. Hannah went along with the experiment and reported that about one-quarter of the people in the waiting room looked at her when she tried to communicate her thought about her giraffe head. Although she still thought it was possible that she could communicate her thoughts to others, she agreed that maybe she wasn't able to. Her children helped her come up with an alternative self-statement when she became concerned that others could read her thoughts: "I sometimes feel uncomfortable in social situations, but that doesn't mean people can read my thoughts or I can communicate my thoughts to them."

• *Work within (and not against) your relative's beliefs.* Sometimes the most important approach you can take to help your relative cope with persistent psychotic symptoms is to work *within* her belief system rather than against it. This tack is most important to take when the symptom interferes with something, but other efforts to bypass or reduce it have not been successful. Working within your relative's belief system involves acting, at least temporarily, as though her delusions might be true, and then seeing whether the obstacle posed by the beliefs can be resolved together.

Adam, age 40, had lived at home with his mother for 15 years. Adam had a long-standing delusion that he was married. This delusion usually had little impact on his behavior, however, although he sometimes talked about his wife. His mother, Carolyn, decided that after so many years of living together she wanted to move into her own apartment and therefore needed to find new housing for Adam. When Carolyn presented this plan to Adam, he objected to the idea of moving into another apartment alone, pointing out that he was married and he should really move in with his wife. No amount of talk-

ing about Carolyn's desire to have her own place, or the absence of Adam's wife in his life up to this point, was successful in changing Adam's refusal to consider moving into his own apartment.

To resolve this impasse, Carolyn suggested they try to find Adam's wife. Adam agreed with this idea. Because he didn't have a clear idea of where she lived, they met with a real estate broker to get some possible leads. The broker suggested some neighborhoods to check out, and Carolyn and Adam proceeded to drive around them to see if anything looked familiar to Adam. They spent one afternoon doing this, without luck, and agreed to try looking another afternoon, in a different neighborhood. After having similar luck on the second afternoon, Carolyn commented to Adam on the way home that they were having trouble finding his wife. She suggested that maybe it would make sense for them to look for an apartment for him in case they couldn't find his wife. Adam agreed, and they began to go apartment hunting the next day.

Putting Psychotic Symptoms in Perspective

Of all of the symptoms of schizophrenia, the psychotic ones are the most difficult to understand because they represent a break in the reality that most people share. Considering how illogical psychotic symptoms seem, it should be no surprise that logical efforts to persuade your relative of the errors in his thoughts or perceptions are not especially effective—and can be downright counterproductive. Accepting this fact is crucial to dealing effectively with your relative's symptoms and to reducing the distress and additional problems these symptoms may cause.

Fortunately, there are many more effective ways of dealing with these symptoms. A good place to start is by empathizing with how your relative feels as a result of psychotic symptoms; this response shows that you care about her feelings and want to help. Connecting with your relative in this way establishes the basis for working together to deal with the obstacles and distress imposed by the psychotic symptoms. In the long run, you'll be most effective if you focus your efforts on reducing the problems associated with your relative's psychotic symptoms, rather than trying to change the symptoms themselves. Even when people with schizophrenia have odd beliefs and unusual perceptual experiences, they are capable of adjusting well and enjoying their lives, including their relationships with family members.

Resources

Deegan, P. (no date). *Hearing voices that are distressing: Self-help resources and strategies (Parts I and II)*. Lawrence, MA: National Empowerment Center. Helpful guides to resources and strategies for dealing with auditory hallucinations, by someone with personal experience. Available at *www.power2u.org/articles/selfhelp*.

Fowler, D., Garety, P., & Kuipers, E. (1995). *Cognitive behaviour therapy for psychosis: Theory and practice*. Chichester, UK: Wiley. A readable book on how to understand psychotic symptoms, help someone cope with those symptoms, and explore alternative explanations to delusional beliefs.

Freeman, D., Freeman, J., & Garety, P. (2006). *Overcoming paranoid and suspicious thoughts: A self-help guide using cognitive behavioral techniques*. London: Constable and Robinson. This useful guide for coping with fears about others is written in a clear and accessible style by several leading international experts.

Hayes, S. C., Strosahl, K. D., & Wilson, K. G. (1999). *Acceptance and commitment therapy: An experiential approach to behavior change*. New York: Guilford Press. Describes how people can articulate their values and goals and gives strategies to prevent problematic thinking and feelings from interfering with one's life. Skim or skip Chapter 2, which provides theoretical and philosophical underpinnings of the approach.

Hearing Voices Network, located in Great Britain, provides support and understanding for people who hear voices. It develops and promotes self-help groups, organizes training sessions for mental health workers and the general public, provides a telephone helpline, and produces four newsletters a year. Their website is *www.hearing-voices.org*.

Kingdon, D. G., & Turkington, D. (2005). *Treatment manual for cognitive therapy of schizophrenia*. New York: Guilford Press. A very practical book on helping people with schizophrenia deal with psychotic symptoms; contains useful educational handouts and worksheets.

Morrison, A. P., Renton, J. C., Dunn, H., Williams, S., & Bentall, R. P. (2004). *Cognitive therapy for psychosis: A formulation-based approach*. New York: Brunner-Routledge. Describes how to understand the origins of psychotic symptoms and how to help people reduce their distress and improve their quality of life.

Tarrier, N. (1992). Management and modification of residual positive psychotic symptoms. In M. Birchwood & N. Tarrier (Eds.), *Innovations in the psychological management of schizophrenia* (pp. 147–169). Chichester, UK: Wiley. Provides a framework for systematically assessing and teaching coping strategies for dealing with psychotic symptoms.

Works Cited in This Chapter

Johns, L. C., Nazroo, J. Y., Bebbington, P., & Kuipers, E. (2002). Occurence of hallucinatory experiences in a community sample and ethnic variations. *British Journal of Psychiatry, 180*, 174–178.

Ohayon, M. M. (2000). Prevalence of hallucinations and their pathological associations in the general population. *Psychiatry Research, 97*, 153–164.

Persistent Psychotic Symptoms

Coping Assessment

Instructions: Complete a separate copy of this form for each psychotic symptom that you and your relative agree to work on. Record your answers in the second column.

1. Describe the symptom as specifically as possible.	1.
2. What is your relative's reaction to the symptom? What feelings does the symptom cause?	2.
3a. At what time of day does the symptom occur most often or is the most severe?	3a.
3b. At what time of day does the symptom occur least often or is the least severe?	3b.
4a. In what situations is the symptom most likely to occur or is the worst?	4a.
4b. In what situations is the symptom least likely to occur or is the least troubling?	4b.
5a. What strategies has your relative tried in the past to cope with the symptom?	5a.
5b. Which of these strategies have worked? Which have not?	5b.
6a. What strategies is your relative currently using to cope with the symptom?	6a.
6b. Which of these strategies are helpful? Which are not?	6b.
6c. How often are the helpful coping strategies used?	6c.
7. Are there any positive consequences of having the symptom, such as avoiding unpleasant tasks or situations?	7.
8. Are there any negative consequences, such as not being able to enjoy a movie?	8.

Coping Skill Rating Scale

Coping skill being practiced: _____

Date	Time	How helpful was the coping skill? 1 = not helpful 2 = somewhat helpful 3 = very helpful
		1 2 3
		1 2 3
		1 2 3
		1 2 3
		1 2 3
		1 2 3
		1 2 3

CHAPTER 18

━━━━━━━

Negative Symptoms

A s described in Chapter 2, negative symptoms such as apathy, social avoidance, and blunted affect (diminished emotional expressiveness) are the hallmark of schizophrenia. Because they tend to persist over time and often appear in mild form several years before the full syndrome of schizophrenia, you're probably very familiar with them. You may also be well aware of their impact on the quality of life for your relative, you, and your family. Learning how to cope more effectively with these symptoms can improve your family relationships and your relative's ability to achieve personal goals and enjoy life.

Evaluating Your Relative's Negative Symptoms

Negative symptoms are defined as the *absence* of doing, thinking, or feeling things that other people ordinarily do, think, and feel. Not laughing at something most people think is funny, not enjoying activities or relationships, and not having much to say in a conversation are examples.

There are many different ways of categorizing negative symptoms. One of the most widely used approaches was developed by Nancy Andreasen, MD, PhD, at the University of Iowa, who identified five types of negative symptoms: *blunted* or *flattened affect* (diminished facial or vocal expressiveness), *alogia* (diminished speech or thought), *apathy* (lack of motivation or interest), *anhedonia* (lack of pleasure), and *inattention* (difficulty paying attention). We discuss the first four types of negative symptoms in this chapter, and we address inattention (along with other common cognitive difficulties) in the next chapter. Use the Negative Symptoms Checklist (Worksheet 18.1 at the end of the chapter) to determine which negative symptoms your relative has.

Distinguishing Negative Symptoms from Other Problems

Although negative symptoms are a primary feature of schizophrenia, they can also be caused by other factors. Knowing what is behind these symptoms can help you and your relative resolve them to whatever extent is possible. Lack of enjoyment from activities (anhedonia), for example, can be part of depression. Social avoidance or lack of enjoyment can come from anxiety. The primary distinction between negative symptoms and depression or anxiety is your relative's mood: If your relative feels blue and talks about feeling down, depression may be a problem; if your relative reports feeling anxious, anxiety may be a problem.

Medication side effects can also sometimes be mistaken for negative symptoms. As discussed in Chapter 10, high levels of medication can cause drowsiness, lethargy, and low energy levels, making the person appear apathetic and uninterested. One common side effect of conventional antipsychotic medications is *akinesia*, or diminished expressiveness. Akinesia and blunted affect can be difficult to distinguish from one another without altering the person's dosage or type of medication. Fortunately, this side effect is much less common with the newer novel antipsychotic medications that are most often used. If you're concerned that your relative may be experiencing medication side effects, however, consult her doctor.

Psychotic symptoms can also contribute to negative symptoms. For example, if your relative avoids contact with others when hallucinations worsen, or if persistent delusions interfere with her ability to enjoy herself, these psychotic symptoms could cause negative symptoms such as social withdrawal and anhedonia. This does not mean negative symptoms are *necessarily* caused by psychotic symptoms, only that it's possible. It's also possible that both types of symptoms are independent or even that the negative symptoms are contributing to the psychotic symptoms. For example, if your relative avoids people and is engaged in few structured activities (negative symptoms), this lack of meaningful stimulation and opportunities for reality testing can increase her vulnerability to psychotic symptoms such as hallucinations and delusions.

If you think some of your relative's negative symptoms may be related to one of these factors, consider trying the strategies for reducing depression (Chapter 21), anxiety (Chapter 20), medication side effects (Chapter 10), or distress caused by psychotic symptoms (Chapter 17). If you think your relative's negative symptoms are primary, or if negative symptoms persist despite your attempts to address other underlying factors, applying strategies for coping with specific negative symptoms may help.

Coping with Specific Negative Symptoms

Many people with schizophrenia are aware of their negative symptoms, but they vary as to how bothersome they find them. In contrast, their relatives frequently are distressed by these symptoms, finding them a greater strain than psychotic symptoms. The best strategies for coping with negative symptoms are those that reduce your distress *and* help your relative compensate for, or overcome, the limitations imposed by his symptoms.

Blunted Affect (Diminished Emotional Expressiveness)

Most people with blunted affect are surprisingly unaware of their lack of emotional expressiveness, and it's generally not a source of significant distress for them. It can, however, lead to misunderstandings between your relative and others.

People with blunted affect often *experience* emotions just as strongly as other people, but they don't *convey* these feelings in their facial expressions or tone of voice. The fact that your relative may not appear interested when you're talking with him, or may not appear to enjoy watching a movie doesn't mean that he *isn't* actually interested in your conversation or enjoying the movie. Therefore, the best way to avoid misunderstandings is to get in the habit of checking with your relative about how she feels instead of assuming that you know her feelings without asking.

Alogia

Alogia means an inability to speak or think, but the most common problem associated with it is what is known as *poverty of speech* (not talking much). A less common problem is *poverty of speech content*–saying things that don't add up to much. If your relative says little, he is probably aware of it but not distressed by it. You, on the other hand, may have found it frustrating to communicate with someone who has so little to say.

The most important first step toward coping effectively with alogia is to remember that your relative is not choosing to speak so little, and that not saying much doesn't mean she doesn't like or care about you. Many people with schizophrenia have this problem, and it may be related to the cognitive impairments associated with the illness (see Chapter 19). They are not to blame for it and don't mean anything personal by the behavior.

Fortunately, there are ways of making conversations with your relative easier and more comfortable. One strategy is to make a special point of doing things together where the focus is not on talking. When you go shopping, to the movies, or on nature walks together, your relative can talk at a pace that is less taxing and permits many breaks. Not only is the overall experience more enjoyable for both of you, but you end up with topics for later conversation.

Apathy and Anhedonia

Most people who have *apathy* (lack of interest in pursuits such as school, work, or relationships) also have *anhedonia* (not enjoying things). Fortunately, the same coping strategies tend to be effective for both symptoms.

Of all the symptoms of schizophrenia, relatives often find apathy the most frustrating. We've heard many family members express the same sentiment as Bob's father: "I know Bob has schizophrenia and can't help that, but if only he could go to his program regularly or get a part-time job!" Many family members assume mistakenly that apathy is under their relative's control. Like hallucinations, delusions, or alogia, however, apathy is a symptom of schizophrenia and is not directly under your relative's control.

As with alogia, the first step toward coping effectively with apathy is acceptance. Realizing that apathy is part of your relative's illness will help you avoid blaming her for this symptom and may lead you to establish more realistic expectations. Family members who cope effectively with apathy often have developed a positive mental attitude reflected in positive self-statements that enable them to maintain a good relationship with their relative:

- "I know he's doing the best that he can."
- "I understand that her difficulty doing things and following through is a part of her illness."
- "He's not lazy; this is just a symptom of schizophrenia."
- "I can't change her behavior, but maybe I can help a little."

Accepting apathy as a part of your relative's illness doesn't mean there's nothing you can do to help. Consider exploring these strategies:

- *Include your relative in daily activities*. Left alone, people with apathy and anhedonia may just sit around the house doing nothing. By including your relative in activities with other family members, you can often engage her in conversation and sometimes stimulate her interest. These activities can include mundane tasks such as grocery shopping and going to the bank or dry cleaner as well as fun activities such as going out for pizza, to the museum, or to the movies.

When inviting your relative to join you, avoid placing expectations on his behavior. Simply invite him to come along and allow him to participate to the extent desired. With no demands on his behavior, he may become more willing to join you. People with schizophrenia often have trouble anticipating what it will be like to engage in a particular activity, so they have little interest and expect not to enjoy it. Getting your relative involved in actual activities circumvents his negative expectations and provides experiences that sometimes turn out to be more fun or interesting than he expected.

- *Regularly schedule enjoyable activities*. Because apathy and anhedonia often involve negative expectations about how enjoyable an activity will be, it's important to schedule specific recreational activities each week so that your relative can learn how to anticipate and enjoy activities such as going to the movies, going out to eat, bowling, visiting art galleries, and walking in the park. When people with schizophrenia get into the habit of participating in a recreational activity on a regular basis, their enjoyment of the activity gradually grows.

At first, you may need to do most of the work in selecting an activity you think your relative may enjoy. You may also need to convince her to participate. And, to repeat an important point, once your relative agrees to come along, remember to *place as few expectations on her behavior as possible*. After the activity is over, ask her what the experience was like for her. Don't expect her to report that she found the activity very enjoyable the first time; it may take several occasions before she really enjoys it. However, if you can stick with doing an activity together over a period of time, chances are good that your relative will begin to enjoy it and become able to anticipate these positive feelings. If one activity doesn't seem to work over a period of time, try another.

Selma was interested in practically nothing and reported being unable to enjoy anything. Her parents decided to try scheduling a regular activity with her to see whether they could decrease her apathy and anhedonia. After discussing it together, they agreed to eat dinner out once a week (they chose Wednesday night). Selma was not very interested in coming out to dinner with her parents, but with some encouragement she agreed. At first, they went to the same restaurant each week, so that Selma could become familiar with it. For the first 6 weeks, Selma ordered the same meal each week: a cheeseburger and fries. After the first time, she seemed to find the dinners a little more enjoyable. Gradually Selma began to try different selections from the menu. On Thursdays, Selma's mother would bring up the topic of the last meal they had eaten out, to get Selma's impressions; on Mondays or Tuesdays Selma's mother would talk about what she was thinking of eating. One week, after a few months of eating out, Selma indicated to her mother on Tuesday that she was thinking of trying a chicken dish. Selma had begun to look forward to their night out. Eventually, the family agreed to begin trying different restaurants on their night out to expand the range of their experience.

• *Identify former recreational activities.* At the core of apathy and anhedonia is the expectation that activities won't be enjoyable. Identifying potentially pleasurable activities might therefore be difficult, but you could explore what your relative used to enjoy doing. People sometimes give up hobbies, sports, or other interests because of the disruption caused by their schizophrenia (psychotic symptoms, hospitalizations, family conflicts), not from lack of enjoyment. Your relative may not have positive expectations for these activities because it's been so long since he tried them or because they remind him of the time before he became ill. By helping your relative identify these activities and form a plan to try them again, you can help him experience some unanticipated enjoyment. Bear in mind that your relative may need to become reacquainted with the activity over a period of time before he truly enjoys it again.

Pedro had been an avid sports enthusiast as a teenager and as a young adult before he developed schizophrenia. He had been an excellent baseball player, playing throughout high school and then in a local league after he graduated, and had frequently attended games and followed several sports on TV and in the papers. These interests seemed to fall by the wayside after he developed schizophrenia; he didn't even know how his favorite baseball team had done the previous year and showed no interest in anything. His wife, Marissa, and son, Jesus, remembered his love of sports and decided to see if this interest could be revived. After talking it over, Pedro agreed to try watching some baseball games on the TV with them. The first several times he couldn't watch the whole game, although he admitted enjoying some of it. Over time he became able to watch an entire game on TV, and he and his son went to a local minor league game. Later that year, Marissa gave him a subscription to a sports magazine, and he began reading occasional articles from the magazine.

• *Break down big goals into small steps.* Your relative may have vague ideas of how she would like things to be different, but not of how to achieve these changes. Apathy and anhedonia may result from this difficulty in pursuing goals that are meaningful to her. By talking about these goals with your relative, you can help her identify small steps that could be taken toward the goal, without pressuring her to take those steps. With each step she does take, you can praise her for the progress and remind her that the step contributes to her longer-term goal. Strategies for solving problems can be useful in helping your relative make progress toward goals (see Chapter 15).

• *Increase daily structure.* Just as increased structure can have beneficial effects on psychotic symptoms, it can be helpful for apathy and anhedonia—which can be a by-product of inactivity. Doing nothing can lead to caring about nothing, which can worsen the tendency to do nothing. This vicious circle can be broken by ensuring that your relative is engaged in at least some structured activities on a daily basis, such as part-time work, classes, a peer support center, or a volunteer job. Planning specific activities to do over the weekend can help to structure this time, such as taking a walk, going to the store, doing chores, or visiting a museum.

• *Focus on the future, not the past.* For some people with schizophrenia, apathy and anhedonia are caused by their own awareness of how they've changed. They may feel discouraged and demoralized and conclude that the effort is not worthwhile. Reminding your relative of how she used to be different can contribute to this feeling of being a "failure." Focusing instead on the future, helping your relative develop a personal vision of recovery (see Chapter 3), and identifying and pursuing recovery-oriented goals can prevent unnecessary and discouraging comparisons with the past and provide realistic hope for change and a good quality of life.

Facing the Challenge of Negative Symptoms

Many family members find that the negative symptoms of schizophrenia, such as apathy and anhedonia, are the most difficult ones to cope with because they *seem* to be under the individual's control, even though they are not. People with schizophrenia themselves often battle these symptoms, which can have a major impact on many different areas of their functioning: at work, in school, as a parent, and in personal relationships. Although coping with negative symptoms is a formidable challenge, you and your family's efforts, in collaboration with your relative, will be rewarded. The strategies described in this chapter, combined with other strategies described in Part VI of this book, provide a solid foundation for taking on the challenges of negative symptoms. Through teamwork and persistence you and your relative can overcome the effects of negative symptoms, and in so doing, improve the quality and enjoyment of his life.

Resources

Negative symptoms in schizophrenia (1995). Rochester, NY: Wheeler Communications Group. This film was created by Nancy Andreasen, MD, PhD, and her colleagues at the University of Iowa Hospitals and Clinics. It provides an explanation of the nature of negative symptoms in schizophrenia, their possible causes, and their management.

Mueser, K. T., Valentiner, D. P., & Agresta, J. (1997). Coping with negative symptoms of schizophrenia: Patient and family perspectives. *Schizophrenia Bulletin, 23,* 329–339. This article describes different coping strategies people with schizophrenia and their relatives use to deal with negative symptoms.

Negative Symptoms Checklist

Instructions: Place a checkmark next to each negative symptom that you have observed in your relative over the past month.

	Check below
Blunted Affect	
1. Diminished or absent facial expressiveness during interactions with others	
2. Unchanging, monotonous, or inexpressive voice tone when conversing	
3. Lack of gestures when conversing	
Alogia	
4. Little said during interactions	
5. What is said in conversation doesn't add up to much	
6. Stopping in the middle of a sentence and forgetting what was to be said	
Apathy	
7. Difficulty initiating or following through on activities	
8. Lack of interest in doing things	
9. Sitting around doing little or engaging in activities requiring little effort (such as watching TV)	
Anhedonia	
10. Lack of enjoyment from recreational activities	
11. Inability to feel close to others, such as friends or relatives	
12. Difficulty experiencing pleasure from anything	

CHAPTER 19

Cognitive Difficulties

Problems with thinking (*cognitive difficulties*) are a common feature of schizophrenia that can have a major impact on your relative's day-to-day functioning, such as in social relationships, the ability to work or go to school, and the ability to take care of himself. By understanding the nature of these cognitive difficulties, you can begin to pinpoint specific problems related to thinking skills, which can help you develop strategies to address those problem areas.

The Nature of Thinking Difficulties

Most people with schizophrenia experience some problems in cognitive functioning. Studies of people with schizophrenia have found that a decline in thinking skills occurs early in the illness and is related to social, educational, and employment difficulties. Cognitive difficulties are usually relatively stable over the course of schizophrenia, although some medications may improve thinking, and work is under way to develop rehabilitation programs for improving thinking skills.

Thinking difficulties take different forms in people with schizophrenia. Some of these difficulties may be readily apparent, such as having trouble paying attention or taking a long time to respond in conversation. Other problems may be less apparent at first, such as the ability to grasp a concept or to solve a problem. The areas of cognitive functioning in which they have the most strengths and weaknesses vary among individuals with schizophrenia.

What Is Thinking?

Thinking involves the ability to perceive and process information from the environment and to use that information to identify goals and make plans for achieving them. You'll have a better grasp of your relative's cognitive difficulties if you understand the different types of thinking skills, which can be broken down into five general categories: *attention and concentration, information processing speed, memory and learning, executive functions,* and *social cognition. Lack of insight* into having an illness, or any disability at all, is a sixth type of cognitive difficulty that is particularly important to schizophrenia. Chapter 24 provides strategies for dealing with insight problems in your relative.

Attention and Concentration

Attention is the ability to focus on something, such as looking up a number in a phone book without getting distracted by unrelated things, such as the sound of a truck passing on the street outside. *Concentration* is the ability to sustain attention long enough to complete some or all of a task. Problems with attention are at the core of many of the cognitive difficulties experienced by people with schizophrenia. Being unable to pay attention leads to problems in social situations (such as not tracking the conversation), task-oriented situations (such as work), and self-care situations (such as basic hygiene).

People with schizophrenia may have difficulties with attention and concentration for a number of reasons. Sometimes they are distracted by their symptoms, such as hallucinations or delusions. For example, auditory hallucinations are distracting because they draw the person's attention away from the external world and toward the voices. Similarly, a person can be preoccupied with a paranoid delusion that makes it difficult to focus on the real world around her. People with schizophrenia also experience heightened sensitivity to stimuli in general, such as sounds, which can make it difficult to stay focused on something. The sound of a radio or TV in the background could make it hard for your relative to focus on a conversation, a job task, or a basic self-care skill.

> *Ethan had serious problems with attention and concentration. Without his mother's supervision, his grooming and hygiene were spotty, leaving him looking quite disheveled. His hair might be uncombed or half combed, his shirt not be buttoned up correctly, or he might shave only half of his face. Ethan had a job stocking merchandise at a local warehouse, which his supported employment specialist had helped him get. He was able to work only short periods of time and often needed prompting to stay focused on his job. During conversations, Ethan frequently lost track of what the other person was saying and appeared "spacey." People often needed to repeat things to him so he could follow what was said. Ethan had few leisure or recreation activities. He sometimes watched TV, although even when doing this his attention would drift away from what was happening on the show.*

Information-Processing Speed

Information-processing speed is the speed with which a person can absorb and process (or understand) new information. One very common challenge for people with schizophrenia is that they process information at a slower speed than others. Thus they require longer periods to solve problems and complete tasks, which can lead to social difficulties. The person may be slower to respond to others, and it may appear that he is not involved and doesn't care about the other person, even when he does.

Gwendolyn, a 23-year-old woman with schizophrenia who is married and has two children, does not complete chores in a timely fashion, such as laundry or meal preparation, and her conversations with other people usually seem to lag. Her slower conversational pace feels awkward to people who don't know her, but her family members have come to accept it and are comfortable with it. Gwendolyn has a good sense of humor about it, and her relatives recognize that she's usually on track and accurate, even though it takes her a bit longer to react to things and get her point across.

Memory and Learning

In order to learn, we must have the capacity to remember information. People with schizophrenia often have difficulties with memory, which can make it harder for them to learn new things. It's not that they don't want to learn, but more time and effort are often required—which takes patience for everyone involved.

Problems with memory may be readily apparent. Your relative may forget appointments, people's names, or previous conversations. Difficulties with memory can also be disguised as other problems such as poor job performance, slow skill acquisition, or apparent lack of attention to simple requests made by others.

Problems with learning and memory are common in people with schizophrenia for many different reasons. At least part of the problem is related to poor attention and concentration: Learning new information and skills is difficult for someone who can't pay attention in the first place. Research on memory shows that people with schizophrenia have difficulties in both short-term (or *working*) memory and longer-term memory. Problems with long-term memory can also occur when the person does not view particular information and skills as personally relevant or important. Or the individual may be preoccupied with other concerns (e.g., delusions or hallucinations), making it harder to remember. Difficulty organizing information in a way that facilitates long-term retention is also typical. In a common memory test that requires people to learn 25 words, each word belonging to one of five categories (e.g., fruit, animals, furniture), those with schizophrenia tend to recall fewer words, in part, because they are less able to identify the different categories.

Ruth's memory problems are often apparent to her relatives and friends. Ruth's mother sometimes asks her to pick up something at the grocery store, and she forgets or picks up the wrong thing. Ruth's case manager often has to say things several times for Ruth to remember the points; he is sure that Ruth has remembered something only when she can repeat it back to him. Ruth's a job at a grocery store gives her difficulty because she has to retrieve items from storage, but forgets which items to get unless she writes them down. Similarly, she has trouble remembering the names of her coworkers. Ruth often forgets to take her medication, even though she understands its benefits. Ruth's mother constantly reminds her to take her medication.

Executive Functions

The term *executive functions* encompasses a broad range of complex cognitive skills that are critical to many aspects of daily living: the ability to plan, to solve problems, to grasp concepts, and to reason logically. These cognitive functions are considered "executive" because they require the organization of information that is critical to implementing plans and rely on the more basic cognitive functions of attention and concentration, information processing speed, and learning and memory. Like an executive in a company who relies on her employees but must nevertheless make management decisions that influence the whole company, executive cognitive functions are responsible for decision making while also relying on the work of more basic cognitive skills.

Problems in executive functions can lead to a variety of different life challenges. Poor planning ability can lead to problems with money management, a failure to anticipate the consequences of certain actions (such as using drugs or alcohol), and an inability to identify and take steps toward personal goals. The inability to plan ahead can also interfere with problem solving (see Chapter 15). Difficulties in executive functions make it harder to grasp concepts. For example, an individual with limited executive functions may have more difficulty grasping the expression "the customer is always right" and using it appropriately at work. Difficulties with abstract thinking can make it harder to succeed in some school-related subjects, especially mathematics and science. Difficulty grasping concepts may also make your relative unaware of his problems or of having the illness of schizophrenia, a subject taken up in detail in Chapter 24.

Social Cognition

Social cognition (also called *social intelligence*) refers to the cognitive processes involved in effective social behavior, such as the ability to "read" someone else's feelings through facial expression and voice tone, to perceive another person's intentions or perspective, to "take a hint" during an interaction, and to understand common social rules (such as not trying to start a conversation with someone who is busy doing something else). Social cognition skills depend on all the other cognitive skills described above and are critical to successful social experiences. Because people with schizophrenia often have limited social cognition skills, social problems are not uncommon.

Dominick is a young man with schizophrenia who lives with his father and two sisters. When he talks with his family members and friends, he is prone to misunderstanding their feelings about him and often thinks that they're angry with him when they're not. Family members have learned that Dominick isn't always quick to pick up on hints, such as that his sister's telling him he smelled meant he needed to use deodorant. People who are close to Dominick have learned to compensate for some of his difficulties in understanding social situations. However, these problems often produce socially awkward moments with people whom Dominick does not know well, because he is not always aware of common social conventions. For example, when meeting a new person, Dominick sometimes gives very personal information about himself, such as detailed descriptions of digestion problems, which can make the other person feel uncomfortable and reluctant to continue the conversation.

Worksheet 19.1 at the end of the chapter includes a checklist of cognitive difficulties commonly experienced by people with schizophrenia. Complete this checklist to identify the areas of cognitive functioning that may pose coping challenges for your relative. We explore strategies for coping with these challenges in each domain later in this chapter.

Factors That Can Contribute to Cognitive Impairment

Difficulties in cognitive functioning are a cardinal feature of schizophrenia, and the factors identified in the stress–vulnerability model can influence cognitive functioning—which means that reducing factors related to stress and vulnerability may improve your relative's thinking skills. Specifically, medication, alcohol and drug use, and stress can all impede cognitive functioning, and the possible effects of each should be given serious consideration.

Medication Effects

Antipsychotic medications can have both positive and negative effects on cognitive functioning in people with schizophrenia. One common side effect is sedation, which can slow the speed at which your relative understands and responds to information. At the same time, antipsychotics are effective at reducing distractions due to psychotic symptoms and may modestly improve attention, concentration, and the more complex cognitive skills such as learning, memory, and executive functions.

Some research evidence suggests that novel antipsychotics have more beneficial effects on cognitive functioning than conventional antipsychotics. One reason for this difference may be that conventional antipsychotics often produce uncomfortable *parkinsonian* side effects (such as tremors and restlessness) that are frequently treated with *anticholinergic* medications (such as Cogentin), which may interfere with memory. Novel antipsychotics are much less likely to produce parkinsonian side effects and are therefore less likely to require anticholinergic medications.

Substance Use

The use of substances such as alcohol, marijuana, and cocaine can have a prominent effect on cognitive functioning in anyone, but as discussed in Chapter 22, people with schizophrenia have an increased sensitivity to the effects of drugs and alcohol, which can include more thinking problems. Different types of commonly abused substances have a variety of effects on cognitive functioning, as summarized in the following table. In addition to the direct effects of substances on cognitive functioning, having an addiction leads to a preoccupation with obtaining more of the substance, and this preoccupation can distract the person from paying attention to work, going to school, or taking care of herself. Similarly, people with addictions typically crave substances, which can make it more difficult to focus on accomplishing necessary functional tasks. In addition, people may

Cognitive Effects of Commonly Abused Substances	
Substance	Cognitive effects
Alcohol	• Slowed reaction times • Drowsiness • Difficulty concentrating • Acting impulsively (not thinking ahead) • Memory difficulties
Cannabis (such as marijuana, hashish)	• Drowsiness
Stimulants (such as cocaine and amphetamines)	• Hyperalertness • Increased distractibility • Difficulty planning ahead
Sedatives (such as benzodiazepines)	• Sedation • Slowed reaction times • Problems with attention and concentration
Hallucinogens (such as LSD, PCP)	• Distortion in perceptions • Increased distractibility • Memory problems
Narcotics (such as heroin or prescription painkillers such as Vicodin and Demerol)	• Sedation • Decreased ability to concentrate • Slowed reaction times • Difficulty planning ahead

develop depression, anxiety, and irritability because their lives are out of control due to their substance use, and they feel at a loss as to how to make any changes.

Stress

As Chapter 11 explained, managing stress in people with schizophrenia is critical to preventing relapse. But stress also can amplify cognitive disorganization, making your relative less able to concentrate, remember things, and solve problems. If subtle worsening of cognitive functioning begins to show up as problems at work, in self-care, or in conversing, your relative may be suffering from stress that threatens to precipitate a relapse and you should take steps together to identify and deal with possible stresses and impending relapse (see Chapters 11 and 12).

Strategies for Coping with Cognitive Difficulties

A variety of strategies can minimize the impact of cognitive impairments on your relative's day-to-day functioning. In some cases, coping strategies can actually improve thinking skills. In other cases, coping strategies may reduce distress and interference caused by the cognitive problem. As with coping strategies for other symptoms and problems, most people find it useful to develop and practice several different coping strategies for a particular problem.

Attention and Concentration Problems

Having a short attention span and difficulty concentrating can interfere with your relative's ability to perform job-related tasks, take classes, or hold conversations with others. Several strategies may be helpful in minimizing the effects of limited attention on daily functioning.

• *Schedule regular rest breaks.* Tasks that require focused attention for extended periods of time can be taxing for people with schizophrenia. When a person loses his concentration, time is required to refocus attention and reorient to the task at hand—which can be frustrating. Scheduling regular rest breaks is a practical way of avoiding or minimizing this problem.

Everyone needs to take a break when concentrating on something for a long time. People with schizophrenia benefit from more frequent breaks, and scheduling such breaks gives them greater control over their ability to concentrate when needed. The frequency and duration of the breaks need to be determined individually, because some people benefit from breaks every 10 or 15 minutes whereas others may be able to go as long as half an hour or an hour. Rest breaks can last from a couple of minutes to 10–15 minutes, depending on how long the person has been concentrating.

Your relative can do whatever she pleases during the break. Often people find it helpful to leave the work area. Some people like to practice relaxation exercises, whereas others may prefer a brief walk or munching on a piece of fruit. Scheduled rests can facilitate work and school performance and make accomplishing these critical tasks easier and more enjoyable.

• *Remove distractions.* Your relative may be sensitive to distractions in his environment, which can draw his attention away from doing tasks. Removing these distractions or minimizing them makes it easier for your relative to focus. Common distractions include noise (people talking in the background, TV) and activity (people entering and leaving the room). Sit down and talk with your relative about how to minimize distractions. Aside from removing distractions or finding a more peaceful work area, your relative may be able to use ear plugs to dampen the distracting effects of any remaining (and unavoidable) noises.

• *Shape attention span.* You can work with your relative to gradually increase the duration of her focused attention. First, you and your relative need to determine how long she can focus at a time, and then schedule regular breaks. Then, when a comfortable schedule of work and breaks has been established, start gradually increasing the duration of work periods. Don't try to increase the duration of attention too quickly or you may overtax your relative's attention span and discourage her. Each time you increase the length of time for paying attention you should maintain the schedule of work and breaks for anywhere from several days or weeks, depending on what feels comfortable and manageable to your relative. The same approach to shaping attention can also be used to help your relative learn how to decrease sensitivity to distractions. In this case, you and your relative need to work together to identify ways of focusing on a task in the absence of distractions and then to gradually reintroduce those distractions so that your relative can practice remaining focused.

Charlene, 35, has schizoaffective disorder and lives with her partner, Monica, and her two children, ages 5 and 7. One of Charlene's household responsibilities is to cook dinner for the family. Monica works a regular job during the day, so she is usually not around to help Charlene with the cooking. Although Charlene is a very good cook, she had trouble focusing on the tasks involved in preparing meals and often got distracted, resulting in problems such as an unset table, burned food, or unprepared courses. Monica and Charlene decided to work together to see whether they could help Charlene improve her ability to focus on preparing dinner each night.

To begin, Charlene and Monica agreed it would be helpful for Monica to observe what happened when Charlene worked on preparing a meal so that they could better understand where her problems lie. Charlene prepared dinner Saturday night while Monica sat in the corner of the kitchen and took notes. After dinner had been prepared and the children put to bed, they sat down to talk about Monica's observations. Monica started by praising the meal that Charlene had made. She then said she had observed that Charlene had difficulty paying attention to preparing the meal for more than 10 minutes at a time and sometimes was distracted after even briefer periods of time. Charlene had a portable TV in the kitchen and was often distracted by it. Her children also frequently called her out of the kitchen. When Charlene became distracted, it took her several minutes to remember where she was in preparing the meal, and sometimes she would start to do tasks over again.

After talking over these observations, Charlene and Monica decided on three changes. First, to decrease the distracting effects of the TV in the kitchen, Charlene agreed to leave it off. Second, Monica and Charlene decided to prohibit the children from watching TV during the afternoon (they usually watched TV all afternoon and were bored by it by dinnertime, which is why they often interrupted Charlene) but to allow them to watch a special show while Charlene prepared dinner. Third, Charlene and Monica decided it would be helpful to schedule breaks during meal preparation. They agreed that 10 minutes was a good period of time for Charlene to work before taking a break. Using a timer, Charlene would take a 5-minute break after the timer went off and return to preparing the meal for another 10 minutes. Fourth, to help Charlene remain organized in preparing the meal, she and Monica came up with a list of the different steps involved, and at each break time Charlene would note where she stopped so that it would be easier to resume her task after the break.

Charlene and Monica put this plan into effect and agreed to talk over how it was going the following week. The next week Charlene reported that taking the scheduled breaks had worked very well and that she didn't feel as stressed as she used to about preparing dinner every night. Charlene also indicated that she thought she could focus her attention longer, so they agreed to increase her time periods for preparing meals to 15 minutes before taking a break. Charlene and Monica continued checking in every week about the plan, troubleshooting minor problems that came up, and exploring whether to increase the length of time that Charlene spent preparing dinner before taking breaks. After several months, Charlene was able to focus on meal preparation for 30 minutes at a time before taking a scheduled break.

- *Play computer games.* Your relative may enjoy playing computer games, which can also be a way of increasing his attention span. Going to a store and selecting a computer game together or finding a game you can play online is a good way to explore this option. As with shaping attention span, your relative may find it helpful to play the computer game for brief periods of time, taking breaks before returning to the game and gradually increasing his attention to focus on it.

Slowed Information-Processing Speed

Slowed information-processing speed can increase the time required to complete tasks, making it harder to get things done on time. In general, slowed information-processing speed is one of the more stubborn difficulties experienced by some people with schizophrenia. Nevertheless, there are strategies you and your relative can use to minimize the effects of this problem.

- *Don't rush it.* Despite a slowed processing speed, your relative may be very articulate in what he says and very competent in the tasks he performs. Rushing your relative by finishing sentences or cajoling him to finish his bathroom routine in the morning more quickly can make him feel more uncomfortable and self-conscious about this limitation. Give your relative the time he needs and show that you're comfortable and confident in him and that you accept his way of doing things. This attitude can ease tension and make you more comfortable with each other.

- *Allow time to complete tasks.* If your relative wants to work or is working, it's important that she have the flexibility and time to complete tasks at a comfortable pace. For example, being a cashier may not be a good job for someone with slow information-processing speed, whereas working as a grocery stocker might be a better job because the same time pressure usually does not apply.

- *Overpractice.* *Overpractice* means practicing a task again and again to the point where it becomes automatic. If it's important to be able to complete certain tasks more quickly, either at home or at work, your relative can improve the speed at which she completes these tasks by practicing them extensively. It may take a great deal of practice, but once your relative has gotten good at particular task, she can often do it without even thinking about it.

Rubin, a 52-year-old man with schizophrenia, and his sons Edward (17) and Dwight (25), moved to a new apartment in a large city. Their apartment door had three locks on it, and it took Rubin about 10 minutes to open the door each time he came home. He found this frustrating, so Dwight decided to work with his father to help him get into his apartment more quickly. First, Dwight and Rubin clearly labeled all three keys and locks with numbers so that it would be easy for Rubin to know which key unlocked which lock. Second, they reviewed how each lock worked (two required a single turn, one required two turns). Third, with Dwight's encouragement, Rubin practiced locking and unlocking the door. The first time, he practiced unlocking the door three times in a row; the average time it took him to unlock the door was 3½ minutes. Rubin took a rest. Then Rubin agreed to try unlocking the doors five times in a row. This time he was able to unlock the doors in an average of 2 minutes and 15 seconds. The next day Rubin practiced five more times in a row and got even faster: an average of only 1 minute and 50 seconds to unlock the door. After one more practice session, Rubin required only 1 minute and 30 seconds to unlock the door—which pleased him rather than frustrated him.

Learning and Memory

Problems related to memory difficulties can be minimized by developing compensatory strategies. The same strategies for dealing with memory limitations in people who don't have schizophrenia are also useful for those who do.

- *Use memory aids.* The easiest way to compensate for memory limitations is to use memory aids, such as keeping a calendar, writing lists of things to do, and always having a paper and pencil handy to jot notes. Keeping a calendar is a good organizational strategy for remembering appointments. Teaching your relative how to maintain a calendar can help him avoid missed appointments and other important events. Using a pocket calendar is especially helpful, because your relative can carry this wherever he goes. Some people also like to keep a yearly calendar hanging on the wall near the telephone, because many appointments are made on the phone.

Keeping lists of things to do can minimize the chance of forgetting to do something important and ensure that items are not forgotten when the person goes shopping. There are many different strategies for keeping lists. We suggest using a master "to do" list that includes all the things your relative wants to remember to do. Then, based on this list, she can construct daily or weekly "to do" lists that include the things that need the most immediate attention. Another approach is to keep a small notebook in her pocket or purse that contains daily "to do" lists. Any uncompleted task can be carried over to the next day's "to do" list. When your relative is learning a new routine or skill, writing down the steps and posting them in a prominent place (such as the refrigerator) can make it easier for her to acquire the skill.

- *Develop a daily routine.* Developing a daily routine allows habits to be formed that make it easier to attend to basic tasks without having to think of each one. Getting up at a regular time, eating breakfast at a regular time, tending to daily hygiene needs, taking medication, and going to work, school, a rehabilitation program, or some other activity can become part of a routine. Other activities of daily living can also be built into the routine. Helping your relative find a standard place to put keys, wallet (purse), glasses, and other personal items may make it easier for him to find these items when needed and minimize stress and time spent looking for them. Creating an orderly living environment— for example, learning to put soiled laundry in a particular place—can also minimize the effects of memory limitations and disorganization for people with (and without!) schizophrenia.

- *Practice, practice, practice!* Similar to improving information-processing speed, one of the most effective ways of overcoming memory limitations is to practice new skills and retrieve new information to the point of overlearning them (i.e., they become automatic).

- *Use memory-sharpening strategies.* Numerous self-help books have been written for people who want to improve their memory. These books describe practical strategies that people can use to enhance memory. For example, most forgetting occurs within just a few seconds of learning new information; if we aren't paying attention, the information never enters our short-term memory and is therefore not available for long-term storage. Teaching your relative to repeat critical information to herself as soon as she learns it can ensure that the information goes into short-term memory—which, in turn, increases the chances that it will be retained over the long term. So repeating someone's name to herself right after she has met that person can increase the chances that she will remember the person's name later.

Executive Functions

By working with your relative, you can minimize the effects of his planning and problem-solving limitations on his daily functioning.

- *Schedule problem-solving meetings*. Meeting regularly with your relative to identify and take steps toward achieving goals and to brainstorm solutions for problems she is experiencing can be an effective way to compensate for limitations in executive functioning. By talking with your relative about goals, planning together how to achieve them, monitoring progress, and troubleshooting as necessary, you and your relative can overcome difficulties she may have in planning ahead. These meetings can also be useful times to identify problems that need to be addressed. Many families find that meeting on a weekly basis prevents problems from accumulating.

- *Avoid the use of metaphors*. People with limited executive functions often have difficulty grasping the meaning of metaphors. For example, your relative might understand the saying "The apple doesn't fall far from the tree" in a literal way. Such language can be confusing and is best avoided if your relative has difficulties in this area.

- *Match daily tasks to your relative's cognitive skills*. Difficulties planning ahead and solving new problems are most troublesome if your relative is working or involved in other daily activities that frequently involve new and challenging problems. One approach is to help your relative find work or other daily activities that are appropriately matched to his ability to plan and solve problems. For example, Duana's schizophrenia made it hard for her to plan meals and cook for the family, so she and her husband, Geoff, agreed that he would do the cooking and Duana would set the table and do the dishes.

Social Cognition

A variety of different strategies can be helpful in minimizing or compensating for your relative's problems in social cognition (such as difficulty recognizing others' emotions accurately). In general, these strategies involve either helping your relative develop better social cognition skills or improving how you communicate with your relative.

• *Practice recognizing facial expressions*. A useful strategy for helping your relative improve her skills in recognizing facial expressions is simply to practice with her. There are a variety of ways to do this. You can go through magazines and cut out pictures of people with different facial expressions, or go through them together without cutting out the pictures, and ask your relative to identify the different expressions. Sometimes it may be helpful to focus just on people's facial expressions. At other times it may be helpful to talk about the situation or context as well as the facial expressions, since the situation can provide important cues as to what each person is feeling. If your relative names an inaccurate or unlikely emotion, you could provide your perspective and explain why you think the person might be experiencing a different emotion. Your relative may need to practice once or twice a week for several months.

Another strategy for helping your relative hone his emotion recognition skills is to watch TV or movies together and to talk about the different emotions characters are portraying. Soap operas are particularly useful for this strategy because the emotions displayed by characters are dramatic and the storylines can be engaging. Try watching TV with the sound turned down and discuss what each of the different characters appears to be feeling and why. If you're watching a videotape or DVD of a movie or TV show, you can then replay it, this time with the sound on, and discuss what you saw.

Yet another way to practice identifying different emotions is to play "Name That Emotion," with your relative alone or with other family members too. Write down the names of a number of different emotions—*anger, fear, joy, pleasure, disgust, surprise, annoyance,* and *sadness*—on pieces of paper and put them in a hat, shake the hat, and take turns pulling out a piece of paper from the hat. The person who is "it" then tries to communicate that emotion to the other person *without using words* (only facial expressions and gestures). The other person (or people) tries to guess the emotion. After demonstrating each emotion, talk about it and discuss how different emotions are expressed with different facial expressions. This exercise can help your relative practice recognizing emotions as well as communicating specific emotions with her facial expressions and gestures.

• *Use explicit feeling statements*. You can also make communication easier with your relative by not assuming that he knows how you feel. Instead, use clear "feeling statements" such as "I'm upset because you didn't do the dishes," "I was worried when you didn't call," "I'm proud that you got a job," or "I'm happy to see you." Avoid giving hints, which require the other person to infer what you want. Being direct can avoid the problems that often occur when your relative has trouble picking up on a hint. Rather than saying "There sure are a lot of dirty dishes," try saying "I could use some help with the dishes. Do you mind pitching in?"

• *Discuss social norms with your relative*. Your relative may find it helpful to discuss the social norms of situations she encounters. For example, if she wants to get to know some of the other people at a local YWCA where she exercises, discussing possible topics of conversations with her and how much to reveal about herself may be helpful. If your relative is starting a new job, talk about how to respond to instructions, feedback, or criticism from the boss. When discussing social norms, you can matter-of-factly tell your relative about important unwritten social rules, such as not talking about very personal matters to people you don't know well or not asking coworkers at a new job out on a date. You can also elicit your relative's understanding of those situations, her thoughts about what those unwritten rules might be, and provide your perspective as needed. Discussing social norms can help your relative avoid the embarrassment caused by violation of these norms and feel more comfortable in new social situations.

Cognitive Rehabilitation

Over the past 20 years numerous advances have been made in the *cognitive rehabilitation* (or *cognitive remediation*) of those with brain injury. Rather than accepting brain injuries as permanent and unchangeable, these approaches aim at restoring lost cognitive functioning through the systematic use of cognitive training procedures. In more recent years, these advances have been adapted and applied to improving the cognitive skills of people with schizophrenia.

Cognitive rehabilitation programs for schizophrenia typically involve a combination of different activities designed to improve cognitive functioning. Computer-based training programs have been developed to help people sharpen their attention and concentration, information-processing speed, memory, and problem-solving skills. These programs usually provide (1) practice on a combination of tasks with gradually increasing levels of difficulty, (2) games designed to improve thinking skills in entertaining ways, and (3) assignments to use newly developed cognitive skills in regular daily life. Group meetings designed to improve social cognition skills (such as recognizing others' emotions, solving interpersonal problems, trying to understand others' intentions) through practice, discussion, and home assignments may also be included. In addition, individual sessions may be used to help people develop personalized strategies for overcoming or compensating for the effects of cognitive limitations on functioning, such as at work.

Research on the effects of cognitive rehabilitation programs indicates that they can help people with schizophrenia make modest improvements in their cognitive functioning. There is some evidence that, combined with other rehabilitation approaches such as social skills training (see Chapter 25) and supported employment (see Chapter 26), cognitive rehabilitation can help improve other areas of functioning such as social relationships and work. While much research still needs to be done, the results thus far are promising and it is likely the field will continue to see advances in this important area. Cognitive rehabilitation programs for schizophrenia are not widely available in the United States, but they are increasing in their availability. There may be such a program at your local community mental health center or somewhere in your community.

Coping Effectively with Cognitive Problems

Difficulties in thinking are common in schizophrenia and affect all aspects of functioning, including living independently, performing at work or school, and social relationships. Although cognitive difficulties tend to be relatively stable over time, by working together you can help your relative develop effective coping strategies. The key to coping successfully lies in focusing your efforts as specifically as possible: Pinpoint the areas of functioning that are problematic for your relative (such as accomplishing specific self-care tasks, work or school assignments, or parenting tasks). Explore how cognitive difficulties contribute to these problems. Develop strategies that are specifically tailored to address these problems. Don't feel daunted by this task; sometimes even very simple solutions for cognitive difficulties can profoundly improve functioning!

Resources

Lorayne, H., & Lucas, J. (1974). *The memory book: The classic guide to improving your memory at work, at school, and at play.* New York: Ballantine Books. Excellent, practical guide for improving memory that has been used successfully for many years.

Medalia, A., & Revheim, N. (2002). *Cognitive dysfunction associated with psychiatric disabilities: A handbook for families and friends of individuals with psychiatric disorders*. New York State Office of Mental Health, 44 Holland Avenue, Albany, NY 12229. Available at the New York State Office of Mental Health website: *www.omh.state.ny.us.* This is a useful booklet that describes the nature of cognitive difficulties experienced by people with mental illness and strategies families can use to help their loved ones manage these problems.

Small, G. (2002). *The memory bible: An innovative strategy for keeping your brain young.* New York: Hyperion.

Note. See the Resources section of Chapter 15 for recommended books on improving problem-solving skills.

Instructions: Check boxes below that apply to your relative's behavior

Attention and Concentration	No	Somewhat/ sometimes	Yes
Loses track of the conversation or gets off topic easily			
Does not complete, or requires frequent prompting to complete, basic self-care skills (grooming, hygiene)			
Does not pay attention when given instructions			
Performs poorly at school or work because of not completing tasks			
Complains frequently about being distracted			
Unable to read anything more than one or two paragraphs long			
Has difficulty watching a TV program or a movie			
Has difficulty doing basic housework or homemaking tasks such as cooking, laundry, washing dishes, etc.			
Information–Processing Speed	**No**	**Somewhat/ sometimes**	**Yes**
Shows delayed responding during conversations with others			
Speaks more slowly than other people			
Requires a long time to complete self-care tasks despite focused attention on them			
Requires longer time to complete work or school tasks			
Needs other people to talk more slowly to understand what they're saying			
Memory and Learning	**No**	**Somewhat/ sometimes**	**Yes**
Forgets to take medication			
Forgets appointments (e.g., with doctors, case manager, therapist, family, friends)			

Memory and Learning	No	Somewhat/ sometimes	Yes
Does not attend to basic self-care skills, such as dental hygiene, bathing, and use of deodorant, despite stated intentions			
Forgets simple things such as people's names, conversational topics, and agreements reached with other people			
Performs poorly at work or school on tasks that require remembering things (or extensive studying or practice to learn relevant information)			
Has difficulty remembering leisure and recreational activities			
Does not remember basic information, such as about his/her psychiatric illness and its treatment			
Executive Functioning	**No**	**Somewhat/ sometimes**	**Yes**
Has difficulty managing money (e.g., runs out of money before the end of the month)			
Has problems resolving conflicts with others			
Engages in impulsive behavior without apparent regard to its consequences			
Has problems formulating goals and making plans to achieve them			
Requires frequent assistance to handle new job responsibilities			
Has trouble thinking creatively when established solutions don't seem to work			
Has difficulty understanding abstract concepts			
Social Cognition	**No**	**Somewhat/ sometimes**	**Yes**
Has difficulty perceiving others' emotions from facial expressions and voice tone			
Lacks empathy and understanding of how others feel			
Has trouble picking up on hints from others			
Behaves inappropriately or says awkward things because of poor understanding of social norms			

CHAPTER 20

Anxiety

Estimates vary as to how common anxiety problems are among people with schizophrenia. It's safe to assume, however, that most people experience at least some difficulties with anxiety during their lives, and for some individuals, anxiety is debilitating and interferes with daily functioning and quality of life. It's also common for relatives of people with schizophrenia to have anxiety related to their loved one.

On the positive side, there are many ways you can help your relative cope with and overcome anxiety. There are also effective strategies that can help you prevent anxiety from harming your own well-being and your relationship with your relative.

Understanding Anxiety in Schizophrenia

For some individuals, increases in anxiety are an *early warning sign of a relapse*. In these cases, anxiety may be a temporary problem that, if responded to quickly, can be reduced or eliminated (e.g., by increasing medication dosage; see Chapter 12). *Psychotic symptoms* such as auditory hallucinations can also cause anxiety, particularly when the person hears voices that are insulting, predict terrible occurrences (such as the impending end of the world), or order the person to hurt himself or others (*command hallucinations*). Command hallucinations are often unpredictable and may intensify if the person tries to combat them. People who experience command hallucinations often feel in a terrible bind: They feel anxious about the consequences of either ignoring these voices or complying with them. Delusions can be equally anxiety provoking. Imagine how you would feel if you thought someone was trying to hurt you or others could read your mind.

Your relative could also feel anxious because she is haunted by *unpleasant memories* related to becoming psychotic and receiving treatment. The memories can create a sense of vulnerability in your relative, especially if your relative has recently developed schizophrenia; she may fear that these events will recur. This fear can lead your relative to avoid situations associated with those memories or to be unwilling to make any changes in her life (thus becoming immobilized). The anxiety may even prompt your relative to deny that she has an illness or any problems and to refuse to participate in treatment.

After experiencing some bouts with depression and then a decline in functioning, Abdul began to develop psychotic symptoms, including the belief that he was a special messenger from Allah who had been sent to reunite the world in peace. Abdul believed that, because of this special relationship, he would be protected by Allah no matter what he did. In the midst of an argument with a friend about this point, he sought to prove it by driving his car off the side of an elevated highway. Fortunately, the car landed in the top of a large tree, and they were not injured. When the police and ambulance came, they recognized that Abdul had a mental illness and took him, against his will, to the local psychiatric hospital. There he was given medications—also against his will—and on several occasions he was restrained or secluded when he became disruptive. While Abdul was in the hospital, he was afraid to come into contact with other people with psychotic symptoms. One person threatened him, saying "If you don't stay out of my mind, I'll show you a thing or two."

With medication, Abdul's psychotic symptoms subsided, and he was discharged from the hospital. In the weeks and months after he returned home he became increasingly anxious when he thought back on his experience. He was mortified to think that he had almost killed himself and his friend in his psychotic state, and he had unpleasant and intrusive memories of being held down and forced to take medication. When he looked back, he also remembered his contacts with other patients on the ward as being very scary, and he wondered if everyone now thought he was "mental." He didn't think he was "mental," and he attributed his psychotic episode to smoking pot. He often refused to take his medication and attend aftercare appointments at the clinic, which led to frequent arguments with his family.

Another source of anxiety for your relative may be *uncertainty about the future.* By its very nature, schizophrenia sometimes involves episodes in which the person loses control over his thinking and feeling and even his future. Before a person with schizophrenia has learned how to manage his illness, he is likely to experience unpredictable relapses and hospitalizations as well as difficulties working and taking care of himself, leaving him dependent on others. This dependence contributes to anxiety, especially if the person lives with his parents, who will not be able to provide care indefinitely.

Your relative may have anxiety problems for reasons unrelated to schizophrenia. Four fairly common anxiety problems in people with schizophrenia are *social anxiety* (fear in social situations), *posttraumatic stress disorder* (PTSD; anxiety due to recurrent memories of past upsetting events), *obsessive–compulsive disorder* (OCD; anxiety around mental obsessions and/or repeated "checking" behaviors or other "safety" behaviors such as handwashing or hoarding), and *panic disorder* (panic attacks that can lead to avoiding situations). Each of these disorders is more common in people with schizophrenia than in the general public.

Helping your relative manage anxiety effectively can have many benefits, the most obvious of which is reducing distress. Another benefit is acquiring the ability to deal with potentially anxiety-provoking situations, rather than avoiding them, which may be important in achieving long-term goals (such as in work or in closer personal relationships). A final benefit of less anxiety is an improved relationship with your relative because anxiety often makes people difficult to get along with and irritable.

Symptoms of Anxiety

Mild levels of anxiety are associated with thoughts of worry or concern, whereas with more severe anxiety the predominant state is one of fear or terror. Avoidance of anxiety-provoking situations is a common response that can be so great that your relative is afraid to do almost anything. Anxiety is also usually accompanied by increased physiological arousal, such as greater perspiration, shortness of breath, heart palpitations, muscular tension, trembling, and agitation.

Assessing Anxiety in Your Relative

If you have observed signs of anxiety in your relative but are unsure of his feelings, talking with him openly can be helpful. It's easy to mistake behaviors such as social avoidance or agitation for anxiety when other possible explanations exist, such as an increase in psychotic symptoms. When talking, it may be helpful to use a number of different words to refer to anxiety, such as *scared*, *afraid*, *uneasy*, *worried*, or *concerned*. The Symptoms of Anxiety Checklist (Worksheet 20.1) at the end of the chapter may be helpful to complete with your relative.

Once you know your relative has problems with anxiety, you can gather more information about her fears. When talking with your relative, be empathic, avoid saying that the fear or concern is not valid, and try to get specific information about what your relative is afraid of. Talking about your relative's concerns will help you understand the circumstances under which your relative feels anxious—and why.

Helping Your Relative Cope with Anxiety

First, you need to evaluate whether your relative's anxiety is an early warning sign of relapse. If not, you need to develop specific methods for helping your relative deal with his fear. These methods depend on what your relative is afraid of and how the fear affects his behavior and functioning. Following are strategies for handling anxiety that arises from four common sources in people with schizophrenia: psychotic symptoms, specific situations, memories of past psychotic episodes and negative treatment experiences, and the future. We also briefly discuss three common anxiety problems in the general population as well as in people with schizophrenia: social anxiety, PTSD, and OCD.

Anxiety as an Early Warning Sign of Relapse

Each person with schizophrenia has a unique pattern of early warning signs of relapse that typically involves a combination of changes in mood, thinking, and behavior. Increased anxiety is a common early warning sign that is often accompanied by depression, difficulty sleeping, and social avoidance. The two most important clues to whether your relative's anxiety is an early warning sign of relapse are whether it developed or worsened over a relatively brief period of time (such as several days or weeks) and whether past relapses have been preceded by similar bouts of anxiety. If you think your relative's anxiety may be a sign of relapse, follow the relapse prevention plan developed by you and your relative (Chapter 12).

Anxiety Related to Psychotic Symptoms

You may have already had difficulties trying to deal with your relative's anxiety in response to her psychotic symptoms. The initial reaction of most family members is to try to persuade their relative that her delusional beliefs or hallucinations are not real. Such attempts invariably fail because the very nature of delusions and hallucinations is that they *seem* real to the people who experience them.

Rather than trying to convince your relative that he shouldn't or needn't be anxious, try to understand and empathize with his feelings and then explore ways of reducing those unpleasant feelings. The best way to show you're concerned about your relative's feelings is to listen and then imagine how you would feel if you had the same experiences. Let your relative know what you heard by reflecting back his description: "I can see that it must be very upsetting to hear these voices yelling at you all the time."

By reflecting back your relative's concerns, you validate her feelings, help her feel understood, and avoid making unnecessary judgments about the nature of the concerns. If your relative is fearful about delusions, you may find it helpful to view these beliefs as being similar to the more common phobias. Objectively, it doesn't make sense to be terrified of being in a high building, in a closed space, or of most snakes and spiders, yet to people with these phobias the anxiety is quite real.

Once you've shown your understanding and concern, you can explore ways of reducing this anxiety with your relative. Some people reject offers of help; others readily accept. Your relative may shy away from accepting help with anxiety about psychotic symptoms because of a strong sense of privacy. Keep trying gently. If your relative accepts your help, you can talk together about how to deal with the anxiety. The following three general strategies are useful for coping with this type of anxiety.

• *Improve coping with the psychotic symptoms.* Helping your relative develop strategies for minimizing the disruptive effects of psychotic symptoms (see Chapter 17) can decrease the anxiety associated with those symptoms. For example, using distraction techniques, positive self-talk, and social engagement can reduce anxiety related to auditory hallucinations.

• *Use relaxation and other stress-reduction techniques.* Relaxation techniques such as progressive muscle relaxation, breathing exercises, and pleasant imagery can directly reduce anxiety (see Chapter 11 for stress reduction techniques).

• *Identify ways to manage difficult situations.* The anxiety related to psychotic symptoms may be worse in some situations than others. By identifying problematic situations, you can help your relative develop a plan for minimizing the accompanying stress. For example, a family gathering involving many relatives might be hard for a person with paranoid thoughts. The person could handle this situation by spending a half-hour at a time at the gathering and taking breaks to rest and relax before returning. Taking a problem-solving approach to helping your relative manage these problematic situations can be quite effective (see Chapter 15).

Anxiety Related to Specific Situations

Your relative may find certain situations anxiety provoking—it may not always be clear why—and therefore avoid them whenever possible. However, the fear associated with these situations can actually increase each time your relative avoids one, leading to even more avoidance. This vicious circle increasingly impedes your relative's functioning and pursuit of long-term goals.

You can help your relative cope by encouraging him to gradually expose himself to the situations that cause anxiety so he can overcome the fear associated with them. Talk over the idea with your relative to make sure he agrees with you about the advantages of conquering the fear. Then work together to identify related situations. Using that list, you can rate the situations by how much anxiety each situation causes.

The idea is for your relative to start with a situation that causes a low level of fear and to repeatedly confront this situation until she no longer feels anxious. Then she moves on to the next situation, which is only a little more anxiety-provoking than the first. Once again, repeated exposures to the situation will decrease the anxiety, at which point your relative can go on to a slightly more anxiety-provoking situation. Over time this exposure will gradually reduce your relative's fear.

Duane felt very anxious about riding on public transportation, and over the past year he had refused to go on any buses or subways. As a result of Duane's anxiety his mother had to drive him to his day treatment program a few miles away, and he was unable to participate in a peer support program across town. After Duane and his mother talked it over, he agreed to try to work with her on decreasing his anxiety about riding public transportation. Even the idea of riding public transportation caused Duane to feel anxious, so they agreed to start on some situations that wouldn't involve actually getting on the bus or subway. Then they began to work on more challenging situations. Duane's mother agreed to accompany him in some of these situations to make them less anxiety provoking. The situations that they started working on included (in the following order):

1. *Waiting at the bus stop closest to home with his mother and watching three buses go by.*
2. *Waiting at another bus stop with his mother and watching three buses go by.*
3. *Waiting at the bus stop closest to home alone and watching three buses go by.*
4. *Waiting at another bus stop alone and watching three buses go by.*
5. *Riding one stop with his mother on the bus closest to home and then one stop back home.*
6. *Riding three stops with his mother on the bus closest to home and then three stops back home.*
7. *Riding one stop and back alone.*
8. *Riding three stops and back alone.*

When these situations were mastered and Duane could use the bus for short trips close to home, they began to work on traveling farther away from home and decreasing his anxiety about riding the subway. Gradually, over several months, Duane overcame most of his anxiety about riding on public transportation and began to be able to take advantage of opportunities he had previously avoided because of his anxiety.

Anxiety Related to Past Psychotic Symptoms

If your relative has experienced psychotic symptoms only during acute episodes, he may be troubled by intrusive, unpleasant memories of these symptoms, which can be anxiety provoking. Sometimes the anxiety is related to a particular situation in which the psychotic symptoms occurred, resulting in fear of that situation.

While Don was experiencing a relapse of psychotic symptoms, he went to a baseball game and became terrified that other fans were looking at and talking about him. Family members were alert to Don's early warning signs of relapse and were able to arrange an appointment with his psychiatrist, who adjusted his medication and averted a relapse. However, Don continued to remember his experience at the baseball game after his psychotic symptoms had abated, and he no longer wanted to go to games because of the anxiety he felt about them. This anxiety even spread to riding the subway line that he had taken the day he had had trouble with his psychotic symptoms.

At other times your relative's anxiety may be due to memories of losing control, being frightened by bizarre thoughts, feeling afraid for her life or her loved ones' lives, or being overtaken by hallucinations. These fears are more diffuse and not attached to particular situations. Rather, the anxiety reflects the person's emotions about the memory of the disturbing symptoms and her concern over whether the symptoms will return. This concern can be so great that your relative is afraid to do almost anything for fear of "rocking the boat" and bringing on a relapse.

There are several ways to help your relative overcome anxiety related to past psychotic symptoms. If your relative is anxious about a specific situation, try the gradual exposure strategy described in the previous section. Don and his family worked toward helping him gradually overcome his fear of the subway and baseball games so that he was able to enjoy going to games again. If your relative feels anxious that his symptoms will return, you can help by talking about how to minimize the chances of a relapse. Taking medication, participating in daily structured activity, being alert to stress and handling it effectively, and monitoring early warning signs of relapse can all greatly reduce the possibility of a symptom relapse. Understanding how these steps can prevent future relapses will increase your relative's feeling of control and reduce his feelings of vulnerability and anxiety.

When anxiety stems from memories of past psychotic symptoms, gently encourage your relative to talk with you about the memories. If your relative is willing to talk, be supportive and empathic, let her talk as long as she wishes, and avoid jumping in too quickly to try to "solve" the problem. Just the process of talking about the unpleasant memories with someone who is supportive can reduce anxiety and make it easier to live with the memories. Your relative may need to talk about the memories more than once before the anxiety is sufficiently under control.

Anxiety Related to Memories of Negative Treatment Experiences

When people become psychotic and lose contact with reality, they often must be hospitalized involuntarily. Furthermore, when in the hospital, they may be subjected to involuntary treatment; secluded or restrained when their behavior is aggressive, self-injurious, or disruptive; and exposed to other people who are psychotic or disorganized. All of these experiences can be terrifying and may lead to unpleasant and recurrent memories—and efforts to avoid any reminders of those events.

Involuntary hospitalization and treatment can be a traumatic experience for everyone involved, but especially for the person with schizophrenia. The most important tack you can take to help your relative cope with anxiety due to memories of negative treatment experiences is to encourage him to talk about those memories as you listen with full attention. It may be hard for you to listen to the painful events your relative endured, and for your relative to talk about them, but over time it will become easier and your relative will become less frightened. It's important to refrain from giving advice and from making any corrections or judgmental statements when you're listening to your relative. Rather, simply show that you care and understand. Then, as you talk about the memories, you can work together toward taking steps to prevent another relapse and to ensure that if a relapse begins to happen, additional treatment can be provided in a less traumatic way. That is:

1. Review with your relative the principles of relapse prevention (such as taking medication, minimizing substance use, and reducing stress).
2. Develop a relapse prevention plan (Chapter 12).
3. Complete an advanced psychiatric directive, which specifies the type of treatment your relative wants if a hospitalization becomes necessary in the future (Chapter 13).

Fortunately, dehumanizing practices such as routinely handcuffing people who are being committed involuntarily to a hospital and using restraints have been decreasing steadily in recent years, in part through mental health consumer advocacy efforts. However, these practices continue in some places, and the traumatic nature of involuntary hospitalization probably cannot be avoided altogether. So, helping your relative talk about memories related to such experiences can reduce associated anxiety and help prevent their recurrence in the future.

Over a period of several months, Louise began withdrawing from her husband and children and spending more time in her room alone, acting bizarrely and talking to herself. Her husband and children grew increasingly concerned but didn't know what to do. Eventually Louise refused to eat food prepared at home and accused her family of trying to poison her. After several days of this behavior, Louise's husband felt he had no choice but to contact the police, who told him how to file a petition for a warrant that would require her to receive a psychiatric evaluation.

When Louise saw the police coming to her home, she thought they were plotting with her family and barricaded herself in her room. The police broke down the door and Louise tried to fend them off with a kitchen knife. Fortunately, no one was hurt, and she was subdued. The police then handcuffed her and took her to the psychiatric hospital, where she was evaluated and admitted. Louise remained paranoid and highly agitated for several weeks, disrupting activities on the ward, lashing out at others, and accusing the staff of plotting against her. On several occasions she was held down and injected with medications that made her feel stiff and woozy, and a number of other times she was secluded and physically restrained to a bed.

Eventually Louise's symptoms were controlled by the medication, and she became her old peaceful self again. She was discharged, prescribed an antipsychotic medication, and given an aftercare appointment at the local community mental health center. However, soon after returning home, Louise stopped taking her medication, and she went to only one appointment at the mental health center. She refused to go to any more aftercare appointments, despite her husband's pleas. When they tried to talk about it together, Louise explained that she didn't want to think about it and that the whole experience was a nightmare she wanted to forget. Taking medication and going to the mental health center only reminded her of the experience.

Louise's husband decided to shift the focus of their talks to trying to better understand what her experience had been like. He told her he knew she had been through a lot and it was hard to talk about but that he really wanted to understand what had happened to her in the hospital and to support her as her husband. In response to this accepting and caring attitude, Louise began to talk about what had happened. She described how terrified she had felt when the police came, how she thought her husband was trying to hurt her, and then that the police were going to hurt her. She described being in the hospital as like a nightmarish blur, but as she talked more about it, her memories of specific events became clearer, such as a time she was forcibly given medication after she overturned a table in the recreational area. With her husband's encouragement, Louise also talked about the experience of being restrained. This was especially frightening to Louise because it reminded her of when she had been sexually abused by her stepfather as a child. Talking about these experiences was hard for Louise, and on several occasions she broke down and cried, and her husband held her and comforted her. But talking also helped Louise process and understand the experiences, which, in turn, reduced her anxiety about her memories. Eventually Louise and her husband were able to begin talking about how they could prevent a relapse from happening in the future. Taking this step made them both feel more comfortable and in control over their lives.

Anxiety about the Future

Many people with schizophrenia are concerned about their future, including where they will live, how they will support themselves, and who will be there to help them. If your relative is dependent on others to get her basic needs met, her anxiety about the future can almost be expected. However, each person's perception of the future is unique, and some people have great difficulty looking ahead. If you think this concern may be contributing to your relative's anxiety, check it out with her.

Anxiety about the future is best allayed by beginning the difficult process of planning with your relative. Even if you can't be precise about all future plans, the more you talk about it and the more information you get, the less anxiety your relative is going to feel; see Chapter 30.

Specific Anxiety Disorders

As noted, social anxiety, PTSD, OCD, and panic disorder are the four anxiety disorders especially common in people with schizophrenia. The symptoms they cause are the same for those with and those without schizophrenia, but these disorders often go undiagnosed in routine care for schizophrenia. They may intensify other symptoms of schizophrenia, such as psychotic symptoms, as well as contribute to additional thinking difficulties due to their distracting effects. Anxiety disorders can also interact with the symptoms of schizophrenia as follows.

Social anxiety involves feeling extremely uncomfortable in social situations and having a constant fear of being evaluated harshly. Extreme social anxiety can lead people to avoid being with others, even though they may desperately want friends and close relationships. Social anxiety in schizophrenia is often compounded by delusions and paranoia, such as the belief that others are talking about the person or laughing at him or that others "have it in" for him. Difficulties in social skills that are common in schizophrenia (see Chapter 25) can result in awkward social interactions, further increasing social anxiety.

PTSD can develop after someone has been exposed to traumatic life events, such as being physically or sexually abused or assaulted, witnessing someone being hurt or killed, or being in an accident or natural disaster. People with schizophrenia are more likely to have been exposed to traumatic events, and when they develop PTSD they often experience intrusive memories of what happened and try to avoid reminders of the events (as Abdul and Louise did). Memories of traumatic events in people with schizophrenia can be so vivid they are hard to distinguish from hallucinations (such as intrusive images from witnessing the accidental death of a sibling), and some hallucinations have related themes (such as one Korean War veteran with extensive combat exposure who heard voices of fallen comrades calling to him). Delusions may also have some of their roots in traumatic experiences. For example, research by Max Birchwood, PhD, and his colleagues at the University of Birmingham has shown that the experience of having been bullied in childhood is related to paranoid delusions and perceiving voices as having power over oneself in people who later develop schizophrenia.

People who have *OCD* hoard useless objects (such as old newspapers) and can't bear to throw things away, or feel compelled to perform certain actions over and over again (such as repeatedly washing their hands because of a fear of contamination) or engage in certain thoughts (such as counting) even though they realize the behavior doesn't make sense. OCD symptoms can overlap with schizophrenic delusions. For example, those with OCD in the general population usually know their fears of contamination are unrealistic, though they still feel compelled to wash their hands, while someone with schizophrenia and OCD may hold the delusional belief that contamination is likely.

Panic disorder involves experiencing intense, sudden fear that one is having a heart attack, losing control, or going crazy and is usually accompanied by a rapid increase in physiological signs such as a pounding heart, chest pain, sweating, and muscular tension. These panic attacks often seem to "come out of the blue" and can be so frightening that they result in the person refusing to leave home alone (called *agoraphobia*). People with schizophrenia and panic disorder often report that their panic symptoms developed around the same time as their psychotic symptoms, and the two types of symptoms may worsen one another.

Antidepressant medications are effective in treating anxiety disorders in the general population, although little research has evaluated their effects in people with schizophrenia. Cognitive-behavioral treatments have also been developed, and although research is still in its infancy, there is growing evidence that these treatments can be adapted successfully for anxiety disorders in those with schizophrenia. The adaptations in these treatments for schizophrenia usually involve working at a slower pace, closely monitoring the person's stress level, and simplifying instructions and homework assignments to practice skills taught in sessions.

Treatment for social anxiety generally involves helping people identify and challenge problematic beliefs they think others hold about them, and practicing social skills. Treatment for PTSD usually involves helping people confront their fears, both memories and real situations, and challenging inaccurate beliefs they may have developed in response to the traumatic events. Treatment for OCD involves helping people refrain from engaging in compulsive behaviors so that they can see that nothing terrible will happen. Treatment of panic disorder involves helping people understand that panic symptoms are signs of physiological overarousal (or overactivation) and developing and practicing strategies for lowering their arousal level when the first signs appear, such as by using breathing exercises.

To find someone who can help your relative, contact your local mental health center or look for a private cognitive-behavioral therapist. In addition, self-help books, such as the ones listed in the Resources section at the end of this chapter, are available to help people cope with and overcome these anxiety disorders.

Dealing with Your Own Anxiety

The nature of schizophrenia can give rise to anxiety in anyone who lives with or is close to someone with the illness. The sheer unpredictability of your relative's disorder—from fluctuating symptoms to the limited, and varying, effectiveness of treatments—may leave you feeling helpless and understandably anxious. Naturally you are also concerned about your relative's future. Fortunately, you do have control over your own anxiety. Dealing effectively with it is crucial to increasing your own satisfaction with life and enhancing your relationship with your ill relative, as well as with other family members.

In reading this book, you are already taking the most important step toward overcoming your anxiety about your relative. By becoming informed about schizophrenia and developing strategies for handling stress, communication problems, and specific symptoms, you are exercising control where some control is possible, increasing your ability to anticipate and modify your relative's behavior. In the long run these efforts will make you feel less helpless and reduce your anxiety. Meanwhile, you can also use short-term strategies for reducing anxiety, such as the methods described in Chapter 11 for managing stress and those described in this chapter.

Facing Anxiety

Trying to escape feelings of anxiety and the situations that evoke them is one of the most common methods people use to deal with anxiety. Unfortunately, anxiety chases us down and grows in the process. Eventually, conquering anxious feelings means learning how to accept them and face them head on. Understanding the nature of your relative's anxiety as well as your own is the first step toward dealing with it. You have many options at your disposal for helping you and your loved one deal with anxiety so that it does not dominate your lives. Trying the coping strategies outlined here will empower you both to overcome anxiety and its effects on your lives.

Resources

Bourne, E. J. (2003). *The anxiety and phobia workbook* (3rd ed.). Oakland, CA: New Harbinger. In addition to providing strategies for coping with anxiety and phobias, this book contains several worksheets to help people apply the information to their own situations.

Foa, E. B., & Wilson, R. (2001). *Stop obsessing! How to overcome your obsessions and compulsions* (rev. ed.). New York: Bantam. A world expert on the treatment of OCD (Foa) describes how to confront and overcome obsessions and compulsions.

Hyman, B. M., & Pedrick, C. (1999). *The OCD workbook: Your guide to breaking free from obsessive–compulsive disorder.* Oakland, CA: New Harbinger. This self-help guide to coping with and overcoming OCD contains useful worksheets.

Jeffers, S. (1992). *Feel the fear and do it anyway.* New York: Fawcett Books. A classic in self-help for anxiety problems.

Schiraldi, G. R. (2000). *The post-traumatic stress disorder sourcebook: A guide to healing, recovery, and growth.* Los Angeles: Lowell House. This book helps people understand, cope with, and overcome their reactions to traumatic events.

Locating a Psychotherapist for Anxiety

Albert Ellis Institute, 45 East 65th St., New York, NY 10021; (212) 535-0822; (800) 323-4738; *www.rebt.org.*

Association for Cognitive and Behavioral Therapies (formerly called the Association for Advancement of Behavior Therapy), 305 Seventh Ave., 16th floor, New York, NY 10001; (212) 647-1890; *www.aabt.org.*

Symptoms of Anxiety Checklist

Instructions: Place a checkmark next to each symptom that your relative has had over the past month.

	Checkmark
Mood and Thinking	
Worry or concern	
Fear	
Irritability	
Difficulty concentrating	
Behavior	
Avoidance of feared situations	
Escape from unpleasant situations	
Trembling	
Agitation (e.g., pacing)	
Increased Arousal	
Perspiration	
Heart palpitations	
Muscular tension	
"Butterflies" in stomach	
Mild nausea	
Dizziness	
Shortness of breath	

CHAPTER 21

Depression

Most people who have schizophrenia experience some problems related to depression. And, as a result of the stress and strain of having a loved one with a mental illness, family members may also feel its effects. Depression can have a far-reaching impact on your relative's functioning and quality of life, often contributing to lost productivity, relationship problems, and the inability to enjoy life's pleasures. That's why helping your relative cope with depression is of critical importance. For you, these mood problems may compromise your enjoyment of life as well as your ability to help your relative. You'll find strategies in this chapter for helping your relative and yourself deal with the disabling effects of depression.

Depression in Schizophrenia

Depression and schizophrenia are closely related; in fact depression is often one of the first signs of schizophrenia, frequently developing months or years before psychotic symptoms emerge. Depression also continues to be a problem for many people with schizophrenia.

Depression may also be a natural response to disturbing hallucinations and delusions. Hearing voices that criticize them, call them names, or exhort them to hurt themselves or others; believing that others are watching them or attempting to control them; thinking their body is malfunctioning; or believing that they or the world are not real can leave people with schizophrenia feeling helpless, hopeless, and worthless—key ingredients of depression.

Some people are also acutely aware of how their illness has affected them and their families, the limitations the illness has imposed on their ability to achieve their goals, and the differences between themselves and their siblings and peers without schizophrenia. People with insight into their illness may be more aware of the stigma associated with mental illness—and hence more vulnerable to depression.

Depression in people with schizophrenia can lead to thoughts about hurting or even killing themselves. About half of all people with schizophrenia make a suicide attempt at some point during their life, and about 1 in 20 dies from suicide. This risk of suicide is higher than in the general public and is similar to the risk of suicide in people with other serious disorders, such as bipolar disorder. Most people who have suicidal thoughts or who make suicide attempts have problems with depression. Chapter 13 provides strategies for evaluating your relative's risk for suicide, taking steps to prevent suicide attempts, and responding to an imminent threat of suicide.

As a result of depression, your relative may find it difficult to pursue work or social relationships. Hopelessness is the ultimate enemy; feeling it, people give up and are unable to enjoy even the simple pleasures of life. Helping your relative cope effectively with depression involves creating a sense of optimism and belief that the future can be better. Identifying and pursuing personal recovery goals, as described in Chapter 3, can help manifest this better future. In addition, fostering a positive mental attitude in your relative can improve both the quality of her day-to-day experiences and the course of her illness.

Symptoms of Depression

Melanie, who lives with her mother and two of her children (ages 4 and 7), often seems rather down. Her facial expression, although blunted somewhat, is sad, and she speaks and moves slowly. Melanie doesn't seem very interested in doing much and complains about having low energy and not finding much pleasure in anything other than eating. She tries to help out with her children, but her mother ends up doing most of the work. Much of Melanie's day is spent eating and sleeping. Sometimes her mother finds her crying alone in her room. When she asks what's wrong, Melanie often replies that everything seems hopeless, the voices she hears put her down, and her life just doesn't seem to be worth living.

The most common symptoms of depression can be divided into three broad categories: mood disturbances, negative thoughts, and physical and behavioral changes.

Mood Disturbances

The most common mood is one of sadness—a sense of loss or hurt that is constant over time. Sad or "blue" feelings are often (but not always) reflected in the person's facial expressions and voice tone. Sad feelings may be accompanied by feelings of guilt; your relative may ruminate excessively over mistakes made in the past. If your relative has severe depression, he may experience feelings of dread—a horrible feeling that is difficult to describe but contains elements of pain, fear, and despair. These feelings can make it difficult to face the day each morning. People with depression may also feel anger, which may be directed at themselves or others, and irritability, although some feelings of sadness usually are also present.

Negative Thoughts

Negative thinking and mood problems go hand in hand. Some of the most common negative thoughts include those around hopelessness, helplessness, and worthlessness. Your relative may be overly self-critical and perfectionistic, which quickly results in discouragement and giving up, and she may ruminate about negative topics such as death and suicidal thoughts.

Physical and Behavioral Changes

Depression often involves changes in eating and sleeping habits, as well as self-care, energy, and activity level. A very common sign is loss of appetite, often accompanied by weight loss, although some people have the opposite problem of eating too much. Your relative may have difficulty getting enough sleep and feel chronically tired as a result. Some people wake up early in the morning (such as 4:00 or 5:00 A.M.) and are not able to get back to sleep. Others have the problem of sleeping too much; family members and friends may worry that the person is sleeping his life away. People also report a loss of energy, which is accompanied by slowed activity and social withdrawal. Sometimes, however, depression is reflected by an *increase* in activity level in the form of agitation.

Distinguishing Depression from Other Common Problems in Schizophrenia

Evaluating whether your relative has depression can be complicated by a number of factors, as described in the following pages.

Negative Symptoms

Negative symptoms are easily mistaken for depression. For example, if your relative has *blunted affect* (flattened facial expression, inexpressive tone of voice), talking with her may leave you with the impression that she is depressed because of the apparent lack of enjoyment or engagement in the conversation. Similarly, if your relative has anhedonia (less enjoyment from recreational activities or social relationships), you might conclude that this is due to an underlying depression. In both of these cases, your relative may be experiencing negative symptoms, depression, or both. The confusion arises from the fact that these two types of symptoms overlap. People with depression *do* experience less enjoyment from activities and relationships, and they are often less expressive when interacting with others. However, anhedonia and blunted affect in a person with schizophrenia do not necessarily indicate depression—they may be due solely to negative symptoms.

The best way to understand what your relative is feeling is to ask. If your relative reports feeling sad, guilty, or hopeless, he is probably depressed.

Medication Side Effects

In addition to negative symptoms, two side effects of antipsychotic medications can easily be mistaken for depression (see Chapter 10 for further information about treating these side effects).

Akinesia is a side effect that reduces spontaneous movements, such as facial expressions and gestures, and makes it harder to initiate the usual activities. Akinesia is very difficult to distinguish from blunted affect. However, akinesia can be improved by altering the dosage or type of antipsychotic medication or side effect medication. Just as it may be easy to mistake blunted affect for depression, akinesia may be mistaken for depression. Talking with your relative about how she feels is the best strategy for assessing depression. If you're concerned that your relative may have akinesia, consult her physician.

Akathisia causes feelings of restlessness, usually accompanied by pacing or rocking behavior. Akathisia is a very upsetting side effect for many people, and it can make them appear unusually agitated. Fortunately, akathisia occurs much less commonly with the newer novel antipsychotics than with the conventional antipsychotic medications. The primary distinction between akathisia and depression is that in akathisia the person's distress is due mainly to the feeling of restlessness, whereas in depression distress stems from feelings of sadness and hopelessness. Once again, talking with your relative is the key to understanding whether he has depression. Akathisia can be treated effectively by modifying the dosage or type of medication. If you're concerned that your relative may have akathisia, consult his physician.

Physical Problems

Symptoms of depression can also occur as a result of physical conditions such as anemia, thyroid gland malfunction, and diabetes. Furthermore, certain medications used to treat heart disease and hypertension can produce mild symptoms of depression. One class of drugs used for heart disease, beta-blockers (such as Inderal), can produce some symptoms of depression. Beta-blockers are also occasionally used in the treatment of schizophrenia and antipsychotic medication side effects. Encourage your relative to get a physical exam to help determine whether her symptoms of depression are the result of a physical condition.

Assessing Depression in Your Relative

The Symptoms of Depression checklist (Worksheet 21.1) at the end of the chapter can help you and your relative get a better idea of whether he is depressed. No set number of symptoms must be present for you to conclude that your relative has depression. The more symptoms, the more likely it is that depression is a problem.

Depression as an Early Warning Sign of Relapse

Increases in depression can be an early warning sign of relapse. Changes in mood may be subtle, but to family members who know the person well, they can be quite apparent. It's therefore important to recognize when an increase in depressive symptoms is an early warning sign of relapse and a cue to put into action your plan for responding to early warning signs (see Chapter 12). This chapter focuses on strategies for helping your relative cope with persistent depression that is not an early warning sign of relapse but a daily state of being.

Helping Your Relative Cope with Depression

No single strategy is best for helping your relative cope with and overcome feelings of depression. In fact, people often benefit from trying a number of different methods. Most important is helping your relative identify which strategies are most effective for her.

Before implementing any strategies, however, you need to talk over the matter with your relative to see whether he views depression as a problem and can be motivated to work toward improving it. People with depression often lack energy and motivation. Therefore, it's best to try small steps and establish modest goals at the beginning, to avoid overwhelming your relative and expecting more effort from him than he can muster. You can be of greatest help in your discussions by showing your relative that you understand and are concerned with his feelings and by instilling some hope that change is possible.

Specific Coping Strategies

There are several strategies for helping your relative cope with depression.

Scheduling Pleasant Events

When people are depressed, they often stop engaging in activities they used to enjoy. A stressful event or a difficult situation can interfere with a person's usual routine, including recreational activities, and often the person does not resume these activities. People with schizophrenia are especially prone to developing depression because of the chaotic effects of their disorder. For example, people's daily routines are greatly disrupted every time a relapse and hospitalization takes place so it's not surprising that they have difficulty reestablishing their routines following discharge.

Assisting your relative in making specific plans to engage in enjoyable activities can help lift her out of depression. Planning to take a 1-hour walk in the park on Thursday afternoon and going out to a movie on Friday night are examples of scheduling specific times for pleasant activities. Your relative may find it hard to schedule and follow through on these activities on her own. Meeting regularly with your relative to talk over and schedule activities will foster her ability to plan and participate in activities on her own. Chapter 28 contains more tips for helping your relative develop leisure and recreational pursuits.

Increasing Activity Level

People often become inactive and lethargic when they are depressed. In turn, these feelings of lethargy can worsen the depression. People with schizophrenia may be especially vulnerable to depression that arises from inactivity because they have a limited degree of stamina and are prone to lethargy, even when they are not depressed. Helping your relative increase his activity level, such as by walking, jogging, bicycling, or aerobics, can markedly improve his mood. Even less strenuous types of exercise, such as walking up the stairs instead of taking the elevator, can help.

Engaging in exercise regularly or modifying daily habits can be hard, even for people who do not have a psychiatric disorder. Naturally, these difficulties are even greater for a person with schizophrenia. The following are a few pointers for helping your relative increase her activity level.

1. *Set small, attainable goals*. By helping your relative set manageable goals that he is likely to achieve, you "program success" and encourage your relative's efforts to change. For example, the two of you might set a goal of taking a 10-minute walk once a week.

2. *Work gradually toward long-term goals*. After your relative achieves success with the first small goal, think of a new one that is one step closer to the long-term goal. For example, after a few weeks of taking one 10-minute walk per week, take two walks per week, working toward the long-term goal of walking or jogging daily.

3. *Build in rewards for following through*. Talk over with your relative ideas for rewarding her for following through on her plan. Rewards can involve only your relative (e.g., watching a favorite TV show, taking a nap) or both of you (cooking a special meal, renting a movie to watch together).

4. *Record progress on a regular basis.* Encourage your relative to mark down on

a calendar, a record book, or a notebook every time he engages in the planned activity to show progress over time. These records can be reviewed routinely to point out increases in activity and to troubleshoot when the activity has been missed.

5. *Include others in the activity.* Explore with your relative whether doing the activity with others would make it more enjoyable or easier. Your relative can consider asking you, a friend, or another relative to come along or could do the activity with an organized group (such as the YMCA) or in a public place (such as a park).

Correcting Unhelpful Thinking

How and what we think about the world around us has a tremendous bearing on our mood. For example, if we think that the world is a cruel, cold, unforgiving place, we will no doubt experience unpleasant feelings. Our thoughts shape our feelings. Certain thinking styles are self-defeating because they reflect only the bad side of things; feelings of depression follow in their wake. By challenging and correcting unhelpful thoughts, a person can decrease feelings of depression. In fact, there is a great deal of evidence from research that helping people recognize and change their thinking styles has a beneficial effect on the symptoms of depression.

If your relative has problems with depression, the chances are high that she has some unhelpful thinking patterns aside from any delusions she may have. Helping your relative change her thinking can improve her depression. One way of accomplishing this improvement is to help your relative challenge her beliefs about how the world "should," "must," or "ought" to be, because such beliefs are often inconsistent with the real world. People with schizophrenia are especially prone to these types of beliefs, because they are saddled with the burden of a severe illness that occurs randomly and is not "fair." Helping your relative recognize and challenge self-defeating beliefs can improve her mood by providing a more realistic and adaptive way of thinking about the world and her circumstances. Examples of self-defeating beliefs and more adaptive alternatives are provided in the table on the next page.

Another way of helping your relative correct unhelpful thinking is by recognizing *common problematic thinking styles* (also called *cognitive distortions* or *maladaptive thinking*) that lead to depression. Erroneous and self-defeating conclusions are the result of the different ways people incorrectly process information about the world around them. For example, people sometimes jump to conclusions when they experience a setback, and the conclusion can make them feel helpless and depressed.

Bob was depressed because he was recently turned down for a part-time job. When he talked it over with his wife, he revealed that he believed he would never be able to get a

Self-Defeating Beliefs versus Helpful Thoughts	
Self-defeating belief	Helpful alternative thought
"I *must* be liked by everyone."	"It would be nice if everyone liked me, but I know that's not possible."
"My relative *shouldn't* give me such a hard time."	"I would prefer it if my relative didn't give me such a hard time. What can I do to change this problem?"
"I *have to* get this job."	"I would like to get this job, and I'll try my best to get it. If I can't, I can always try getting another job."
"It's *unfair* that I have to suffer like this when I don't deserve it."	"I don't like having to suffer this way; nobody likes to suffer. Is there something I can do to improve this situation?"

job–a depressing prospect. His wife empathized with his disappointment about not getting the job and then raised the question of whether he really had enough information to know that he would never *get a job. When they explored this conclusion together, Bob admitted that he had looked for only one other job in the past few months and agreed that he might be "jumping to conclusions" when he thought he would never get a job. By correcting this common problematic style of thinking, Bob felt better about his employment prospects.*

Examples of common problematic styles of thinking are provided in the following table. You can help your relative adjust his common problematic styles of thinking by reviewing this list together and practicing catching and correcting instances of when these problematic thinking styles occur.

Additional Strategies for Specific Symptoms

Some symptoms are very troubling and persist over long periods of time. You can help your relative manage these symptoms by encouraging him to try the coping strategies described in the table on the facing page.

Professional Treatment for Depression

Coping strategies can be very effective at reducing or eliminating depression in people with schizophrenia. However, you may also want to consider seeking professional help. Two types of treatment deserve attention: pharmacological treatment and psychotherapy.

Medication Treatment

Antidepressant medications are effective for treating depression in the general public, and they can also help people who have schizophrenia. Not everybody with schizophrenia who is depressed benefits from antidepressants, but it may be worth a trial if your relative has not received one. If you and your relative are interested in this approach, explore it with her doctor.

Psychotherapy

Psychotherapy is also very effective for treating depression in the general population, especially three types: cognitive-behavioral therapy, problem-solving therapy, and interpersonal therapy. *Cognitive-behavioral therapy* assists people in challenging unhelpful thinking patterns (as just described) and setting and pursuing personal goals. *Problem-solving therapy* teaches people a structured set of skills for solving problems (similar to those described in Chapter 15) and helps them use these skills to resolve problems and pursue personally important goals. *Interpersonal therapy* helps people identify and resolve conflicts they have with other people, which are presumed to contribute to feelings of depression. If your relative is

Examples of Common Problematic Thinking Styles	
Problematic style of thinking	Example
All-or-nothing thinking	Seeing things in "black and white"; for example, "If I can't get the job I really want, it's not even worth looking at something else."
Overgeneralization	Viewing a single negative event as indicating a never-ending pattern of defeat; for example, "I'm a failure because I was just hospitalized again."
Mental filter	Focusing only on the negative and ignoring the positive; for example, "I don't think I'm getting anywhere; I still don't have a job" (despite having stayed out of the hospital 6 months and having improved self-care skills).
Overpersonalizing events	Interpreting an event as personal when it is not; for example, "I don't like to ride the bus because the bus driver doesn't like me; he scowls at me" (when the bus driver scowls at everybody).
Jumping to conclusions	Drawing conclusions based on inadequate information; for example, "I know you think I'm lazy when I don't get up on time," or "If I call up one of my old friends, she won't be interested in getting together with me because it's been so long since we've seen each other."

interested in pursuing therapy, you might consider exploring whether your local community mental health center could provide one of these approaches; if not, and if you have the financial resources, you could investigate the availability of a private practitioner.

Dealing with Your Own Depression

Depression can be contagious. If your relative has problems with depression, his blue mood can lead to similar feelings in you. Or you may feel depressed because of your struggle with your relative's illness. If you feel depressed and have the symptoms described earlier in this chapter (see Worksheet 21.1), try to deal with this problem. Depression can sap your energy, dampen your ability to solve problems, and make you less able to help your relative.

You may find some of the strategies described in the previous section helpful. Scheduling pleasant events and increasing your activity level, including exercise, may be useful strategies. For many relatives, the strain of having a close family member with schizophrenia is so great that they stop taking care of their own needs, relinquishing recreational and health pursuits as they focus all their atten-

Strategies for Coping with Specific Symptoms of Depression	
Symptom	Coping strategies
Loss of interest, lack of energy, slowed activity level	• Set goals for daily activities. • Take small steps to structure a full program of constructive activity. • Pinpoint small areas of interest that you can pursue easily and build upon them. • Avoid comparing your current interest or energy level with the past.
Loss of appetite	• Eat small portions of food that you like. • Take your time eating. • Avoid eating with others if you feel pressure to finish. • Drink plenty of fluids, especially fruit juices or smoothies, protein shakes, and high-calorie drinks like Ensure.
Sleep disturbance	• Go to bed at your usual time. • Avoid sleeping during the day. • Reduce caffeine intake (coffee, tea, colas) to not more than two or three per day and not for several hours before going to bed. • Don't lie awake in bed for more than 30 minutes; get up and find something to do. • Try relaxation exercises.

tion on trying to help their relative. The upshot is that depression ensues, often mixed with feelings of resentment. You can combat this depression by setting aside time for yourself to pursue activities that you enjoy, such as taking an art class, joining a fitness program, doing needlework, or going fishing.

Just as common problematic styles of thinking and self-defeating beliefs can play a role in depression in your relative, they may also influence your mood. Taking the time to notice your thoughts and beliefs about your relative's illness may help you identify unhelpful styles that contribute to your depression. By challenging these types of thoughts, you can take control of your own thinking and thereby improve your mood.

One common problematic style of thinking noted in the table on page 325 is *all-or-nothing (black-and-white) thinking*. For example, you might think "My loved one has no life because she has schizophrenia." This is a distortion of reality because, although your relative's life may be greatly affected by the illness, she nevertheless does have a life and is capable of feelings, accomplishments, and connection with others, including family, friends, and the community (see Chapter 3). Another common problematic style of thinking in family members is *overgeneralization*. For example, you might catch yourself thinking, "My relative has nothing going for her," even though she works part-time at a volunteer job and helps out around the house. In each case, the common problematic style of thinking reflects a grain of truth that is then exaggerated to an unhelpful—and untrue—degree.

Similarly, self-defeating beliefs about your relative's illness can contribute to depression. For example, you may often think "It's unfair that my relative has schizophrenia—we didn't do anything to deserve this!" It is true that neither you nor anyone else caused your relative's illness, and it's not "fair" for anyone to suffer with such a problem. However, this is a world in which bad things happen to people who don't deserve them, and dwelling on the unfairness of the world only interferes with your ability to cope more effectively with the illness.

Another example of a common self-defeating belief is "My relative should show his love for me; I can't stand it if he doesn't." It would be nice if your relative showed more love for you, and it's disappointing when he does not, but you can live with this situation and even maintain a decent, sometimes rewarding, relationship with him. Challenging these types of beliefs can enable you to develop a more helpful way of thinking about your relative's illness and see it as something you can deal with.

The shock and disruption caused by the development of schizophrenia in a relative frequently results in family members keeping more to themselves and seeing friends less often. This self-imposed isolation can stem from the social stigma felt by family members (see Chapter 29), the amount of time devoted to caring for the relative, or both. Social relationships are an important source of well-being and support for most of us, and without these relationships all of us are more vulnerable to depression. Increasing the time you spend with close friends or making new friends can strengthen your social support network and thereby reduce symptoms of depression.

The experience of having a close relative develop schizophrenia can seem devastating to family members. Parents often find they need to adjust their expectations for their daughter's future, including her career options, her ability to live independently, and marriage and children. Many family members have said that having a relative develop schizophrenia is like experiencing the loss of someone close to them. This is an understandable reaction, but by learning strategies to better manage the illness and improve its course, family members can find reasons to be more optimistic. Focusing on improving your relative's strengths and abilities, as outlined in Part VI of this book, often leaves you feeling less overwhelmed by the limitations imposed by the illness.

Even with improved coping, however, you may continue to grieve over the effects of schizophrenia on your relative. If you experience strong, persistent feelings of depression that are difficult to escape, you may have unresolved grief about the loss of your relative as you knew him—a common reaction. *Unresolved grief* is usually a mixture of persistent feelings of sadness, anger, and frustration about having a relative with schizophrenia, which the person has not fully expressed and which weighs him down. If you're feeling unresolved grief, the best way to deal with it and get on with your life is to talk about it with someone who can be supportive—a close friend, a relative, a group of other relatives with similar experiences, a therapist, or a member of the clergy. The grieving process takes time, and you may need to talk about your feelings repeatedly before you feel ready to move on. Recognizing your need to grieve and allowing yourself the time to do it can enable you to get over your depression, accept your relative's illness, and enjoy your relative for who he is.

Maintaining Hope

Depression is commonly experienced by people with schizophrenia and can rob them of the hope they need to pursue their goals and enjoy life. Similarly, depression is common among family members and others who have close relationships with the person with schizophrenia, and it can interfere with their efforts to help their loved one and to enjoy her company. Although the world may seem hopeless when you're depressed, and you may feel helpless at the prospect of improving your life, you and your relative do not have to buy those negative thoughts—it's the depression talking and not reality. The fact that you *feel* hopeless and helpless doesn't mean you really *are*! Challenging self-defeating (and incorrect!) beliefs is the most crucial step you can take toward combating passivity, overcoming depression, and beginning again to enjoy life for what it has to offer.

Resources

Books on Depression

Burns, D. D. (1980). *Feeling good: The new mood therapy.* New York: Avon. Another classic self-help book that teaches people how to correct common styles of thinking that can lead to depression.

Burns, D. D. (1999). *The feeling good handbook* (rev. ed.). New York: Plume. A best-selling follow-up to Burns's previous book on correcting thinking styles that can lead to depression.

Ellis, A., & Harper, R.A. (1999). *A guide to rational living: Thoroughly revised for the 21st century* (3rd ed.). North Hollywood, CA: Melvin Powers Wilshire Book Company. This is a classic self-help book that teaches people how to correct common self-defeating beliefs that contribute to depression.

Locating a Psychotherapist for Depression

Albert Ellis Institute, 45 East 65th St., New York, NY 10021; (212) 535-0822; (800) 323-4738; *www.rebt.org.*

Association for Cognitive and Behavioral Therapies (formerly called the Association for Advancement of Behavior Therapy), 305 Seventh Ave., 16th floor, New York, NY 10001; (212) 647-1890; *www.aabt.org.*

Symptoms of Depression

Instructions: Check the boxes below that apply to your relative's behavior.

	No	Somewhat	Yes
Mood symptoms			
Sadness			
Guilt			
Dread			
Irritability			
Anger			
Unhelpful thoughts about . . .			
Hopelessness			
Helplessness			
Worthlessness			
Death			
Suicide			
Physical and behavioral changes			
Loss of appetite			
Sleep problems			
Slowed activity level			
Agitation			

CHAPTER 22

Alcohol and Drug Abuse

Almost everyone knows someone who has problems with alcohol or drugs and has seen the havoc they can wreak on people's lives. Many of the problems associated with substance abuse are even greater in people with schizophrenia, whose biological vulnerability makes them more sensitive to the effects of alcohol and drugs. If your relative drinks excessively or uses drugs, you already know how this substance use complicates treatment.

What you may not realize is how common these problems are in people with schizophrenia. A large survey conducted in the United States by the National Institute of Mental Health (NIMH) found a 47% rate of substance use disorders in people with schizophrenia—a rate similar to that found by other studies. This is much higher than the rates the NIMH study found in the general population: 16.7% had experienced an alcohol and/or drug use disorder at some time during their lives.

This chapter describes how you can help your relative overcome a substance abuse problem. Substance abuse can be quite severe in people with schizophrenia, and the struggle is a very long one for some. However, by becoming more informed about the problem, available treatment options, and strategies for managing it, you can play an important role in helping your relative regain control over her life and begin to escape the powerful hold of alcohol and drug abuse.

First, though, it's important to know what we mean by *abuse* versus *dependence*. A person whose substance use interferes with working, social relationships, or health or exposes him to dangerous situations has an alcohol or drug *abuse* disorder. A person who is also physically dependent on the substance or has difficulty controlling his use and gives up other activities to use substances has an alcohol or drug *dependence* disorder. Physical dependence is defined as having withdrawal symptoms (such as headaches, nausea, or tremors) when the substance is not taken or developing tolerance to the substance (needing larger amounts to achieve the same effects).

The Effects of Substance Abuse on People with Schizophrenia

People with schizophrenia have extremely sensitive nervous systems due to their biological vulnerability to the disorder. As a result of this vulnerability, even small amounts of substances can worsen symptoms and hasten relapses and rehospitalizations. Using substances can also have harmful effects on day-to-day functioning, such as causing conflict in close relationships and interfering with work, school, or self-care. Alcohol and drug use can also lead to legal problems (arrests for public intoxication, possession of illegal drugs, driving under the influence of alcohol), housing instability (such as being evicted from one's apartment), money problems, and health problems (such as infectious diseases contracted via unsafe use of drugs or unsafe sex or the physical effects of chronic substance abuse).

The Effects of Substance Abuse on the Family

If you're familiar with the effects of substance abuse on your relative, you probably also know its impact on you and your family. Frustration is one of the most common reactions. Family members often understand that having schizophrenia is beyond the person's control, but they have more difficulty seeing excessive drug or alcohol use as also beyond their relative's control. It is frustrating to see a relative on a path of self-destructive substance abuse, which is made all the worse when the abuse occurs in flagrant violation of household rules and disrupts the tranquility of the home. You can use Worksheet 22.1 at the end of the chapter to identify the possible consequences of your relative's substance abuse.

Another common reaction among family members is anxiety and fear. Substance abuse can make people prone to hostile or angry outbursts, social withdrawal, or suicide attempts. The fear associated with this unpredictability can be compounded when the person has stolen from family members or has a history of violence.

Anger, helplessness, and despair are all feelings you and your family may be experiencing if your relative has a substance abuse problem, and everyone reacts differently to these emotions. Some family members may disengage themselves from the fray, whereas others get involved in frequent arguments. When your relative lives at home, these tumultuous feelings can result in a tense family atmosphere that is unpleasant for all. Helping your relative overcome his substance use problems will improve the outcome of his illness *and* reduce tension in your family.

Patterns of Substance Abuse

Many different substances can be abused, some legal and others illegal. Here we focus on substances that can worsen the course of schizophrenia, such as alcohol and "street drugs"; cigarette smoking is addressed at the end of this chapter.

Types of Abused Substances

As summarized in the table below, the most commonly abused substances can be grouped into six categories: alcohol, cannabis (marijuana), stimulants (cocaine), hallucinogens, sedatives, and narcotics. People with schizophrenia are most likely to abuse alcohol, marijuana, and cocaine, although abuse of other drugs is common as well. Most people with substance use problems abuse more than one substance.

Accessibility often determines which substances are used. In most settings alcohol, marijuana, and cocaine are most commonly available, although in some areas other drugs may be more popular, such as amphetamines or heroin.

Social Situations

Because drugs are usually obtained from other people, drug abuse tends to take place in social settings. Alcohol can be obtained easily and consumed alone, so about half of all alcohol abuse by people with schizophrenia occurs alone.

Who Is Most Likely to Develop Substance Use Problems?

People who have problems using substances, whether or not they have schizophrenia, are more likely to be male, young, and single, with lower levels of educa-

Commonly Abused Substances and Their Effects	
Type of substance	Effects
Alcohol: beer, wine, "hard" liquor	Drowsiness, slurred speech, loss of motor coordination, slowed reaction time, relaxation, depression
Cannabis: marijuana, hash, THC	Mild euphoria, relaxation, anxiety or panic, perceptual distortions, racing or paranoid thoughts
Stimulants: cocaine, "speed" (amphetamine)	Alertness, energy, feeling "high," anxiety, nervousness, psychotic symptoms
Hallucinogens: LSD, Ecstasy, PCP, MDA, mescaline, peyote	Perceptual distortions or hallucinations, impaired judgment, feelings of unreality
Sedatives: Valium, Librium, Seconal	Drowsiness, slurred speech, loss of motor coordination, slowed reaction time, relaxation, depression
Narcotics: heroin, morphine, codeine	Euphoria, drowsiness, relaxation, "high" or "spacey" feelings, slowed reflexes

tion. Substance use problems are also more common in people with schizophrenia who have family members who have experienced substance use problems. Research studies indicate that, similar to schizophrenia, vulnerability to substance abuse is partly genetic.

The substance use problems of many people with schizophrenia occurred before the onset of the illness, although others do develop these problems after they become ill. Drug abuse can also trigger the onset of schizophrenia in vulnerable people at an earlier age than for people who don't use drugs. There are no clear symptom differences between people with schizophrenia who are prone to substance abuse, although there is some tendency toward higher levels of depression and anxiety.

Assessing Your Relative's Substance Use

You may already know whether your relative has an alcohol or drug problem. If you don't, you can discuss the issue with him and also use your powers of observation.

People often give accurate information about their substance use when asked in a straightforward, matter-of-fact way. Take a nonthreatening approach that avoids putting your relative on the defensive. An admission is likely to be accurate, but a denial may not be, especially if your relative has used substances in the past.

Of course "secret" substance abuse may be readily apparent if your relative carelessly leaves empty bottles of alcohol or drug paraphernalia lying around. "Drug paraphernalia" includes items such as pipes (marijuana, crack cocaine), rolling papers (marijuana), cut plastic tubes (snorting cocaine, speed, or heroin), vials or small bags (for storing drugs), or needles. You may smell marijuana or crack cocaine smoke from your relative's room or notice alcohol missing from your supply.

The most important clues to substance abuse if such objects aren't in view can be found by observing your relative's symptoms and level of functioning. Substance abuse may explain relapses or severe symptoms that cannot be accounted for by medication nonadherence or identifiable life stressors. It could also be behind problems in functioning, such as failing to meet expectations that were formerly met (oversleeping and being late for a job or program, not doing agreed-on household chores), conflict in close social relationships (including family members), or neglect of self-care. A recent deterioration in appearance (appearing disheveled, tired, or anxious) could be caused by substance abuse, as could becoming more withdrawn or more agitated and irritable.

Other behavioral signs include associating with a different crowd—people who seem "tough," who always want to "party," who don't work, or who appear interested in your relative's money. Or your relative may have started to have noticeable health problems, such as a bad cough, severe headaches, stomach pain, or "the shakes."

Another possible sign of covert substance abuse is your relative's inability to manage money. Or you may notice that cash or valuables are missing. Given that most individuals with schizophrenia have very limited funds, those who develop a serious substance abuse problem may steal to support their habit, including stealing from their own families. In one family the 25-year-old son with schizophrenia repeatedly sold his relatives' possessions (such as their TV set) to support his crack cocaine addiction.

Clinicians who work with your relative may be aware that he has a problem with alcohol or drugs, but many are not. Try to create open channels of communication with your relative's treatment team about his substance use (with your relative's permission) so you can all share information and perspectives.

Understanding Your Relative's Substance Use

From your perspective the negative effects of substance abuse may be so apparent that you are bewildered by your relative's use of drugs or alcohol. From your relative's perspective, however, substances have positive effects, and these—enhancing socialization, helping him cope with symptoms, providing pleasure, and simple habit—are what drive his use. Understanding these reasons can make it easier for you to help him overcome the problem.

Socialization

People with schizophrenia often have limited social outlets and fewer opportunities for meeting their social needs. Using substances is an easy way of connecting with people for those who have few friends. In addition, many people with schizophrenia began using substances with friends before they became ill, and continue to use to maintain these friendships. Drinking and using drugs with others can make people feel more "normal" and less stigmatized by their illness; they may feel accepted by others, gain a sense of group identity, and gain self-esteem.

Maryjo had always been shy and awkward around other people, even when she was a child and adolescent. She didn't have any close friends but confided to her parents and a school counselor that she wished she had some. In her senior year of high school Maryjo began to keep to herself even more, and then to talk about aliens controlling her mind. Maryjo was hospitalized and diagnosed with schizophrenia. Medications reduced her symptoms, but she was still rather awkward socially. She got her own apartment and started a supported education program. Near her apartment she met some young people who invited her to a party. She accepted, and at the party she was introduced to drugs, including marijuana and cocaine. The people at the party seemed to like her, and they didn't care that she went to the mental health center. She began spending more and more time with them—which meant using more drugs. She often had money problems and began

Body negative effect

to have conflicts with her landlord because of the parties she held at her apartment. She became addicted to crack cocaine, which worsened her symptoms and led her to engage in casual sex when she was high. Maryjo felt conflicted because she liked her friends and felt they accepted her, but her life was a mess in terms of her finances, her housing, her symptoms, and her relationship with her parents.

Before Eric developed schizophrenia he had been a social teenager. In high school he had enjoyed hanging out with his buddies, which often included drinking and smoking pot together. Even after high school, when Eric and most of his friends got jobs or went to a local community college, they continued to spend quite a bit of their free time together, carousing, drinking, and smoking. Two years after graduating from high school Eric began to experience bouts of depression and anxiety and had difficulty concentrating at his job in an auto repair shop. Over the next year his behavior became strange, and his friends talked with his family, who finally persuaded him to see a doctor. An examination indicated that Eric was experiencing symptoms of schizophrenia–including hearing voices and believing that others could control his thoughts–and he was hospitalized. Eric was prescribed an antipsychotic medication, which cleared up most of his psychotic symptoms, although he felt tired and low on energy.

After Eric left the hospital, he returned to his job and to socializing with his friends. He tried to pick up where he had left off with his friends, including using alcohol and smoking pot regularly, but now the effects of those substances were more profound. Sometimes when he drank he became irritable or threatening, and smoking pot tended to bring back his psychotic symptoms. Eric was confused because he had always enjoyed drinking and smoking, but now he couldn't seem to handle either. Even so, he didn't want to stop using because he valued spending time with his friends.

Coping with Symptoms

Many of the symptoms of schizophrenia can be distressing, and some people use substances in an attempt to manage them through *self-medication*. Someone with auditory hallucinations may drink heavily to escape hearing voices; someone with negative symptoms may abuse stimulants to increase his energy level. Any substance may temporarily alleviate feelings of anxiety, depression, or irritability. Particularly for people who have not yet developed personal recovery goals and are not future-oriented, these short-term benefits may seem to outweigh the long-term costs in worsening of symptoms.

Twenty-six-year-old Ivan took medication but continued to have psychotic symptoms, including persistent auditory hallucinations that told him he was no good and should kill himself and delusions that other people could read his "impure thoughts." He also had severe depression, anxiety, suicidal thoughts, and difficulty sleeping. Despite these symptoms, Ivan sometimes played music, drank, and used a variety of drugs with several friends. He was prone to drinking both with them and on his own. He was aware that in the long run drinking seemed to worsen his depression and suicidality. But in the short run he found it gave him some relief from his hallucinations, depression, anxiety, and sleep difficulties; he would often drink until he passed out—which gave him a break from his troubling symptoms.

Pleasure

If alcohol or drugs did not cause pleasurable feelings, these substances would not be addictive. People with schizophrenia are particularly prone to using alcohol or drugs because they often have few other leisure and recreational activities, and they suffer from boredom. Their lack of friends, work, and money may further limit their involvement in enjoyable activities. Using alcohol and drugs provides an immediate source of pleasure that may fill an important gap in your relative's life.

Habit or Routine

Sometimes people use substances for such a long period of time that using becomes a habit important in its own right. If your relative is physically addicted he may use the substance in response to cravings or to avoid unpleasant withdrawal symptoms. He also may use the substance because the routine he has established provides needed structure to his daily life. Everyone has a need for meaning and purpose in life, and for some individuals that meaning is provided by maintaining an addiction to alcohol or drugs.

Edgar was addicted to crack cocaine. Every morning he got up around 7:00 A.M. and went to the local train, subway, or bus station, where he would panhandle for money. By 9:00 or 10:00 A.M. he had usually accumulated enough money to buy some crack, so he would go to a local "crack house," where he would purchase some of the drug and smoke it. After he had finished smoking and the effects of the crack had worn off, Edgar would go to his local mental health center, where he participated in a group. Sometimes later in the evening Edgar would hook up with friends and get some more crack, but not on a regular basis. When he talked over his addiction with his sister, he said he liked the feeling crack gave him—it made him feel alert and "with it." Edgar also said he liked to have something to look forward to, and it gave him a reason to get up in the morning.

Evaluating Your Relative's Reasons for Using Substances

You may already know some of the reasons your relative uses substances from things he has said in the past. You may also find it helpful to broach the topic with him. Remember that, when doing so, your goal is to *understand* why he uses substances, not to pass judgment or change behavior. You can complete the Reasons for Using Substances Checklist (Worksheet 22.2) at the end of the chapter, if possible with your relative, to summarize his most important motives for using substances.

How You Can Help

Your special relationship with your relative puts you in a unique position to help her overcome substance use problems. But first you need to understand the natural change process through which people come to grips with having an addiction and make a personal decision to take back control over their lives.

The Stages of Change

The *stages of change* is a useful concept that describes the process most people go through when they decide to change a problem behavior, such as abusing substances, smoking, or being overweight. The stages of change were described by James Prochaska, PhD, and Carlo DiClemente, PhD, include precontemplation, contemplation, preparation, action, and maintenance. At the *precontemplation stage* the person isn't even thinking about changing her substance use behavior, whereas thoughts about change do occur during the *contemplation stage.* During the *preparation stage* the person has decided she wants to change and starts making plans to reduce or stop using substances. These plans are then implemented in the *action stage.* The *maintenance stage* is focused on preventing relapses of substance use or abuse.

The stages of change underscore the fact that recovery from substance abuse is a gradual process, involving first the development of awareness of the problem, then motivation, and then the skills and support for changing behavior and developing a healthier lifestyle. By identifying which stage of change your relative is in, you can help him progress to the next stage while avoiding alienating him by pushing too hard. The table on the facing page provides specific strategies and suggestions for helping your relative progress through the different stages of change.

Keeping Channels of Communication Open

Talking with your relative about her substance abuse is the first and most important step in dealing with the problem. Most people who abuse alcohol or drugs deny or minimize their problem, so they must see that it's a problem if they are to work toward solving it. Your best chance of helping them do this is by keeping channels of communication open.

When talking to your relative, your immediate goals are to open the channels of communication, express your concerns, and understand your relative's perspective. Your longer-term goals are to help your relative see that his sub-

Tips for Helping Your Relative through the Stages of Change from Substance Abuse to Sobriety

Stage of change	Definition	Helping tips
Precontemplation	Your relative is not thinking about changing his/her substance use.	• Avoid blaming and "guilt-tripping" your relative. • Express your concerns directly. • Ask if your relative is concerned about his/her substance use.
Contemplation	Your relative is thinking about changing his/her substance use.	• Encourage your relative to talk about change without pressuring him/her. • Explore with your relative how his/her life could be better with sobriety. • Ask nonjudgmental questions to help your relative consider possible problems related to substance use (e.g., relapses and rehospitalizations, money problems, difficulties with relationships).
Preparation	Your relative is preparing to change his/her substance use behavior.	• Discuss with your relative the merits and disadvantages of cutting down on substance use vs. abstinence. • Help your relative make plans to deal with high-risk situations for using substances (e.g., symptom flareup, social situations, boredom). • Keep motivation to change high by talking about how sobriety will improve your relative's life.
Action	Your relative reduces or stops using substances.	• Provide lots of support for efforts to change. • Problem-solve together how to handle difficult situations (e.g., offers to use substances, cravings to use). • Don't get too discouraged by your relative's "slips" or "relapses" and understand these as part of the natural recovery process. • Remind your relative of his/her reasons for becoming sober. • Talk with your relative about possible benefits of self-help groups (e.g., AA, dual recovery).
Maintenance	Your relative has changed and wants to remain sober.	• Praise your relative for his/her accomplishments in becoming sober. • Focus attention on other important life areas (e.g., health, relationships, independence, work). • Support involvement in a self-help group (e.g., AA, dual recovery). • Continue to help your relative handle difficult situations, if needed (e.g., offers to use, cravings).

stance use is a problem and develop a plan for dealing with this problem. When talking, express your concerns directly—use "I" statements and "feeling" statements ("I feel worried," "I feel upset," "I feel irritated") and be specific. Try to understand your relative's perspective by being a good listener and using reflective listening skills (see Chapter 14). Be firm rather than meek, but avoid being judgmental or expressing outrage or strong anger. Anger is natural, but expressing it too strongly and blaming your relative may discourage him from talking with you about the problem.

Identifying Advantages and Disadvantages of Substance Abuse

People with an addiction are often reluctant to talk about the negative effects of their substance use before the positive side has been acknowledged. By using Worksheet 22.3 at the end of the chapter, you can help your relative construct a written list of both the advantages and disadvantages of using substances. Seeing a comprehensive written list may make it obvious to your relative that the disadvantages of using substances outweigh the advantages. You can discuss the list with her to see whether it can help her make a decision about changing her substance use habits.

> *Nicholas had experienced problems with drinking and smoking marijuana for several years. With the help of his parents, he made a list of the advantages and disadvantages of using substances. The advantages he identified included:*
>
> 1. *It relaxes me.*
> 2. *It's fun to do with friends.*
> 3. *It reduces boredom.*
> 4. *I sleep better after drinking.*
> 5. *Smoking pot makes me feel "high."*
>
> *The list of disadvantages included:*
>
> 1. *I often run out of money before the end of the month.*
> 2. *Smoking pot sometimes makes me paranoid.*
> 3. *I feel groggy the day after I've been drinking.*
> 4. *Sometimes it makes the voices worse.*
> 5. *It causes tension between me and my parents.*
> 6. *I still feel depressed after drinking or smoking pot.*

Developing Alternatives to Substance Use

Recognizing the disadvantages of using drugs or alcohol may motivate your relative to work on the problem, but only if you acknowledge the need the substance use answers and consider alternatives for getting those needs met. You'll want to think together about alternatives like developing more rewarding relationships, coping more effectively with symptoms, finding enjoyable outlets for spending free time, and having something meaningful to do every day.

Developing alternatives to using substances can be hard work. However, helping your relative develop these alternatives is critical to creating a quality life free from the effects of alcohol and drugs. A combination of strategies described in this book can be useful in developing alternatives to substance use:

- Problem-solving methods (Chapter 15) can be used to brainstorm possible alternative activities and make plans for pursuing them.
- Part V describes a wide range of strategies for helping your relative cope more effectively with different symptoms.
- Chapter 25 addresses ways to improve social relationships.
- Chapter 28 addresses ways to improve leisure time.
- Chapter 26 discusses how to pursue meaningful goals related to work and school.

The following sections provide pointers to consider when helping your relative develop alternatives to substance use.

Socialization

If your relative uses alcohol or drugs with friends, she will have to learn how to socialize with them without using substances or make new friends who don't abuse drugs or alcohol. Learning how to refuse offers of alcohol or drugs from friends requires assertiveness skills, such as good eye contact, speaking in a firm tone of voice, and repeatedly saying "no" if the other person persists. You can help improve your relative's assertiveness by doing brief role plays of social situations. You or other family members can play the role of friends offering or pressuring your relative to use substances. After each role play, provide your relative with specific feedback about what she did well and how her performance could be improved.

Spending time with new friends may be challenging if your relative has close and long-standing relationships with many friends who use alcohol and drugs and knows few people who don't. Developing new friendships might require a major change such as getting a job, returning to school, or living somewhere else, such as in a structured living situation. On the other hand, if some of your relative's friends use substances and others don't, you can focus your efforts on helping your relative decrease contact with some friends while increasing it with others. If your relative's relationships are not very close, developing new friends may be a viable option.

Pleasure

As mentioned earlier, many people with schizophrenia seek pleasure from drugs because it is so rare in their lives. But sometimes they fail to realize they've given up some forms of recreation *because* of their substance abuse. In that case, it may be helpful to explore with your relative which of the activities she used to enjoy might be worth trying again. An important consideration when trying to help your relative develop alternative sources of pleasure is *time*. Drugs or alcohol produce rapid, positive effects, whereas more time is required for other sources of enjoyment. For your relative to continue to be motivated to develop alternative leisure activities, he will need help dealing with the craving for alcohol or drugs. Problem solving with your relative about how to deal with cravings can be helpful in this regard. Strategies include reminding himself of personal recovery goals that are incompatible with using substances, using positive self-statements to promote coping with urges to use, employing imagery to remind himself of the negative effects of substance abuse, using distraction to shift his focus of attention, and getting support from someone who endorses his sobriety.

Coping with Symptoms

Similar to helping your relative develop alternative leisure activities, learning coping strategies can take time. Some of your relative's symptoms may be caused by her substance abuse, either partly or completely, but it's usually impossible to know which symptoms are caused by substances and which by other problems, so exploring coping strategies for distressing symptoms may be useful in any case. In addition, working with your relative to explore whether substances are worsening problematic symptoms, and learning more effective ways of coping with symptoms, can instill hope in your relative that she can live a better life without the illusory crutch of alcohol and drugs.

Involvement in Structured Activities

The more unstructured time your relative has, the more opportunities he has to use alcohol and drugs. If your relative lacks a regular routine and structured activities, work toward structuring his time. Structured activities can add more meaning and purpose to his life as well as reduce the opportunities for using alcohol and drugs.

Understand that your relative may resist suggestions to increase the structure of her day because she's doing what seems natural and may see little reason to change. It might be easier to motivate her if you discuss how involvement in specific structured activities is related to her longer-term goals; for example, her participation in a peer support program or a social skills training group may help her make new friends or get a job (which means more money and greater independence). However, other steps may also be necessary. In the next section we discuss how to use contingencies (positive and negative consequences) to reduce substance abuse and encourage more positive behaviors.

Establishing Contingencies

Even if your relative is not highly motivated to change, you may be able to alter his use of alcohol or drugs by establishing specific *rewards* for abstinence and specific *costs* for substance use (contingencies). The use of contingencies will be most effective if your relative lives at home with you or if you provide significant financial support to him, but most critical is that you follow through systematically.

The principles of establishing contingencies are quite simple, as you saw regarding consequences for breaking household rules (Chapter 16). Positive consequences of a behavior increase that behavior; negative consequences decrease the behavior. These principles are outlined in the table on page 344.

The Samuelson family had a household rule that prohibited smoking marijuana in the house. Oliver, the member with schizophrenia, sometimes liked to smoke marijuana in his room, and his parents could easily smell it. His parents decided to establish the contingency that Oliver would lose $10 per week of spending money if he smoked in the house. If Oliver smoked in the house more than once during the week, he would lose an additional $10 spending money for each instance. His parents agreed that evidence of "smoking" would be determined by smelling marijuana smoke in the house or finding remnants of a smoked joint. When they presented their plan to Oliver, he objected, saying they might find remnants of previous use and think he was currently smoking. After some discussion, he agreed to take responsibility for systematically going through the house and removing any signs of previous smoking.

The first week, Oliver did not take the plan seriously, and his parents smelled smoke or discovered remnants of a joint on three occasions. They calmly spoke to him each time, letting him know that this would result in reduced spending money for the coming week. When they got together for their weekly meeting, his parents pointed out that they would be giving him $30 less in spending money for the coming week. He objected, saying he wouldn't have enough money for personal expenses, but his parents were firm. Over the next month Oliver continued to lose $20 to $30 in spending money per week, but over the course of the next 3 months the instances of smoking gradually decreased, and he had several successful weeks of not smoking in the house. This contingency plan was helpful for addressing Oliver's smoking in the house but did not affect his marijuana use in other situations, for which other strategies were needed, including helping him deal with boredom and lack of social outlets by finding a part-time job in an area of his interest.

Because using contingencies to alter substance use behavior is hard work and takes time, this approach may not be feasible for some families. Getting an accurate assessment of a person's substance use behavior is often a challenge, but without it you won't know whether imposing consequences has had any effect. Some people are also reluctant to make their relative's life any worse (by imposing a consequence like removal of certain privileges), even if only tempo-

Steps in Establishing Contingencies for Relatives with Schizophrenia

Decide which behaviors you want to increase and which you want to decrease:

1. Work at increasing helpful behaviors as well as decreasing unhelpful behaviors.
2. Consider increasing behaviors that are positive alternatives to substance use.
3. Identify one or two behaviors of each type to work on, but not more.
4. Be as specific as possible.

Decide how these behaviors will be measured, when, and by whom:

5. Look for objective measures of behavior (measures that more than one person can verify).
6. Consider possible problems with measuring a behavior.
7. Decide how often and at what times each behavior will be measured.
8. Decide who will monitor and record the behaviors.

Determine consequences for each behavior:

9. Identify positive consequences for behaviors that you want to increase.
10. Choose positive consequences that are valued by your relative, over which you have control, and which are readily available.
11. Try to shape behaviors you want to increase by providing positive consequences for small steps in the right direction.
12. Identify negative consequences for behaviors that you want to decrease.
13. Choose negative consequences that involve the loss of something valued by your relative (such as TV time), are under your control, and will not result in harm to your relative.

Draw up a specific plan to implement the program:

14. Write down the plan, including:
    - Definitions of the behaviors
    - Who will measure the behaviors and when
    - The specific consequences for each behavior, who will provide the consequences, and when
15. Present the plan to your relative. Decide on a time to meet to follow up on the plan (not more than a week later).

Follow up on the plan and modify it as necessary:

16. Meet regularly to evaluate whether the plan is working as intended.
17. Check to see that consequences have been provided as planned.
18. Modify behaviors and consequences as necessary in order to promote more change.
19. If helpful behaviors do not increase, consider:
    - Are the positive consequences really "positive" for your relative? If not, identify different positive consequences.
    - Is too much behavioral change expected? If so, focus on a smaller increase in behavior and shape larger increases gradually, over time.
20. If unhelpful behaviors do not change, consider:
    - Are the negative consequences really "negative" for the person? If not, identify other negative consequences.
    - Is too much behavior change expected? If so, focus on a smaller decrease in behavior and decrease the behavior gradually over time.

rarily. If you feel this way, remind yourself that reducing substance abuse is in your relative's long-term best interest, and that she may not be able to make this change on her own. You could also stick to positive consequences, giving your relative something extra (such as money or use of the family car) for not using substances. Research in the substance abuse treatment field has shown that giving people money for not using substances helps them achieve abstinence.

Participation in Self-Help Groups

A wide range of self-help groups are available to those with substance use problems. Most of these groups, such as Alcoholics Anonymous (AA) or Rational Recovery, are appropriate for anyone with such a problem. Some groups, such as Dual Recovery Anonymous, are designed for people with a psychiatric disorder and substance abuse problems. Many people with schizophrenia find that these groups provide them with support in combating the urge to use drugs or alcohol, though obviously some awareness that substance abuse is a problem is a prerequisite. You and other family members may find it helpful to attend self-help groups for relatives, such as Al-Anon.

Self-help groups do not, however, work for everyone. People with schizophrenia often report feeling awkward at AA meetings, in part because most participants do not have a psychiatric disorder and in part because some people in self-help groups such as AA have an outdated perspective on mental illness and believe that using any form of medication amounts to a continued dependence on substances. Such an attitude can make someone with a psychiatric illness feel uncomfortable and may discourage adherence to prescribed medication. Many of these problems can be avoided if Dual Recovery Anonymous groups are available in your area. The personalities and dynamics of self-help groups for substance abuse problems vary from one group to the next, even within the same organization. If your relative is willing to consider a self-help group, it may be helpful to encourage her to shop around by attending several different groups to find one that is a good match.

Helping Your Relative Get Professional Treatment

Many people with schizophrenia and substance use problems benefit from professional help. Helping your relative become motivated to seek professional help can play a vital role in his recovery.

Integrated Treatment

Until recently, the treatment of people with dual disorders was fragmented, with mental health services provided by some agencies and substance abuse services provided by others. This fragmentation created many problems for people with schizophrenia, who often had difficulty accessing substance abuse treatment services and failed to benefit from traditional, confrontational approaches to these disorders when services were finally obtained. Fortunately, there has been a movement toward integrating mental health and substance abuse treatments so that services for both disorders are provided by the same team of professionals in a coordinated and integrated fashion.

A variety of treatments may be available at your local community mental health center to help your relative address her substance use problems. Individual treatment approaches are aimed at establishing a good therapeutic relationship with the person, developing motivation to work on substance abuse together, and working toward reducing substance use and preventing relapses of substance abuse. Several different group approaches are often used to help people with dual disorders deal with their substance use problems. Some groups are specifically oriented toward helping people develop motivation to work on their substance abuse problems through discussions among group members and education about the effects of drugs and alcohol (*persuasion groups*), whereas other groups focus on helping people stop using and on preventing relapses (*active treatment groups*). Social skills training groups may focus specifically on the social aspects of substance use, such as dealing with social situations in which substance use occurs (e.g., how to respond to pressure to use) as well as developing rewarding relationships with people who do not use substances. Some dual disorder groups combine education, motivational coaching, the prevention of relapses, and social skills training into a single approach.

Family programs may also be a helpful venue for addressing substance abuse in people with schizophrenia and reducing its effects on family members. These programs usually involve teaching family members, including the person with schizophrenia, about the nature of both disorders, the principles of their treatment, and the negative effects of alcohol and drug use on the course of schizophrenia. In addition, family work often includes helping families improve their communication and problem-solving skills and developing plans for supporting sobriety in the loved one.

Detoxification

When a person is physically dependent on drugs or alcohol, detoxification is often required to safely take the person off the substances without adverse medical consequences, such as seizures. Although detoxification can be done safely on an outpatient basis, inpatient detoxification is more common, with most programs lasting between 5 and 30 days. In addition to the goals of getting the alcohol and drugs out of the person's system and attending to medication needs, inpatient treatment can begin the process of instilling motivation in the person to begin working on substance use problems.

Residential Treatment

For people with schizophrenia and severe substance use disorders, residential treatment programs offer promise. Residential programs generally last for at least 3 months and up to a year or more, with the longer programs being more effective. There are several unique advantages to these programs over other available treatments for people with dual disorders. First, such programs provide a higher level of structure than can be achieved in ordinary outpatient settings, which is beneficial for some people with schizophrenia. Second, residential programs remove people from their customary environments, thus decreasing or eliminating their exposure to many of the cues that triggered alcohol and drug use, such as friends, bars, and parties. Third, the focus of residential programs on helping people manage urges to use substances, develop alternative coping strategies, and improve social skills and self-control provides a more intensive treatment experience than would be possible on an outpatient basis.

Residential programs for dual disorders are not widely available, and the private programs tend to be very expensive. Programs for those receiving public mental health services are, however, increasingly being funded through a variety of local, state, and federal agencies, such as the U.S. Department of Housing and Urban Development.

Effective programs for dual disorders differ from those for people with only substance abuse problems in several ways. Like outpatient services for people with dual disorders, residential programs avoid the strong confrontational approaches often employed in programs for primary substance abuse; such approaches can be unduly stressful for people with schizophrenia. Residential programs for dual disorders also attend to participants' mental illnesses as well as their substance use problems, which may involve helping them learn more about their psychiatric disorder and its treatment, develop more effective strategies for coping with symptoms, and improve self-care and social skills to promote independent living. These programs for dual disorders are most effective when they are provided in the same community in which the person lives and involve a gradual transition from the residence back into the community (usually occurring over many months, at a minimum).

Helping Yourself

Living with a relative who has schizophrenia and substance use problems can be strenuous and create tension among family members. In your efforts to help your relative, it's important not to sacrifice your own and other family members' peace of mind. Ultimately, family conflict will only make your relative's problems worse, which will increase the stress on everyone. It's vital that you take measures like the following to attend to your own needs and those of other family members.

Sticking Together

Substance abuse in a family member can have an extremely divisive effect on the rest of the family, at times pitting one family member against another. For example, when the family member with schizophrenia is an offspring, conflicts often arise between the parents about how to handle problems. To avoid the effects of substance abuse in your family, you need to stick together and take a team approach to the problem. A team approach requires family members to reach a consensus about the problem and how to go about dealing with it. It's important to iron out major disagreements between you and other family members *before* you include the person with substance abuse in discussions about how to handle the problem. If this consensus is achieved, you'll be able to present a unified front and avoid sending conflicting messages. Because continued efforts are usually required to have an impact on substance abuse, discussions among family members need to be held on a regular basis.

Considering Alternative Living Arrangements

Some people with schizophrenia who have serious substance use problems are difficult to treat when they are living at home with family members, but improve when they live in the community with supported housing or in a more structured environment, such as a residential program. It's very difficult for family members to closely monitor their relative's substance use at home, and attempting to do so can cause significant friction among members. If your relative lives at home and you've been unsuccessful in altering his dependence on drugs or alcohol, you should consider alternative living situations for him. You may feel as if you're abandoning your relative, but you're actually acting in his best interest, as well as the best interests of the rest of your family.

Striving to Maintain Your Family Relationships

Many people with dual disorders recover from their substance use problems and enjoy a good quality of life. However, some continue to suffer from both problems for a very long time, with either chronic or intermittent substance abuse throughout much of their lives. The effects of substance abuse on family relationships can be devastating; feelings of demoralization, anger, resentment, sadness, and anxiety may dominate. Many of these feelings may be directed toward the person with the dual disorder, although strife between other family members is also common.

When a substance use problem persists for a long time, it's important to take steps to minimize its effects on everyone in your family. This includes trying to accept the fact that substance abuse is a disorder that can be similar to schizophrenia and that your relative may not be able to fully control it. In such situations it's best to strive to maintain a loving relationship with your relative, despite her problems, and to accept the substance abuse as something that is either unlikely to change or will change only very slowly over many years. Accepting your relative may mean taking steps to minimize the effects of the substance use on your relationship. For example, you may choose not to allow your relative to live at home and not to spend time with her when she has been drinking or using drugs, but still try to keep communication open and let your relative know that you love her. Working toward accepting your relative's substance use problems and minimizing strife among other family members may prove invaluable in maintaining your family strengths and commitments to one another.

The Torino family, with parents Giuseppe and Lucia, had been through a lot even before their youngest son, Nino, developed schizophrenia. Problems with substance use ran in the Torino family. Giuseppe's father had died of complications related to alcoholism, one of his brothers had an alcohol disorder, and Giuseppe himself was a recovering alcoholic who had attended AA for years. Lucia's uncle and one of her brothers had problems with alcohol and drugs, and although Lucia had experimented with drugs in her youth, she had stopped using when she had children. Nino's older brother and sister also had their problems with substance abuse; his brother was addicted to alcohol, and his sister was in and out of substance abuse rehabilitation programs. Nino had developed substance use problems early on; he was drinking by the time he was 12 and using a host of other substances, including heroin, by the time he was 16. However, Giuseppe and Lucia were totally unprepared when Nino developed schizophrenia at age 18 and his–and the family's–problems multiplied.

The Torino family spent the next decade in tumult, learning about schizophrenia, trying to set limits on Nino's behavior, and trying to hold their family together. After several years, Giuseppe and Lucia decided that it was too chaotic to have Nino live at home, and too destructive to their relationship, so Nino moved out on his own. Throughout these years, Nino's substance use problems continued unabated, with heroin addiction being his major problem. Nino was in and out of substance abuse programs and tried methadone several times, but always resumed using heroin. Giuseppe and Lucia were concerned about Nino getting infectious diseases, so they got information for him about how to obtain clean needles through the city's needle exchange program.

Despite their many challenges, the Torino family members remained close to each other and continued to see and support each other. The parents maintained contact with their children, including Nino, and often had him over for meals. Nino's parents gradually came to accept his substance use problems while maintaining a loving relationship with him. Lucia said, "I still hope that he's going to recover from this and pull his life back together again, but I'm not counting on it. More important, I know he'll always be my son and that I'll always love him. And I know Giuseppe feels the same way, and that we always have each other." Giuseppe said, "These have been some tough years, and we got a lot of support from other families at NAMI and Al-Anon meetings. I still enjoy Nino, seeing him and laughing with him, and we'll always be a family."

Smoking and Schizophrenia

Cigarette smoking is one of the most common health risks associated with schizophrenia, with approximately 80% of people with the illness smoking, compared with less than 20% of the general population. No one knows why people with schizophrenia smoke so much, although many different explanations have been proposed. Nicotine has stimulating effects, and it has been suggested that people with schizophrenia may smoke partly to improve their attention and concentration. Some people report that smoking helps their negative symptoms, including feelings of apathy, withdrawal, and lack of pleasure. Smoking may also be a way to fill time and to fight boredom.

What we do know is that smoking causes lung cancer and emphysema, exacerbates money problems since cigarettes are expensive, and can be a fire hazard (from falling asleep with a lit cigarette). Because of these problems, many people with schizophrenia and their relatives are interested in stopping smoking.

Helping Your Relative Stop Smoking

Although many people with schizophrenia want to stop smoking, others are ambivalent or not interested. It's important to respect your relative's right to make this decision, but you can still explore his interest in quitting and express your feelings about his smoking without exerting too much pressure.

Many of the strategies for addressing alcohol and drug abuse problems described in this chapter may be useful in addressing your relative's smoking, including the concept of stages of change. Compiling a list with your relative of the advantages and disadvantages of smoking may be helpful in highlighting the advantages of quitting and identifying possible obstacles to quitting. This can set the stage for exploring with your relative other ways of getting needs met that are currently met by smoking.

In addition to the strategies described earlier in this chapter, you can try several strategies specific to smoking cessation.

Self-Monitoring Smoking

One useful way to help people reduce their smoking is to encourage them to self-monitor it by keeping track of the number of cigarettes smoked per day. This can be done by indicating each time a cigarette is smoked in a small record book or by keeping a running tally on the refrigerator or a wall calendar. Information about when cigarettes are smoked can be helpful when it comes to changing one's habits, and it can be used to set daily goals of reduced smoking.

Gradually Cutting Down

Many people with schizophrenia stop smoking by gradually cutting down over a very long period of time. This method works because it involves a minimum of stress, and the person avoids some of the unpleasant symptoms of nicotine withdrawal. Gradually cutting down is most effective when the person sets a goal of reducing the number of cigarettes smoked each day at a comfortable pace—for example, by smoking only one or two cigarettes per hour and then smoking two or three fewer cigarettes per day every week or two. To make this method work, you should collaborate with your relative in developing a system for keeping track of the number of cigarettes smoked each day and then making it inconvenient to smoke more than intended. For example, each morning (or the night before) you can set aside the designated number of cigarettes for that day.

Saving Money in a Special Account

Another strategy for building incentive to reduce cigarette smoking is to help your relative establish a special account for money that would otherwise be spent on cigarettes. Watching the account grow provides a tangible reward for the efforts involved in cutting down. It also might help to plan with your relative how she would like to spend some of that money.

Michael, who had schizoaffective disorder, smoked about a pack and a half a day, and his wife, Barbara, really wanted him to quit. She was bothered by his smoking at home, partly because of her concerns over exposure to secondhand smoke for their two daughters. She was also concerned about Michael's health; he often had a hacking cough in the morning and easily ran out of breath, even though he was only in his early 40s. Michael also wanted to stop smoking because of its effects on his health and his family. Michael and Barbara talked about his cutting down, and they decided together to build an additional incentive into the plan. Michael enjoyed playing the guitar, and he wanted to get a new guitar. Barbara suggested they set aside half of the money Michael would have spent on cigarettes for a new guitar. Each week they would meet to review how the account stood. After 4 months of cutting down, and a month of not smoking at all, Michael had saved enough money to buy the guitar he wanted.

Using Pharmacological Aids

Many people stop smoking with the assistance of nicotine replacement therapy. The nicotine patch or gum can help satisfy the physical dependence on nicotine while your relative works on breaking the behavioral habit. Then, as he conquers the habit of smoking, he can gradually reduce his physical dependence on nicotine.

Certain medications can also help. Specifically, the antidepressant bu-proprion (marketed with the brand names of Wellbutrin and Zyban) has been shown to help people stop smoking. Medication can also be combined with nicotine replacement methods.

Joining a Quit-Smoking Group

People often benefit from the social support they receive when they choose to quit smoking with a group of other individuals. Quit-smoking groups typically follow a stepwise plan that takes place over a period of a few months and includes increasing motivation for stopping, making a plan, cutting down gradually, and maintaining a smoke-free lifestyle—conducted in the context of a mutually supportive, structured group of individuals. A wide range of quit-smoking groups are available in most communities. Doing research on the Internet, contacting a local hospital or the American Lung Association, or checking in the newspaper are easy approaches to finding a group. Quit-smoking groups that are designed specifically for people with a mental illness may also be available at your relative's local community mental health center.

Pursuing Other Health-Related Concerns

Sometimes the best way for a person to get motivated to work on smoking is to get involved in improving another aspect of her life. Many people get interested in quitting smoking after they've made headway in conquering drug or alcohol problems. Others may become motivated to work on smoking as they attend to health concerns involving diet, exercise, and weight or as they begin to participate in a sport. Exploring health concerns with your relative may indirectly spur her interest in working on smoking.

Eunice had been a cross-country runner in high school before she developed schizophrenia, started smoking, and began living a sedentary lifestyle. Although she knew smoking was bad for her, she was not interested in cutting down. Eunice's brother, Liam, knew how happy she had been as a runner in high school, and he began talking about running with her. Gradually, Eunice became interested in running again. With Liam's help, she developed a plan that involved slowly building up her distance–starting with alternating walking and running laps. After 2 months Eunice was beginning to get into shape, and she no longer alternated walking with running. However, she complained to Liam that she ran out of breath easily and, after talking about it with him, concluded that her smoking was interfering with running. Eunice began to cut down from almost two packs a day; then, after a month, she decided to go "cold turkey" and stop altogether. Stopping smoking helped Eunice with her running, and the next year she began entering local races.

Rising to the Challenge

Substance use problems are among the most common difficulties experienced by people with schizophrenia, and they can be perplexing to family members and professionals alike. Despite the many problems associated with drug and alcohol use, such as relapses and rehospitalizations, people with schizophrenia often continue to use. Similarly, cigarette smoking is extremely common in people with schizophrenia despite its well-established health consequences.

Don't get discouraged by the challenge of helping your relative conquer his substance use problems. Recovery from addiction is possible and all the more likely with the love and support of family members. Following these five steps will likely help your relative tackle his addiction:

1. Open a dialogue so you can talk about using substances with your relative in a nonblaming, nonjudgmental way.
2. Try to understand why your relative uses substances.
3. Enhance your relative's motivation to stop using by exploring how quitting will help her achieve personal goals.
4. Help your relative develop new ways of getting his basic needs met, such as coping with symptoms, socializing, enjoying himself, and having a meaningful daily structure.
5. Explore possible resources at your community mental health center (such as groups) or in your community (such as AA or Dual Recovery Anonymous) that may help your relative maintain her sobriety.

Resources

Books

Daley, D. C., & Spear, J. (2003). *A family guide to coping with dual disorders: Addiction and psychiatric illness* (rev. ed.). Center City, MI: Hazelden. How to maintain a relationship and help a loved one struggling with an addiction and mental illness.

Mueser, K. T., Noordsy, D. L., Drake, R. E., & Fox, L. (2003). *Integrated treatment for dual disorders: A guide to effective practice*. New York: Guilford Press. This is a comprehensive guide to the treatment of substance abuse in people with major mental illnesses, such as schizophrenia.

Prochaska, J. O., Norcross, J. C., & DiClemente, C. C. (1994). *Changing for good*. New York: Avon Books. This book is about changing one's health behavior and is written by the experts who formulated the concept of stages of change.

Washington, A., Moll, S., Pawlick, J., & Goldberg, J. O. (1997). *Smokebusters: An approach to help people with a mental illness move closer to a smoke free lifestyle*. Hamilton, Ontario, Canada: CSVR Foundation. Available from Smokebusters, c/o Hamilton Program for Schizophrenia, 102–350 King St. East, Hamilton, Ontario, Canada, L8N3Y3.

Self-Help Organizations

Al-Anon. This organization is related to AA and is designed for relatives of people with substance use disorders. *www.al-anon.alateen.org*.

Alcoholics Anonymous (AA). This is the most widely available self-help organization for people with alcohol problems, with meetings held in public places (such as local churches) in local communities. Similar organizations exist for other substances, such as Narcotics Anonymous. *www.alcoholics-anonymous.org*.

Dual Recovery Anonymous. This organization is based on the principles of AA, adapted for people with a major mental illness. *www.draonline.org*.

Substance Abuse Effects Checklist

Instructions: Check off the consequences of using substances that your relative has experienced.

Consequences of substance use	Check below
Symptom relapses	
Psychiatric rehospitalizations	
Interpersonal problems with family or friends	
Money problems	
Getting in trouble with the law	
Increased anger or aggression	
Problems with depression or suicidal thoughts	
Infectious diseases such as hepatitis C	
Interference with school, work, or parenting	
Use in dangerous situations	
Spending large amounts of time using or obtaining substances	
Repeated unsuccessful efforts to cut down	
Using more than intended	
Development of tolerance to substance(s)	
Withdrawal symptoms or cravings	
Blackouts or lapses in memory when using	

Reasons for Using Substances Checklist

Instructions: Check off the reasons for substance abuse that your relative has demonstrated or expressed to you.

	Check below
Socialization	
Substance use in social situations	
Substance use with peers before onset of illness	
Desire to be with other people	
Limited other social opportunities	
Coping with Symptoms or Side Effects	
Substance use when alone	
Persistent, distressing symptoms (e.g., hallucinations)	
Severe depression or anxiety	
Medication side effects (e.g., restlessness)	
Pleasure	
Few leisure activities	
Lack of close relationships	
Boredom; not working	
Other Reasons	
Prevent withdrawal symptoms	
Craving	
Habit	
Gives structure and meaning to his/her day	
Something to look forward to	

Advantages and Disadvantages
of Using Drugs or Alcohol

Instructions: Write down all of the advantages you can identify for using drugs or alcohol and all of the disadvantages. Try to think of every possible advantage and disadvantage.

Advantages	Disadvantages
1.	1.
2.	2.
3.	3.
4.	4.
5.	5.
6.	6.
7.	7.
8.	8.
9.	9.
10.	10.
11.	11.
12.	12.
13.	13.
14.	14.
15.	15.

CHAPTER 23

Anger and Violence

A lthough people with schizophrenia are more likely to be withdrawn than aggressive, problems with anger and violence do occur more often than in the general population. And when aggression or violence does occur, family members are most likely to be the victims. For these reasons, family members need effective strategies for dealing with anger, minimizing the possibility of violence, and protecting themselves and others in situations where violence is possible.

Anger and Violence in Schizophrenia

Angry feelings are a relatively common problem in people with schizophrenia, and they can create special challenges for family members and other caring individuals. Anger is a natural emotion that is a response to frustration or the belief that one has been wronged. People with schizophrenia have many things to feel frustrated about. They may hear voices that put them down or distract them and can interfere with engaging in "normal" life pursuits such as working and having close relationships. Feelings of depression and anxiety may abound, making it hard to pursue goals. Negative symptoms may sap their energy and squash their motivation to pursue goals and better themselves, even when they have the necessary skills and resources. Cognitive difficulties may make it hard to concentrate or solve problems, leading to more frustration.

People with schizophrenia may also be unhappy because it's harder for them to enjoy the fruits of a good life, such as working at a rewarding job, earning significant amounts of money, living in a nice house, and having fulfilling relationships. Their lives are more difficult than the lives of others, which can lead to the belief that the world is unfair and that they've been wronged. Furthermore, the stigma of mental illness can lead to angry feelings when they are rejected or feared by others who don't even know them. It's easy to understand why having schizophrenia can be a frustrating experience.

Recognizing Anger in Your Relative

Your relative may express his anger in a number of different ways; he may be irritable, easily annoyed, or prone to outbursts. He may avoid other people, especially those with whom he's angry, rather than expressing his feelings directly. Or he may appear sullen or uncooperative and act dejected. Anger can also be mixed with other emotions such as anxiety or depression. Finally, anger may be masked by other symptoms. For example, someone who is very paranoid may keep his anger to himself, and relatives may not notice until he blows up in an aggressive outburst. In general, if your relative is angry, he is more difficult to get along with, and this added difficulty can be stressful for everyone in your family.

Worksheet 23.1 at the end of the chapter lists common signs of anger. Complete this checklist to see which signs you have observed in your relative.

Violent Behavior

Violence involving physical aggression toward others is much less common than anger but can still be a significant problem in some people with schizophrenia. How often people with schizophrenia are violent has been a topic of much debate among scientists. Some studies, especially those conducted in the United States, suggest that schizophrenia has only a small effect on increasing the potential for violence. However, research studies in countries where community violence is much less common than in the United States (such as in Scandinavia) have found much greater risk of criminal behavior, including violence, associated with schizophrenia. Understanding why your relative is angry and has been violent will help you deal more effectively with the anger and prevent future episodes of violence.

Understanding Anger and Aggression in Schizophrenia

As mentioned at the beginning of this chapter, anger and violence can be explained by a number of factors related to schizophrenia.

Anger and Psychotic Symptoms

Delusional beliefs can lead to anger and aggression. If your relative has *delusions of reference*, she might be convinced that the newscaster is talking directly to her or that two strangers walking down the street, conversing and laughing, are talking about her. If your relative has *delusions of control*, she might believe that another person or a supernatural force is taking thoughts out of her head and inserting other thoughts. If your relative has *paranoid delusions*, she might believe that others are working together in some kind of a conspiracy to harm her; for example, that the CIA, the FBI, and the cable company are part of a grand plot to destroy her reputation by spreading false rumors about her sexual thoughts.

Similarly, hallucinations can be a source of anger. People with schizophrenia often hear voices that put them down, threaten them, or tell them to do things they don't want to do. Such experiences can be annoying and frustrating. Sometimes people respond to these voices by shouting back at them, but it doesn't make them go away.

Psychotic symptoms, and the anger associated with them, can be persistent in some people with schizophrenia (see Chapter 17). For other people, angry feelings that are related to psychotic symptoms can be an early warning sign of relapse. Chapter 12 describes how to identify and monitor early warning signs of relapse and how to create a relapse prevention plan.

Reduced Problem-Solving Skills

As described in Chapter 19, cognitive difficulties are common in people with schizophrenia, especially in areas of thinking that require flexibility and creativity to address new problems. Anger is a natural reaction to a frustrating situation that a person cannot figure out how to resolve. As discussed later in this chapter, helping your relative solve problems may be an effective strategy for addressing anger related to those problems.

Social Cognition and Social Skills

Problems in social cognition and social skills can also lead to angry feelings. *Social cognition* involves the ability to accurately perceive the social information communicated during interactions with others. As we've mentioned, people with schizophrenia often have difficulty recognizing other people's facial expressions, picking up nuances in social interactions, and understanding other people's motives—all of which can lead to misunderstandings and conflict with others. Your relative may think you're angry with her when you're not, and then respond back in an angry way, creating tension between the two of you.

People with schizophrenia are also less socially skilled in dealing with conflict. Your relative may be less likely to acknowledge your perspective, less able to explain his own perspective, and less able to suggest compromise solutions to shared problems. In these ways, poor social skills can contribute to conflict between people and to angry feelings on both sides.

Fear, Anxiety, and Depression

The "fight–flight" response describes how people and animals respond to a perceived threat: They either attack or flee the situation. Your relative's anger may be a defensive reaction to feelings of fear and anxiety—and there are many things that your relative could fear. Fear of social situations is common in people with schizophrenia, who may become angry when forced to be in such situations; likewise, they may fear seeing their doctor because of past unpleasant or traumatic experiences.

Depression is also common in schizophrenia, and when people are depressed, they often feel irritated. Depression occurs for a variety of reasons, such as persistent symptoms, poor housing, lack of rewarding relationships, and difficulty keeping a job.

Stress and Tension in the Family

Stress and tension both within and outside the family can contribute to feelings of frustration in people with schizophrenia, which can lead to angry feelings and aggression. Stress and tension can come from many different sources. For example, financial dependence on family members can result in frustration, as can relatives' attempts to set reasonable limits on a loved one's behavior. People with schizophrenia may also feel frustrated and angry when they're insecure or unable to meet other people's expectations of them. Their perceptions of what others expect may or may not be accurate, but whichever is the case, they may become angry with others as a defensive reaction to their fear of disappointing them.

Substance Abuse

Alcohol and drug use problems can contribute to angry and violent behavior in several ways. First, alcohol and drugs can have *disinhibitory effects*, making people more likely to express and act on angry feelings. In the general population alcohol abuse has been linked to many different types of violence, including fights, domestic violence, and child abuse. Second, the physical need for a substance that comes with addiction can leave a person irritable and hostile because of withdrawal symptoms or intense cravings when the need is not met. In some circumstances, people may become aggressive and intimidate others, including family members, into giving them money to support their addiction.

Third, drug and alcohol use may contribute to angry feelings in people because of the negative effects of these substances on their lives. People with schizophrenia are highly sensitive to the effects of alcohol and drugs, which can destabilize their symptoms and lead to problems with the law, housing, and relationships with others. People with schizophrenia and substance use problems often get frustrated and angry about their out-of-control lives, and this anger can be misdirected at others, particularly family members.

Impulsivity

People who behave impulsively and don't think about the consequences of their behavior before they act are more prone to expressing anger through aggression. This is true both for people with schizophrenia and for those without it. Impulsivity can lead to problems when people fail to consider the social consequences of their aggressive behavior. As described in Chapter 19, people with schizophrenia often have difficulty anticipating others' behavior and planning their own behavior, and consequently they are often impulsive.

Lack of Empathy

People with schizophrenia often have difficulty understanding other people's feelings and experiencing empathy for others. This limitation can be a problem in many ways, particularly in developing and maintaining close relationships. Low empathy might make it more difficult for your relative to notice when you're hurt, emotionally or physically. People tend to stop what they're doing when they perceive that it's hurting someone else, but if your relative can't recognize when you're being hurt, she might not stop her behavior.

Physical Illness

Scientists studying animal behavior have found that an animal given an electrical shock will attack any other animal close by. This phenomenon, called *pain-induced aggression*, appears in humans as well. When people are hurting inside, they are more likely to strike out at others, especially when they don't know why they're in pain.

Your relative could have anger problems due to a medical condition that causes physical pain. People with schizophrenia are often in poor physical health and unable to care well for their own medical needs—partly due to their difficulty in recognizing the source of their discomfort or pain. The result is that people with schizophrenia are more likely to have undiagnosed medical problems, which can lead to discomfort and pain and possibly anger and violence.

Reciprocal Aggression

When people are attacked by others, they often respond by attacking back. If your relative lives in an environment in which verbal abuse or physical fights are common ways of resolving conflict, he may respond in kind. In these situations, effectively addressing your relative's anger and aggression involves changing how everyone resolves conflict, because your relative's behavior is just one part of a more complex social problem involving others.

Strategies for Coping with Anger

A number of strategies are available for dealing with anger in a relative:

Validating Angry Feelings

It's important to validate your relative's angry feelings by showing her concern and understanding. This validation is a critical first step in dealing with anger, even when the cause of these feelings doesn't make sense to you. You can validate your relative's feelings by reflecting them back in an empathic way that shows that you care:

CARLOS: I'm being controlled, I have no free will! This microchip they implanted can even control my thoughts.

URSELLA: That must be very upsetting. It must be hard to feel you don't have any control over your life.

CARLOS: It is. I get so mad sometimes—that's why I break things.

URSELLA: I can understand. It sounds very frustrating.

CARLOS: Sometimes I feel like giving up.

URSELLA: I'm glad you haven't given up yet. Maybe we could figure out some ways of helping you get a little more control over your life.

CARLOS: I'd like that.

Insisting on Civil Communication

Everyone has the right to be treated and spoken to in a civil, respectful manner. When communication from an angry person includes yelling or shouting, name calling, sarcasm, threats, or insults, it is neither civil nor respectful.

If your relative speaks to you in an uncivil manner, let him know you're unhappy with this behavior and ask him to speak civilly to you. Be as specific as possible: "I don't like it when you speak loudly to me like that. Please, if you want to talk to me, don't speak so loudly." Or "It really bothers me when you call me names. Please stop calling me names or I won't speak to you now." It's important to let your relative know you won't continue to communicate with him at this time if he continues to speak uncivilly. If your relative can't speak to you civilly, despite your requests, don't try to resolve the disagreement at this moment; good communication is a prerequisite for successful problem solving. Telling your relative that you insist on civil communication establishes basic ground rules for resolving differences and gaining an understanding of angry or hurt feelings. Sometimes during a moment of anger it's difficult for people to step back sufficiently from the emotionality to engage in constructive problem solving. If you're unsuccessful in restoring civil communication, *take a time out*. The steps for taking a time out are at the bottom of this page.

Identifying Misdirected Anger

Sometimes anger aimed at you is misdirected, so it's important to talk with your relative to find out whether she is, in fact, angry, and if so, with whom. Giving her a chance to talk for a few minutes about what she is upset about is often enough to identify the true cause of the anger and defuse the situation. When trying to understand your relative's anger, speak directly and in a neutral or concerned tone of voice. Try not to become defensive; focus instead on understanding what your relative is upset about and whether you can help her address the problem. Your relative might be angry with you about something because of a misunderstanding. Or she might be angry with someone else, and you can explore the situation together and come up with some solutions to it.

Problem Solving

Sitting down with your relative, talking about his upset feelings, and problem solving together can be a helpful way of addressing angry feelings, including those related to stress and tension within the family. It may be best to hold this meeting once the situation has calmed down and your relative is no longer extremely agitated. Sitting down together, perhaps with other people who might be helpful in solving the problem, shows your relative you're concerned and want to find a resolution with him.

Steps for Taking a Time Out

1. Tell the person the situation is stressful.
2. Say that it's interfering with constructive communication.
3. Say you need to take a break from the situation.
4. Indicate you will be happy to talk about it at a later time.
5. Remove yourself from the immediate situation by moving to another room or going outside.
6. Do not further engage the person in argument.

Broadly speaking, problem solving can be divided into two parts. First, it's important to talk about the problem in order to understand it and determine whether problem solving is necessary. Sometimes simply talking about a problem reveals and clarifies misunderstandings, making further problem solving unnecessary.

When Jonah came home from his part-time job, he was irritable. Over dinner he snapped at his wife when she asked him how his day had gone. Jonah's wife said, "You sound upset about something. Did something happen at work today?" This question prompted Jonah to explain that his supervisor had criticized him about a task he had done at work, and he felt that he had not stood up for himself very well. They talked about what had happened at work, and Jonah decided to talk to his boss to get more information about what had displeased him. Talking about the problem helped Jonah calm down, and in the long run it led to his getting feedback from his supervisor about how to improve his job performance.

Second, it may be helpful to conduct formal problem solving in which two or more people use the steps described in Chapter 15.

Bridget was angry with her father, who kept pestering her about taking her medication. One evening when her father reminded her to take her medication, Bridget blew up at him, accused him of trying to run her life, and stormed out of the room. Once Bridget had calmed down, her father approached her to express his concern and they agreed to meet and problem solve together about it. Bridget said she was upset and annoyed that her father kept reminding her to take her medication, because it made her feel she was being treated like a child. Bridget felt she was responsible enough to take her medication on her own. Her father expressed his concern that Bridget had stopped taking medication in the past, which had led to relapses and rehospitalizations. They agreed to work on the problem of Bridget's taking her medication without her father reminding her.

Bridget and her father sat down together to have a problem-solving meeting. They came up with a number of possible solutions and agreed on one: figuring out a strategy that would help Bridget remember to take her medications before going to bed every night. They agreed that Bridget would put her pills into the pill box the week before and then put her pill box next to her toothbrush. Bridget and her father also agreed to check in each week for a month to see how the strategy was working and to determine whether any changes needed to be made. The strategy was effective in helping Bridget learn to take her medication by herself, and her father learned that he could trust her to do it on her own.

Addressing Underlying Anxiety

Helping your relative address underlying anxiety may eliminate anger that is self-defensive in nature. Your relative may not be aware that she is anxious about something. Talking openly and listening with a kind and sympathetic ear can help identify what your relative's real concerns are. Sometimes when people are anxious, the basis for their concerns are exaggerated. For example, your relative may feel that others are putting her down or making fun of her or giving her a hard time when a careful look at the situation does not support this. In these situations, it helps to talk about the basis of your relative's concern and to evaluate whether the evidence supports the concern or if your relative is exaggerating or ignoring important evidence.

> *When Brianna got home after her first day on a new job, she was unusually irritable and snapped at her brother and his wife, with whom she lived. Brianna was usually a very mild-mannered person, so her brother and sister-in-law were surprised by her behavior. Over dessert they began to talk about her first day at work, and Brianna said that everyone had been staring at her and talking about her behind her back, saying nasty things. As she talked about it more, her brother and sister-in-law encouraged her to consider alternative explanations for what had happened. Was it possible that anyone new at work would attract attention? How confident could she be that they were saying negative things about her? Did anyone actually do anything to show they didn't like her? As she considered these possibilities, Brianna agreed that perhaps her anger had been exaggerated. In fact, she said she was more worried about whether she would fit in at the workplace than anything else, so they talked a little about some good ways of starting conversations with other employees at her job. Brianna felt reassured after this discussion and more comfortable when looking back at her first day on her new job.*

Sometimes the basis for the person's concern is quite realistic. For example, your relative might be angry because he is worried about losing his apartment. In such situations it's helpful to problem solve how to work toward rectifying the situation. Chapter 20 describes more strategies for helping your relative cope with anxiety.

Addressing Anger Related to Substance Abuse

When anger appears to be related to substance use, it's important *not* to try to resolve it when your relative is high or intoxicated. People often have difficulties sitting down and talking about concerns when under the influence of alcohol or drugs. Instead, set aside time to talk about the problem when your relative is sober. Then try to be as honest and nonblaming as possible. Most people with substance use problems feel ashamed of their addiction, and increasing their sense of shame only interferes with motivating them to work on those problems. Establishing dialogue about substance-use-related problems opens the door for exploring whether problems of anger are related to substance use. Further strategies for dealing with substance use in your relative are described in Chapter 22.

Addressing Anger Related to Delusions

You have two options for dealing with angry feelings based on delusions. First, you can attempt to help your relative address her feelings without trying to evaluate their validity. Helping your relative cope with these feelings doesn't mean you're endorsing or agreeing with her beliefs. It just shows her that you care about her feelings and want to help alleviate them. If your relative feels angry because of paranoid delusions, for example, you can explore strategies such as acknowledging the feelings without trying to change them, attempting to relax as much as possible in light of the fact that no harm has come, and reviewing safety plans so that your relative feels as comfortable as possible.

A second strategy for dealing with angry feelings based on delusions is to gently help your relative consider alternative explanations for them. Avoid any direct confrontation of your relative's beliefs, which is likely to push him into a corner, ultimately increasing rather than decreasing his delusional conviction. Instead, explore the evidence supporting and not supporting the delusions. Your relative may conclude that not all of the evidence supports his beliefs and that perhaps he should modify those beliefs. Sometimes when examining the evidence supporting delusional beliefs, more information is needed. As your relative collects more and more information about his concerns, the beliefs may change, and so will the feelings associated with them. More strategies for dealing with delusional beliefs are discussed in Chapter 17.

Strategies for Coping with Violent Behavior

For some individuals, expressing angry feelings is followed by, or accompanies, violent behavior, such as throwing things, pushing, slapping, punching, and other aggressive acts. The most important predictor of future violence is past violent behavior. If your relative has been violent in the past and her aggressive behavior was preceded by the expression of angry feelings, it's important to take steps to protect yourself from being a target of such violence.

When responding to angry feelings that have the potential for violent behavior, try to extricate yourself from the situation without attempting to resolve it. You can acknowledge your relative's concern and indicate a willingness to talk about it later, when the situation is less stressful. Avoid cornering your relative, which may make him feel threatened. It may also be preferable to avoid direct eye contact, which can be interpreted as hostile or confrontational. Responding to anger that has the potential to become violent is most effective when a plan for dealing with such behavior has been worked out in advance—when possible, with your relative—as described in detail in Chapter 13. If you live with your relative, you need to feel completely safe with him, and any real potential for violence is inconsistent with such safety. Chapter 16 describes strategies for establishing household rules or an agreed-on code of conduct.

Medication for Aggression and Violence

Individuals who have significant problems related to anger, aggression, and violence benefit from the antipsychotic medication clozapine (brand name Clozaril). Controlled research has shown that this medication effectively reduces assaults against other people, as well as other problems related to anger and hostility. If your relative has persistent problems with anger and aggression despite adhering to her medications, consider consulting her doctor about a possible trial on clozapine.

Using Legal Recourses

Some people with schizophrenia get out of control and damage property and threaten or hit family members. These problems tend to be worse in people who deny having a mental illness and refuse to take their medications, although they can also erupt in people who take their medication. Despite the disruptive effects of such aggressive and violent behavior, many relatives are reluctant to obtain the legal protection they need. Family members may refuse to call the police in times of need or choose not to press charges against a destructive or aggressive relative once police have arrived. Understandably, they may worry that their loved one will go to jail or feel guilty that their loved one will suffer more at the hands of the criminal justice system. Although these concerns make sense, they may actually work against your relative's best interests; he may *need* to experience these kinds of consequences to learn how to take responsibility for his behavior.

Throughout the United States, increasing numbers of mental health and criminal justice systems are developing jail diversion programs aimed at helping people with schizophrenia and other severe mental illness stay out of jail and manage their mental illness more effectively in the community. Criminal behavior, including property destruction and violence toward family members, is often caused by treatment nonadherence, and jail diversion programs are effective at getting people to adhere to their treatments, including medication. Some judicial systems can commit people with mental illness to outpatient treatment, which would include taking medication. Using legal recourses if your relative is violent or aggressive may provide the consequences necessary to involve her in treatment and to gain better control over her illness.

Looking to the Future

Anger, aggression, and violence can be serious problems for people with schizophrenia and their families. The most important step you can take in dealing with these problems is to face them—to refuse to be a passive victim in the face of potential threats or actual harm. You have a right to feel safe and peaceful in your home and in your relationship with your loved one, and addressing anger and preventing violence are crucial to maintaining that safety and comfort. By trying to understand the roots of your relative's aggression and how they are related to his illness, and working on strategies for reducing anger and preventing violence, you will help not only yourself and your family but also your relative. Good, strong, mutually respectful family ties contribute to the positive quality of life for everyone by maintaining family support and nurturing close relationships.

Resources

Ellis, A. (1977). *Anger: How to live with and without it*. Secaucus, NJ: Citadel Press. This book helps readers identify how their inaccurate thinking perpetuates feelings of anger and resentment, and provides strategies for correcting that thinking and overcoming anger.

McKay, M., & Rogers, P. (2000). *The anger control workbook*. Oakland, CA: New Harbinger Publications. An excellent, practical, self-help book with numerous exercises for managing anger problems.

Nay, W. R. (2004). *Taking charge of anger: How to resolve conflict, sustain relationships, and express yourself without losing control*. New York: Guilford Press. A helpful book that focuses on anger problems in relationships and how to deal with them.

Rubin, T. I. (1969). *The angry book*. New York: Collier Books. A classic—one of the first self-help books about anger that continues to be useful today.

Schiraldi, G. R., & Kerr, M. H. (2002). *The anger management sourcebook*. New York: McGraw-Hill. Lots of good coping strategies for dealing with the effects of anger and overcoming angry feelings.

Angry Signs Checklist

Instructions: Indicate which of these signs of anger you have observed in your relative.

Sign of anger	No	Possibly	Definitely
Irritable, easily annoyed			
Prone to outbursts (yelling, shouting)			
Sullen, dejected			
Uncooperative			
Anxious			
Depressed			
Destructive to property			
Shouting or cursing to him/herself or the walls			

CHAPTER 24

Lack of Insight

*P*eople with schizophrenia often lack insight into their problems, not believing they are ill or denying having any difficulties whatsoever. About half of all people with schizophrenia lack awareness of, or insight into, their illness, a problem called *anosognosia* in neurological terms. Poor insight can contribute to many problems and can be exasperating for families. Coping effectively with your relative's limited insight is crucial to addressing some of the problems related to it and may help you improve your relationship with your loved one. Before you try to apply the strategies in this chapter, be aware that a collaborative relationship that focuses on finding a common ground for working together and minimizing differences in perspectives caused by poor insight is a must.

Insight and Schizophrenia

Lack of insight in people with schizophrenia manifests itself in many different ways. Psychotic symptoms, by their very nature, often involve loss of insight. People who have auditory hallucinations may refuse to believe that their voices come from inside them instead of from external forces. Similarly, delusions involve a loss of insight into the falseness of the strongly held beliefs.

Many people with schizophrenia acknowledge having some problems, such as difficulties with "nerves" or a mental condition, but they insist they don't have schizophrenia. Others may deny having any problems whatsoever. This blatant denial can be especially challenging to family members and treatment providers, who are acutely aware of the person's difficulties in such basic areas as independent living, work, self-care, and social relationships.

Leon, 24, lives at home with his mother and two younger sisters. Leon graduated from high school when he was 18 and worked as a stocker at a local grocery store for 3 years. He gradually began to withdraw from others and started to experience difficulties on the job, such as behaving erratically and appearing confused at times. Leon then quit his job and began spending most of his time alone in his room, where he often was heard talking to himself and laughing. Leon sometimes accused his family members of spying on him, and he wouldn't let anyone watch TV when he was in the room because he believed the TV characters could read his mind. Leon's mother tried to talk to him about her concerns that he was spending less time with friends, was not working, and was out of touch with his family. She suggested that Leon needed help and maybe they could look into that together. However, Leon vehemently denied that anything was wrong. He said he had quit his job because he was tired of it and he stayed in his room because he preferred keeping to himself.

It's common for people to lack insight into their symptoms or their disorder soon after developing schizophrenia. However, over time and through experience people often develop more understanding of their illness. Many people with schizophrenia become aware of certain psychotic symptoms that are part of their illness and are able to recognize hallucinations or paranoid thoughts as symptoms. In addition, over time, many people learn about the positive effects of medication on reducing symptoms and preventing relapses and begin taking it on a regular basis.

If lack of insight "rings a bell" for you as the basis of some of the problems you're having with your relative, Worksheet 24.1 at the end of the chapter provides a checklist of signs of poor insight in people with schizophrenia for you to complete. Clearly identifying the problems is the first step.

Problems Associated with Poor Insight

People who lack insight into having schizophrenia are more difficult to engage in treatment because they don't think anything is wrong and are not motivated to change. Even if a person is forced into treatment, his denial of the problem makes it far more difficult to form a collaborative working relationship with a clinician. Poor insight or minimization of problems can also interfere with medication adherence. Some people with schizophrenia have insight into their need for treatment but lack awareness of how helpful medication can be. They may also think that when their symptoms have been reduced or temporarily eliminated they won't need to take medication anymore.

Problems with insight can make it more difficult to establish a common language for talking about difficulties with your relative, because she may not accept having an "illness." These problems in communication can lead to conflict, especially when relatives try to convince the person that she has an illness. Conflict among family members over how to help their loved one with schizophrenia may then add another layer of difficulty.

Understanding Poor Insight in Your Relative

Having schizophrenia involves a loss in the ability to reality test—to distinguish what is real from what is not. This difficulty may be related to the styles in which individuals process and interpret information. People with schizophrenia have an extreme cognitive style that leads them to look only for evidence that supports their beliefs and to discount evidence contrary to those beliefs. Although paying attention only to things that support one's own beliefs is a natural human tendency, it can lead to, and even reinforce, delusional thinking when taken to an extreme.

Cognitive styles that lead to delusional thinking in schizophrenia may be determined by impaired brain functions that underlie the disorder. For example, Xavier Amador, PhD, at Columbia College of Physicians and Surgeons proposed that poor insight is related to dysfunction in an important part of the brain for conceptual thinking and the processing of information about oneself and the world: the *frontal lobe* (also called the *frontal lobes*). Disturbances in the frontal lobes are involved in a wide range of cognitive problems found in schizophrenia, especially those related to impaired *executive functioning* skills such as planning, problem solving, and abstract reasoning (see Chapter 19 for more about coping with difficulties in executive functioning). Impairments in the frontal lobes may lead to extreme cognitive styles that make it difficult for your relative to consider evidence that does not support his personal beliefs, including the belief that there is nothing wrong with him.

Some people with schizophrenia have partial insight into the problems they experience in their lives but don't think they have the illness of schizophrenia. For example, when Madison was pressed by her brother to admit she had schizophrenia, she emphatically replied, "I know I have problems. I believe I have a grave disability that makes it hard for me to function emotionally and get along with other people. However, I don't believe I have schizophrenia. I've read descriptions of schizophrenia, and I just don't think it's me." For these individuals, lack of insight may be a way of protecting themselves against the social stigma connected to the illness of schizophrenia. People with schizophrenia are often aware of the negative public attitudes toward this condition, such as the belief that people with schizophrenia are crazy or violent. They may reject the diagnosis because they don't feel that the stereotypes of the disorder are an accurate depiction of themselves and their problems. The logic goes as follows: "People with schizophrenia are crazy, dangerous, and a burden on society. I don't think I'm crazy or violent, and I really am worth something. Therefore, I don't have schizophrenia."

People may also lack insight into their delusional beliefs because they provide some comfort and escape from the harsh realities of their lives. For example, it might be preferable to hold on to the belief that you are a king and have vast wealth than to accept the reality that you have no money, no job, no girl-friend, and no plans for the future.

It's important not to confuse your relative's lack of insight with "denial" of the illness, which suggests that "deep down inside" he "really knows" that some-thing is wrong with him. Your relative has no more control over his insight into the illness than any of the other symptoms of schizophrenia. As you try to under-stand your relative's lack of insight, you may find it easier to empathize with his way of looking at things. Fortunately, your relative doesn't have to have good insight into the illness to participate actively in treatment and collaborate with you and the treatment team.

Coping with Limited Insight

There are several strategies for coping with your relative's lack of insight.

- *Avoid confrontation.* Directly confronting your relative about hallucinations, delusions, and the diagnosis of schizophrenia will not help improve his insight and may even be counterproductive. Although you may be tempted, avoid trying to persuade your relative that delusions are not real or that he has a specific ill-ness.
- *Seek common ground.* The most effective strategy for dealing with poor insight is to seek a common ground with your relative about mutual concerns that you can focus on together. Looking for areas of agreement can involve iden-tifying problems that need solving and desired goals to work toward. Although many people with schizophrenia lack some insight into their problems, everyone can be engaged in identifying personally important goals to work toward. Exam-ples of problems or goals that people with schizophrenia have worked on with their relatives are listed in the table on the facing page. People often find that recovery goals constitute common ground, so you may find it useful to review the strategies for identifying such goals in Chapter 3.

Identifying a common ground with your relative minimizes the differences between your perspective and hers. Focusing on differences only serves to high-light the potential for conflict and does not recognize important values and goals you share with your relative. No two people agree perfectly on anything; you're more likely to achieve productive results by seeking and identifying areas of mutual concern.

Brenda developed schizophrenia in her late teens, after dropping out of high school. She continued to live with her mother and had two children, now ages 2 and 5. Their father was not involved in their care or with Brenda after their birth. Much of the chil-dren's care fell on Brenda's mother. Since her first hospitalization at age 18, Brenda had been hospitalized seven times, several of which were precipitated by cocaine and mari-juana abuse. Brenda had also been arrested twice for possession of drugs and was on pro-

Examples of Problems/Goals That Are the Focus of Collaboration in Families	
• Coping with depression • Coping with anxiety • Addressing medication side effects • Reducing or stopping use of alcohol and/or drugs • Budgeting money better • Creating a more nutritional diet to address poor eating habits • Quitting smoking • Problem solving to address conflict • Helping grandparents • Joining a local organization (such as a nature conservancy group) • Reconnecting with old friends • Learning how to sew, crochet, or knit • Learning how to cook • Taking a vacation • Getting better sleep • Improving concentration • Staying out of the hospital	• Decreasing symptom relapses • Staying out of jail • Repairing relationships with family members • Regaining custody or parenting of children • Living independently • Making friends • Finding an intimate partner • Regaining control over money • Finding new leisure and recreational activities • Attending to religious or spiritual needs • Finding a paid job • Finding a volunteer job • Going back to school • Getting involved in art • Participating in a peer support group

bation. *Brenda received medication and saw a case manager at a local mental health center.*

Brenda's routine involved sleeping past noon, watching TV, and occasionally spending time with friends in the evening. Despite having many of the symptoms of schizophrenia, including hallucinations, delusions, apathy, and some difficulties with attention, she flatly denied that she had an illness and rejected any attempts to convince her otherwise. After numerous arguments in which she tried to convince Brenda that she had an illness, her mother began to take another tack: She began to try to find areas of common concern that could serve as a basis for working together.

Over a period of several weeks Brenda's mother began to engage her in discussions about which parts of her life she thought were going well, which were not, and how things could be better. At first Brenda resisted these discussions, expecting them to turn into the usual arguments about her having an illness, using drugs, or failing to take responsibility for herself. As the discussions continued, Brenda's mother introduced the concept of recovery, encouraging her to talk about what recovery meant for her and the kinds of changes that she wanted to make in her life. Eventually, Brenda identified three changes that she wanted to make in her life. First, she wanted to go back to school and get her high school degree. She said she'd always been interested in becoming a beautician but that most beautician schools required a high school degree. Second, Brenda wanted to be a better role model for her children and to be a more active parent to them. To Brenda, being a parent meant feeding her children, dressing them, and spending more time reading to them and playing with them. Third, Brenda wanted to get better control over her drug and alcohol use. She knew that staying sober was a requirement of her probation, but she still used drugs sometimes when she got together with her friends. Brenda said that she thought her use of substances made her symptoms worse, that it was something she did when she was around friends, and she didn't have any friends who didn't use substances. Brenda said she didn't want her children to use substances and being a good role model for them would require her to become sober. Brenda and her mom decided to work together toward achieving these goals. They began by breaking down each of these long-term goals into smaller steps.

• *Find a common language to talk about problems.* To communicate effectively, you need to use a language for discussing problems that both you and your relative find acceptable. Because many people with schizophrenia reject the diagnosis, finding suitable language to talk about problems related to mental illness can be extremely helpful. Some people accept the term *nervous condition* or *stress reaction*. Some individuals find the concept of a *chemical imbalance in the brain* or the more general term *mental illness* acceptable. Some people reject any term that implies a disorder or illness but accept a more generic euphemism, such as "these kinds of problems." Still others are comfortable talking about specific problems, such as difficulties sleeping or relaxing, as long as no reference is made to a mental illness. Some may reject the notion of having problems but can be motivated by concrete goals such as staying out of the hospital and regaining control over of their money.

• *Work toward acceptance.* It can be helpful for you to appreciate the fact that your relative's limited insight is a part of having schizophrenia—which may or may not improve—and to accept your relative as he is. Acceptance is not the same as giving up on your relative or forgoing a positive relationship with him. In fact, such acceptance may facilitate a more rewarding relationship and improve your ability to enjoy your relative as a loved one. In this regard, the Serenity Prayer most aptly summarizes the importance of acceptance:

> God grant me the Serenity to accept the things I cannot change . . .
> Courage to change the things I can . . .
> And Wisdom to know the difference.

Gaining Insight into Your Relative

Difficulties with insight are a common feature of schizophrenia that often, but not always, improve over time. Family members who want to help their relative but encounter roadblocks every step along the way may become extremely frustrated. If this problem weighs on you, the best solution is for *you* to develop insight into how your relative views the world by trying to understand her experience with schizophrenia. The fruits of such insight will be a greater appreciation for your relative's struggles to cope with this perplexing illness and for her as a person and as your loved one.

Resources

Amador, X., & Johnson, A. L. (2000). *I am not sick, I don't need help! Helping the seriously mentally ill accept treatment: A practical guide for families and therapists*. Peconic, NY: Vida Press. This book by the world's leading authority on insight and mental illness (Amador) provides practical advice for families and professionals about how to work with individuals who have limited insight to involve them in treatment. Both authors have relatives with schizophrenia.

Indicators of Lack of Insight

Instructions: Indicate which of the following signs of poor insight your relative has by checking the appropriate box below.

Indicator	No	Somewhat	Yes
Thinks hallucinations are real			
Thinks delusions are real			
Doesn't think he/she has schizophrenia			
Doesn't think medication helps			
Doesn't think he/she has any problems			
Doesn't think he/she needs treatment			

PART VI

Improving Quality of Life

CHAPTER 25

Social Relationships

*O*ne of schizophrenia's most profound effects is that it makes it more difficult to have good relationships. Chapters 14 through 16 explained how to help your relative improve family relationships. But relationships outside the family are just as important. In this chapter you'll find strategies for helping your relative make friends, get closer to people, and enjoy intimate relationships with others.

The Importance of Social Relationships

For many people, the quality of their relationships is a major factor in personal satisfaction and quality of life. Most people value their friends and family members, and many of their activities revolve around these relationships. Supportive relationships can make us feel good about ourselves and more optimistic about the future—which is especially important to people with schizophrenia, who often have low self-esteem and feel discouraged about their prospects in life.

Supportive relationships also improve the course of schizophrenia because of their role in reducing stress, which can trigger or worsen symptoms. Social support can help your relative manage stress in several ways. First, close relationships may prevent stress from occurring because people are able to talk over potential problems and address them before they evolve into crises. For example, if your relative talks to a friend about strategies for managing money, he might be able to avoid running out of money before the end of the month. Second, having someone to talk to and do things with can help reduce the stress of loneliness and boredom. For example, if your relative likes music and has someone to go to concerts with, he will get out more and enjoy life more. Third, friends can also be helpful in reminding your relative to use coping skills in situations when he might forget to use them. For example, if your relative is feeling under pressure, a friend could remind him that taking a walk usually reduces that stress.

Problems in Social Relationships

Schizophrenia is associated with several problems that make it hard for people to develop and maintain social relationships: psychotic and negative symptoms, poor social skills, and cognitive problems. Understanding how these problems interfere with social functioning can prepare you to help your relative improve her relationships.

Psychotic symptoms can interfere with communicating with others. Hearing voices can be very distracting, making it hard to have a good conversation with someone. When Alonzo was being introduced to a young woman he was interested in dating, he was hearing voices that were putting him down. These voices made it very difficult for him to pay attention to what she was saying and to make a positive impression on her. Paranoid delusions can cause a person with schizophrenia to distrust new people or even to doubt the intentions of old friends. MiLing had delusions that people could read her mind, so she avoided making eye contact with other students in her class because she thought they could see through her eyes into her thoughts. She also believed her grandfather was telling neighbors about her secret thoughts, which made her very angry at him and made it difficult for her to feel close to him.

Negative symptoms, including lack of interest and initiative, can make it hard for people to exert the efforts necessary to develop relationships. Your relative may have trouble thinking of something to do with another person or have problems following through with activities that other people suggest. Daryl, for example, said he wanted to ask women out on dates, but just the thought of calling one up, selecting a movie to see, and figuring out transportation issues was overwhelming.

Many people with schizophrenia are at a disadvantage because they lack the full range of social skills necessary to make friends and develop intimate relationships. There are several possible reasons for this limitation, including the relatively early age at which the illness tends to develop (late adolescence, early adulthood), when many young men and women are first learning and practicing the social skills they need as adults. It's fairly common for people with schizophrenia to be uncomfortable starting conversations, asserting themselves, and dealing with conflicts. Jessica, for example, had a hard time knowing what to say when other people started talking to her, and she would become very uneasy at the first hint of a disagreement.

The cognitive problems of schizophrenia also interfere with relationships. Having difficulties with attention and concentration, for example, is a drawback to having meaningful conversations with a friend or loved one. Slower information processing can also be disruptive to conversations because it results in delayed verbal responses, which can make the conversation lag and the participants feel uncomfortable. For example, Adrianna takes so long to answer a question that the other person often thinks she didn't hear or doesn't want to respond, even though she's very interested in the conversation.

These difficulties associated with schizophrenia lead to four major problem areas in relationships: connecting with people, getting closer to people, using social skills, and managing conflict. Strategies for addressing each of these areas are described in the following pages.

Connecting with People

The first step toward developing a relationship is being able to connect with people. To do this, your relative needs to be able to meet people, have interesting things to say, and be responsive to what others say.

Meeting People

Your relative may be interested in having more people in his life but finds it difficult to meet them. This will be especially true if he spends most of his time at home and is not working, going to school, or involved in regular activities. However, the more your relative gets out and puts himself in a position to encounter others, the greater the chances he will connect with someone who shares his interests. If your relative is interested in meeting other people, you can help him identify promising places to do this.

Some of the best opportunities to encounter others occur in public places where people naturally gather for recreation, to pursue an interest, or to take care of business. Many friendships develop because of common interests, so it will be helpful for your relative to choose places that attract people who might share her interests. For example, if your relative likes to read, going to a lecture at a bookstore or library might be a natural choice; if she enjoys nature, becoming involved in a conservation organization such as the Sierra Club might be attractive. Even if your relative doesn't meet people at first, going to places that interest her is likely to be enjoyable.

You can review Worksheet 25.1 at the end of the chapter with your relative and check off the places he would like to go to to meet people. Some of the places involve making an ongoing commitment, such as enrolling in a class or becoming a volunteer, whereas others can be visited on a casual basis. Once your relative identifies locations for meeting people, you can help him make plans to go there. It's common not to meet people on the first visit, so it's a good idea to help your relative plan several trips to the same location before he decides whether it's a good place for meeting people.

Starting and Maintaining Conversations

Part of getting to know someone is having conversations. Starting and maintaining enjoyable conversations is sometimes difficult for people with schizophrenia because it involves a combination of skills affected by their illness: choosing

someone who might be receptive, having something interesting to say, and showing interest in the other person. If your relative has difficulties conversing with
people and is interested in your assistance, you can help him or her pinpoint the
problem area(s) and then review and practice some of the skills described in the
following material.

• *Select a receptive person to talk to.* To help your relative, consider these basic
points you probably take for granted. If someone is in the middle of doing something, such as talking on the phone or reaching for a book from a high shelf, he
may not want to interrupt that activity to talk to you. On the other hand, if the
person is sitting next to you at a concert, waiting for the program to start, he
might be open to a conversation, especially about the music you are both about
to hear. Realize also that in deciding who to start a conversation with, you probably notice the person's expression. If the person has a neutral expression or is
smiling, he is more likely to be friendly and receptive than someone who is
frowning and has a clenched jaw. A person who is making eye contact is also
more likely to want to talk to you than someone who is purposefully looking away
from you. Review all these points with your relative and perhaps even role-play a
few scenarios in which you play a person with whom your relative is considering
starting a conversation.

• *Choose an interesting topic.* A natural subject to talk about would be one
related to what your relative is doing at the time of the conversation. For example, if she is in an art gallery, she could start a conversation about the paintings
or the artists. If she is at a health club, she might talk about exercising or using
the equipment. While volunteering at a zoo, she could talk about the behavior of
the different animals or which animals she especially enjoys.

Explain to your relative that it's often helpful to start a conversation by asking a question, because doing so shows the other person that the speaker is interested in his opinion and encourages a dialogue rather than a monologue. For
example, if your relative is at a lecture about preserving a local park, he could ask
someone else attending the lecture what he thinks is the best feature of that park
or what step should be taken first to save the park. This might lead to a conversation about enjoying that park and whether he has ever been involved in preserva-
tion efforts.

Your relative could also choose to start a conversation by talking about topics
of common interest, such as the weather, current events, or sports. Talking about
general topics could lead to more conversation, depending on your relative's
interests and what she thinks the other person is interested in. For example, talking about weather could lead to a discussion of the recent rains, which could lead
to conversation about how the rainfall affected gardening and the blooming of
certain flowers. Or talking about rain could develop into a conversation about
what kinds of umbrellas are best to carry while walking on crowded city side-
walks.

If your relative has difficulty thinking of topics around which to start conversations, he might benefit from brainstorming with you or from reviewing the table at the bottom of the page, which contains a list of possible opening topics.

- *Look at the person.* Eye contact is important when talking to people because it indicates interest and attention. If your relative feels uncomfortable making eye contact, she can look somewhere close to the person's eyes, such as the nose or forehead. Explain to your relative that in most conversations the speaker looks directly toward the listener's eyes and the listener moves her gaze around the speaker's face. Also explain that it's important to avoid too much eye contact, such as staring intently at someone without blinking or occasionally looking away.

- *Indicate interest.* Explain to your relative that it can be helpful to let the person know he's listening and interested in what the person has to say. Your relative can show his interest by smiling, nodding his head, or saying things such as "uh-huh," "I see," or "okay." Also explain that showing interest in the other person indicates that your relative doesn't intend to dominate the conversation by doing all the talking and that he is receptive to the other's point of view.

- *Tune in to what the other person is saying.* Explain to your relative that asking questions based on what the other person is saying and responding to comments lets the person know she is interested in her perspective. If the other person seems uninterested, your relative could consider changing topics or politely ending the conversation. Suggest that a good rule of thumb is that each person in a conversation should be talking about the same amount—one person shouldn't be talking 90% of the time and the other only 10%. Although two people in a conversation rarely talk *exactly* the same amount, balance is a good idea to be sure each person gets something out of the conversation.

Possible Topics for Starting Conversations

- Weather
- Sports
- Current events
- Pets
- Books
- Television shows
- Movies
- Music
- Food
- Restaurants
- Hobbies
- Something you are doing together
- Nature
- Favorite seasons
- Art

- *At first, avoid telling things that are too personal.* Explain to your relative that when he's just getting to know someone, he should not reveal very private information about himself. Such information can make the other person feel uncomfortable, which makes it harder to make a connection. Give your relative an example: "Telling someone you just met about a painful hospitalization or a serious medical condition might be more information than he wants to hear at first. When you get to know the person better, he'll feel more comfortable with conversations about more personal topics. In general, people in conversations tend to disclose a similar amount of personal information about themselves. It's a good idea to pay attention to what the other person is revealing about himself so that you can match his level of disclosure."

Getting Closer to People

If your relative wants to get closer to a person that she already knows, she needs to decide what to say to the other person, what to do with and for the other person, and how much and when to disclose personal information about herself. She might be interested in reviewing and practicing some of the following skills with you.

Communication Skills for Increasing Closeness

- *Express positive feelings and give compliments.* As you know, telling someone how you feel about him can help bring the two of you closer. You might explain it to your relative: "One way to express affection is to tell the person that you admire certain qualities he has. For example, you could tell [fill in the name of your relative's friend] that you like his honesty, creativity, or sense of humor, and give specific examples of these traits. Another way to express affection is to let him know that you appreciate the things he says or does. For example, you could tell your friend that you appreciate it when he cooks food you enjoy. Or you could compliment him on his clothing or hairstyle."

- *Ask the person questions about herself.* Getting to know others involves trying to understand more about their thoughts and feelings. Some individuals volunteer information about themselves, but others do not. Explain to your relative that if the person does not naturally volunteer, it's helpful to ask directly about what she is thinking and feeling: "How did you like the movie we just saw?" or "What do you think about your job?" Continue your explanation: "If your friend expresses negative feelings, avoid judging or disagreeing and try to empathize with the feeling she describes. For example, if she tells you she's bored with her job, you could say something like 'I'm sorry you're bored; that must be a difficult situation,' rather than 'You shouldn't be bored; you're lucky to have a job.' "

- *Try to understand the person's perspective.* Explain to your relative that each person's experience and perspective are unique and that to understand some-one's point of view it could be helpful for him to ask himself questions such as:

— "What is the person feeling?"
— "What is the person thinking?"
— "If I were in his shoes, what would I feel or think?"

You might continue to explain to your relative: "When you think you under-stand someone's perspective, it can be helpful to check it out to see if you are correct or not. For example, if your friend has been talking about her concerns over starting a new job, you could say something like 'From what you've said, it sounds like you're a little worried about having new responsibilities on the job. Is that the way you feel?' Let your friend know you're interested in knowing more about her. For example, you could say 'I've never been in that situation before; I'd like to know more about what it's like for you.' "

Getting Closer

• *Do things together.* Identifying activities that your relative can do with the person he wants to get closer to can provide rewarding experiences for both of you. Explore interests your relative has in common with his friend to think of things they can do together. Explain to your relative: "You can ask your friend directly what he likes to do. Doing activities together will give you something to talk about and opportunities to get to know each other better. For example, if you and [name of friend] go on a hike together, it would be natural to comment on the scenery and how it feels to be hiking."

• *Be willing to compromise.* Explain to your relative that in close relationships neither person can always have her own way, and that being willing to compro-mise and negotiate shows she is not selfish and cares about her friend. You might continue: "In a compromise each person generally gets some of what she wants, but she also usually has to give up something. The goal is to reach an agreement that is acceptable to both people. If you and your friend reach an impasse around some issue, try to explain your viewpoint briefly, listen to your friend's view-point, and suggest a compromise that takes both of your perspectives into consid-eration. For example, you and your friend may both want to see a movie, but one of you wants to see an action movie and the other wants to see a comedy. One possible compromise would be to see a comedy tonight and an action film next week. Another compromise would be to choose an action film that has elements of comedy. Still another compromise might involve selecting a third kind of film, such as a documentary or a musical, that might interest both of you."

• *Be there for the person and help out.* Closeness to another person involves being available to him during a time of need. Explain to your relative that we all need help sometimes and it's important to recognize when someone you care about needs you. The person may need hands-on help, such as assistance with moving, or emotional support, such as a shoulder to cry on after losing a loved one. When we are close to someone, we are there through good times and bad and offer help when it's needed.

• *Do things for the other person on a regular basis.* Explain to your relative that in addition to being available in times of need, people who have close relationships are usually interested in making each other happy. For example, if the person your relative is close to likes to go for walks, your relative might offer to go walking with her. If your relative's friend enjoys listening to jazz, your relative might turn the radio to a jazz station during dinner. If the person your relative cares about has a favorite dish, she might cook that dish; if the friend enjoys humor, your relative might repeat a joke or funny story that was told to her.

• *Disclose personal information gradually.* Explain to your relative that as people get closer to each other, they reveal more details about themselves. Deciding how much to tell someone can be tricky: "If you tell too much too soon, the other person may feel overwhelmed and may pull away from the relationship. But if you disclose too little over time, it may be hard to have a truly close relationship."

Strengthening Social Skills

Social skills are the specific behaviors involved in interactions with others that enable people to be effective, to get their point across, and to meet their social needs. People with schizophrenia often have poor social skills, and this limitation interferes with their ability to make friends or deepen interpersonal relationships. Poor eye contact while speaking, lack of vocal inflection and facial expression, slowness when responding to others, and difficulty finding interesting conversational topics are common social skills problems for persons with schizophrenia.

Social Skills Training Programs

Social skills training has become an increasingly popular method used by professionals to systematically teach people skills that will help them improve their personal interactions. People are taught either individually or in groups, with training taking place over several months or even years.

Research on social skills training indicates that people with schizophrenia are capable of improving their social skills and that these improvements can result in better social functioning. Although skills training involves hard work, the positive nature of the practice and the feedback given often make the learning enjoyable. If your relative decides that improving social skills is an important goal, she may appreciate your help in locating a skills training program. Such programs are often available at the local community mental health center.

The specific social skills training programs available may differ from one

---

Steps of Social Skills Training

1. Help your relative select a specific social skill that is related to achieving one of his/her goals.
2. Break down the skill into three or four steps.
3. Briefly discuss the rationale for each step.
4. Model (demonstrate) the skill in a role play (a pretend interaction) and ask for feedback from your relative about how you performed the steps.
5. Ask your relative to practice the skill in a role play.
6. Give specific positive feedback about how your relative performed the steps.
7. Offer a suggestion for how the skill could be improved.
8. Ask your relative to practice the skill again and provide more feedback.
9. With your relative, develop an assignment to practice the skill in a real situation.
10. Follow up to see how the skill worked and decide what to do next.

---

center to another. One training program for people with psychiatric disorders that has become widely available in recent years is the social and independent living skills (SILS) program developed by Robert P. Liberman, MD, and Charles Wallace, PhD, and their colleagues at the University of California at Los Angeles. The SILS program uses written materials and videos in a structured step-by-step approach to improving people's social skills in specific areas, such as conducting basic conversations, communicating in the workplace, and making friends. Another resource used to guide skills training is *Social Skills Training for Schizophrenia*, by Alan S. Bellack, PhD, and colleagues. This book provides instructions on how to conduct social skills groups and includes the steps of 60 specific social skills.

Helping Your Relative Build His Social Skills

You may have difficulty locating a social skills training program in your area, or your relative may be reluctant to participate in a local program. If your relative still wants to improve his social skills, and you're willing to help, you may be able to work together to make some progress in this area. Improving skills takes time and patience, but it's worth a try if other avenues are not available to you. In the table above we list the steps for helping your relative improve a specific social skill.

Taylor's long-term goals were to have friends and a girlfriend. In talking to his parents, he said his major obstacle was feeling uncomfortable starting conversations with other people. He was receptive to his parents' offer to work together on increasing his conversation skills. Taylor's parents broke down the skill of starting a conversation as follows:

1. Choose a topic that might interest the other person.

2. Speak in a voice tone that is neither too soft nor too loud.

3. Look at the other person.

After discussing how each of the steps can enhance a conversation, Taylor's father demonstrated in a role play how he would start a conversation, with his mother pretending to be a fellow student in Taylor's computer class. Taylor observed the role play and then commented on what he had noticed, such as his father's choice of topic, his tone of voice, and eye contact. Next Taylor practiced starting a conversation, with his mother again pretending to be a student in the computer class. Taylor's parents gave him positive feedback by praising his opening topic (the challenge of completing their last homework assignment). Then they suggested it might be even more effective if he spoke more loudly. In a second role play Taylor spoke in a louder voice, and he even did a third role play in which he worked on improving his eye contact.

Together Taylor and his parents came up with the assignment of starting three conversations with students he already knew in the computer class. A week later when he followed up with his parents, Taylor reported that trying to start conversations had gone "all right." He had felt a little nervous at first but became more relaxed when the other person seemed interested. Taylor decided that the following week he would like to try starting conversations with three people, including one individual he didn't already know.

These steps provide just one way of helping your relative improve her social skills. The basic principles of practice, positive feedback, and specific suggestions for improvement can be used in other ways to improve skills and facilitate social interactions. The key to success is a willingness to work together and to take complex skills and break them down into smaller, easier steps.

The table on the facing page contains examples of role plays that you can suggest to your relative when working on specific skills related to improving his relationships.

Dealing with Conflicts in Relationships

Schizophrenia can make conflicts not only more likely but also more upsetting to your relative. Your relative should not, however, avoid relationships just because they might lead to conflict. Relationships are vital to your relative's quality of life and will help her reduce stress and avoid relapses. Therefore, it's critical that your relative learn the strategies for managing conflicts described in detail in Chapters 14 and Chapter 15.

The Power of Love

Your relationship with your relative is the single most valuable asset for helping your loved one get closer to others. Having people in one's life and enjoying

Role-Play Examples for Specific Social Skills

Social skills	Possible role plays to suggest to your relative
Starting a conversation	• You are at the bookstore and notice that someone is reading the same book as you. • You are sitting next to someone at church who is singing the hymns especially well. • You are waiting with several other people for your exercise class to start.
Giving compliments	• A friend has done you a favor. • A classmate or acquaintance is wearing an attractive article of clothing. • Your date has a new haircut.
Finding common interests	• You are taking a class, and a new person has joined. You would like to get to know him/her. • You are having lunch with a person you met on your new job. • You are at a party and you meet an interesting person.
Asking someone for a date	• There is a person with whom you volunteer that you would like to get to know better. • You decide to ask your new neighbor out on a date. • You have a lot in common with someone you met in a class.
Understanding the other person's perspective	• Your coworker just got an assignment that he/she wasn't expecting and is unprepared for. • Your friend's cat has run away. • Your friend tells you about an argument with his/her roommate.
Compromise and negotiation	• Your date does not like the kind of food served at the restaurant you suggest. • Your roommate wants to decorate the living room in a color that you do not particularly like. • Your friend wants to go bowling, but you want to go to get ice cream.

closeness with others, including intimate relationships, is an important part of what makes life worth living. Because of your special relationship, you are in a unique position to help your relative articulate and pursue his interpersonal goals. By loving and supporting your relative, you convey that he has worth and something to contribute to others. Feeling close and loved by another sets the stage for being able to connect with and love others. Through your love and help, your relative can learn how to get closer to other people as well.

Resources

Bellack, A. S., Mueser, K. T., Gingerich, S., & Agresta, J. (2004). *Social skills training for schizophrenia: A step-by-step guide* (2nd ed.). New York: Guilford Press. Contains the steps for 60 different social skills and describes how to set up role plays, give feedback, and develop assignments to practice skills.

Compeer at *www.compeer.org* offers programs and services that promote volunteering as a friend to someone with a mental illness.

Liberman, R. P. *Social and independent living skills (SILS)*. Available at *www.psychrehab.com*, click on "Modules for Training Social and Independent Living Skills." Trainers manuals, client workbooks, and videos to help people improve their social skills in specific areas, including basic conversation, friendship and intimacy, and recreation.

Places to Meet People

Instructions: Review this worksheet with your relative, checking off the places he/she would like to go to meet people.

Places to meet people	Would like to try
Library	
Bookstore	
Class	
Support group	
Volunteer program	
Church, synagogue, temple, mosque, etc.	
Peer drop-in center	
Health club or exercise club, such as the YMCA or private gym	
Park	
Museum	
Concert	
Coffee shop	
Special interest group related to hobby, sports, conservation, nature, recreation, or politics	
Sing-along	
Other:	

CHAPTER 26

Work and School

Work—and the education that prepares people for work and for life—is an important part of the society we live in. Schizophrenia, unfortunately, often has a dramatic effect on school and work performance, with the result that school dropout rates are often high and employment rates very low. We believe people with schizophrenia deserve the opportunity to earn the income and respect and experience the meaningful activities and structure that come from reaching educational goals and having a job.

With determination, the support of loved ones like you, and the assistance of rehabilitation programs, your relative can find meaningful work or complete his education. This chapter describes vocational and educational programs that may benefit your relative and suggests strategies for helping him pursue important educational and employment goals.

Unemployment and Schizophrenia

Employment rates for people with schizophrenia are generally below 20–30%. Yet most people with schizophrenia and other severe mental illnesses express a desire to work. Work gives people something to do; it provides them with a sense of purpose and improves their financial standing. Helping your relative return to work or find a job for the first time is an important step in her recovery for many reasons. In addition, working part-time will usually not affect your relative's medical insurance, and depending on how much your relative works, she may continue to receive disability income.

The Meaning and Importance of Work

Work means many different things to different people, whether or not they have a mental illness. Work gives people something that they need to do and thus helps structure their time. As described earlier in the book, the stress–vulnerability model of schizophrenia indicates that structured, meaningful, but not overdemanding activities can minimize stress and improve functioning. In fact, research shows that when people with schizophrenia work regularly or engage in other structured activities, the severity of their psychotic symptoms, such as hallucinations and delusions, drops significantly.

Involvement in meaningful activity can be a very important benefit of work. Everyone has a need for meaning in his life, and such meaning is often provided by a combination of activities in the realms of interpersonal relationships, work, spirituality, and recreation. Work often gives people something important to look forward to because they feel they are contributing to meeting a particular need. Whether the job involves clerical work, food preparation, serving, computers, art, advertising, cleaning, or animal care, it contributes to the running of a modern society. Having a job that fulfills some basic function helps people feel they are contributing members to society and part of the workaday world. For example, Lauren described the meaning of work as "I have to know that I'm doing something that's meaningful for me, whether it's teaching kids or doing social change. If it's not personal at all, I couldn't do it. I always created my own job" (quoted in Provencher et al.).

Another important benefit of work is the extra money it provides. People with schizophrenia often receive a modest amount of disability income, which can force them to live in substandard housing with limited material possessions; they are often unable to afford amenities such as a nice music system, a car, or costly leisure activities (e.g., playing golf, skiing). Work can have a dramatic effect on their ability to upgrade their lifestyle.

A final benefit of work is that it provides people with social opportunities. We often meet other people at our workplace, and these connections can serve as a basis for developing friendships. While it's important to learn the boundaries between social relationships at work and other, closer relationships, contact with coworkers provides a useful way of getting to know people better. Many of these relationships may be rewarding, even when they don't extend beyond the workplace.

Concerns about Loss of Disability Entitlements

People with schizophrenia and other major mental illnesses are often afraid to return to work because they believe it will threaten their medical insurance and any disability income they receive, such as Social Security Supplemental Income (SSI) or Social Security Disability Insurance (SSDI). Addressing these concerns may be critical to your relative's decision to seek work. Most federal and state benefits programs have work incentive provisions designed to encourage people to go to work. Depending on which benefits programs your relative receives, she can work part-time or even full-time and still retain some cash benefits and/or health insurance coverage. In most cases, your relative will be financially much better off working than not.

However, the benefits programs are complex and difficult to understand, and the specific rules concerning disability insurance and income differ somewhat across states and also across individuals, depending on a host of factors. Therefore, getting expert advice is paramount. Arrange a meeting with a disability benefits counselor, who can explain specific rules regarding your relative's disability entitlements and how work may affect them. Benefits counseling is provided at most community mental health centers. If you have difficulty locating such counseling where you live, try contacting your local office of the Social Security Administration.

Vocational Rehabilitation Programs

A wide variety of vocational rehabilitation programs have been developed for people with mental illness. The core philosophies and approaches to rehabilitation can differ significantly across these different programs. We describe several programs here and then provide a more detailed description of one particularly effective approach to vocational rehabilitation: supported employment.

Psychosocial Clubhouses and Transitional Employment

One of the oldest and most widely used approaches to psychiatric rehabilitation was developed over 50 years ago at Fountain House in New York City, a psychosocial clubhouse still devoted to helping those with severe mental illness reclaim their lives. A fundamental tenet of the clubhouse approach is that work is an important part of daily life and that everyone can benefit from working. To prepare people for the demands of work, many psychosocial clubhouses are based on a *work-ordered day*, in which each member who joins the clubhouse is given specific work assignments involved in running the clubhouse. Such work assignments may include preparing food, washing dishes, cleaning the clubhouse, hosting visitors, or working in the accounting office.

As an individual becomes accustomed to performing jobs at the clubhouse, he becomes prepared to take the next step of working in transitional employment jobs in the community. These jobs are secured by the clubhouse and involve working at a regular job that pays competitive wages. Individuals may work at a transitional job for a limited period of time, such as 3–6 months, before moving on to another transitional job or to an independent competitive job. A variety of transitional jobs may be available, such as working as a cashier, clerical work in an office, delivering interoffice mail, or janitorial work. These jobs are usually entry level.

The transitional employment approach has a number of positive features. Familiarizing individuals with a work routine at the clubhouse prepares them for paid employment. Many individuals with psychiatric disabilities have not worked for a long time, and they are insecure about their ability to work in a paying job. Transitional employment positions offer your relative the opportunity to build her work experience while providing a safety cushion of backup staff if she has difficulties fulfilling her job responsibilities. These positions also can offer her a variety of different work experiences, which may be useful in her deciding which type of job she would like on a more permanent basis.

Work Enclaves

Work enclaves are jobs in which a person with a mental illness works together with other individuals with mental illness in a community setting. These enclaves are usually developed by a vocational rehabilitation agency that obtains contracts to provide specific services for companies and then fulfills the terms of these contracts by employing individuals with disabilities. For example, a work enclave might focus on providing janitorial services to a number of office buildings, with persons with psychiatric disabilities working in supervised crews to provide those services. Most work enclaves pay competitive wages and offer a degree of community integration because the work takes place in the community. At the same time, work enclaves sometimes protect people from stressful demands on their work performance, because the terms of the work are negotiated between the vocational rehabilitation agency and the contractors. One type of work that is usually (but not always) provided in an enclave are jobs from the National Industries for the Severely Handicapped (NISH), which are positions set aside by the U.S. federal government for individuals with disabilities.

Consumer–Operated Businesses

In some communities individuals with mental illness ("consumers" of psychiatric services) own and operate businesses that employ other consumers. A wide variety of such businesses exist, such as coffee shops and clothing stores. Consumer-operated businesses offer the unique opportunity of working for and with other individuals who have psychiatric disabilities and who share the goal of promoting positive public attitudes toward mental illness, including the ability of such persons to work.

Vocational Training Programs

One approach to helping people with psychiatric disorders join the work force is to provide them with prevocational training. Such training focuses on a variety of skills and activities, such as interviewing and job-related skills, developing a regular daily schedule, identifying job-related areas of interest and strength, and acquiring basic social skills for interacting with coworkers, customers, and supervisors. Following the training in these programs, individuals may then receive support in seeking competitive work or may be given work opportunities in sheltered workshops (see next section) where additional training may be provided.

An advantage of vocational training programs is that they provide opportunities to strengthen particular skills and to develop specific plans for pursuing one's vocational goals. A disadvantage of training programs is that they are often time-consuming and do not necessarily lead to gainful employment. Many individuals who express a desire to work want to work *now* and not later and may therefore not be best served by vocational training programs that tend to significantly delay the process of finding a job.

Sheltered Workshops

Sheltered workshops (or sheltered employment) offer work conducted in a protected environment, supervised by a vocational employment agency or mental health agency and free of many of the stresses associated with competitive employment in the community. In this context people typically work at their own pace, are given ample support and encouragement, and are often paid based on what they produce rather than on an hourly wage. In most cases, sheltered workshops pay below minimum wage.

Most sheltered workshops provide some ongoing training and supervision with the goal of helping people move on to competitive employment. The advantage of sheltered workshops is that they provide an opportunity to work in a low-stress environment that is supportive and structured. The disadvantages include the lack of community integration, the low wages, and the fact that sheltered work rarely leads to competitive jobs.

Department of Vocational Rehabilitation

All states have departments of vocational rehabilitation (or departments with similar names, such as the "Bureau for Rehabilitation Services") that provide employment services to people with physical handicaps or medical conditions, to individuals who have been injured on the job and require retraining, to people with psychiatric disorders, and to others with special vocational needs. Depending on the state in which you live, your local department of vocational rehabilitation may provide sheltered workshops, vocational training programs, enclave jobs, and/or supported employment. In addition, these agencies often have funding to support specialized educational programs, for which your relative may be eligible, such as enrollment in a culinary arts program, an auto mechanics program, or a computer class.

The primary advantage of state departments of vocational rehabilitation is that they are widely available and often have funds to support a range of different programs, including educational ones. The major disadvantages are that these programs are often not geared to people with mental illness, they frequently involve long waiting lists and extensive assessment before the person gets a job, and there is often limited coordination between the vocational rehabilitation and clinical treatment. (Your relative's community mental health center is the best source of information on vocational rehabilitation programs.)

In the next section we discuss the supported employment approach to vocational rehabilitation in more detail because of the extensive research supporting it compared to other models of vocational rehabilitation.

Supported Employment

Supported employment is based on the philosophy that people with schizophrenia or other severe mental illnesses are capable of working regular jobs in the community that pay competitive wages, provided that they are given sufficient support. In contrast to other approaches to vocational rehabilitation, supported employment does not assume that people with mental illnesses require either extensive prevocational training or "protected" employment experiences before getting a competitive job. Rather, supported employment programs are based on the premise that people can acquire and keep competitive jobs relatively quickly after joining the program.

In the early 1990s vocational rehabilitation counselor Deborah R. Becker, MEd, and Robert E. Drake, MD, PhD, at Dartmouth Medical School in Hanover, New Hampshire, developed, standardized, and evaluated a program for supported employment in people with severe mental illness. Their earlier studies had shown that many people who had formerly attended day treatment programs were capable of holding competitive jobs in the community when given the necessary support. These studies laid the foundation for later controlled studies of supported employment programs.

In the decade following this early research on supported employment, a wealth of evidence has amassed from studies showing its superiority over other vocational programs (such as skills training, psychosocial rehabilitation, or sheltered work) at helping people with severe mental illness get back to work over 1–2 years. People in supported employment programs are more likely to get competitive jobs, work more hours, and earn more wages from working. Finding a supported employment program is discussed later in this chapter.

Principles of Supported Employment

The core principles of supported employment are briefly described below:

Focus on Competitive Work

Supported employment programs help people find competitive jobs in the community, rather than volunteer work or work that pays less than minimum wage (e.g., in sheltered workshops). Working at a competitive job in the community helps people feel better about themselves and is something that people with psychiatric disabilities are capable of doing.

Rapid Job Search

The goal of a supported employment program is to begin the job search with each person as soon as possible (usually within a few weeks) after referral to the program. This process usually involves meeting with the individual, learning about his job experiences, skills, and interests, and beginning to explore prospective jobs. The speed for starting the job search is set by the individual. Some people start right away, whereas others want to take a slower pace to allow time to visit different job settings and become more familiar with the work world. Rapidly initiating the job search phase of the process is crucial to capitalizing on a person's motivation to work.

Attention to Individual Preferences

Each individual has her own personal preferences about work that need to be taken into consideration. For example, some people like to work with other people, whereas others do not. Some individuals like to work in an office doing clerical activities, others prefer library work, others like cleaning, while still others like a job in the service industry, such as at a fast food restaurant. Matching a job to an individual's preferences can optimize the chances that the individual will perform successfully. Research has shown that people in supported employment programs who get jobs in their areas of interest stay on those jobs an average of twice as long as people who get jobs that do not match their areas of interest.

Individual preferences regarding the type of support provided are also important. Some individuals are willing to allow prospective employers to know about their psychiatric disorder, whereas others prefer not to disclose this information. Some individuals appreciate it when their employment specialists talk directly with prospective employers and help them land jobs and negotiate accommodations. Others prefer the employment specialist to play a "behind the scenes" role to help them find possible jobs, prepare them with job interviewing, and support them in maintaining those jobs.

Follow-Along Supports

In many other approaches to vocational rehabilitation, the role of the program stops when the individual finally gets a competitive job. In contrast, follow-along supports are a critical component of supported employment programs. This phase of support provides a variety of services designed to help people retain their jobs or to help them make a transition to a new job, if needed or desired; on-the-job training, negotiating job accommodations with the employer, doing problem solving with the individual to resolve difficulties at work, providing temporary logistical support in getting to and from work, providing skills training for handling social situations on the job, and offering consultation with the employer to address work-related difficulties. Over time, the degree of support needed declines for many people; some move on to competitive work without support, whereas others continue to need some level of support over the long term.

Integration of Vocational and Mental Health Services

Not surprisingly, mental health issues and vocational functioning are often related to one another. For this reason, supported employment services are integrated with mental health treatment services. The integration of mental health and supported employment services is most effective when it occurs at the level of the treatment team so that both mental health and employment specialists meet together on a regular basis (such as weekly) to discuss their respective concerns.

Gina had been working at a job for 15 hours a week doing clerical work for a small insurance company for the past 4 months. Her work performance had been good and her employer had praised her diligence, but a problem had begun to emerge over the past several weeks. Gina had slept late and had not arrived at work on time on several occasions. Her supervisor expressed concern that Gina was having difficulty keeping up with her tasks, was lethargic, and seemed "spacey" when he gave her work assignments. The employment specialist had also observed that Gina was more disorganized than usual and seemed preoccupied with something else when they talked.

After talking with Gina and getting her permission, the employment specialist shared this information with the treatment team. Upon further discussion the team agreed it was possible that these changes in Gina's work performance might be early warning signs of a relapse. A special meeting was scheduled for Gina and her psychiatrist, who concluded together that these changes were related to a modest increase in her symptoms. Gina's medication was increased temporarily, and this change was successful in warding off a relapse. With Gina's permission, the employment specialist informed her employer that she received an increase in her medication, and they agreed to stay in close touch to monitor her work performance. Gina's work gradually improved over the next few weeks and within a month was back to its usual level. Two months later Gina's medication dosage was reduced to its previous maintenance dose, and her good job performance continued unabated.

Benefits Counseling

Benefits counseling is critical to supported employment. An employment specialist (or other informed professional) can allay fears people have about losing disability insurance and income and help them make informed decisions about how much they want to work. Providing information about the effects of work on benefits can also relieve concerns family members may have about their relative working, thereby freeing family members to offer their fullest support for pursuing this important goal.

Finding Supported Employment Services

As described in Chapter 5, supported employment services can often be accessed through your relative's local community mental health center. Some mental health centers provide supported employment services within their own program, so your relative may not need to go elsewhere to get those services. Other mental health centers may have working relationships with separate vocational rehabilitation agencies that provide supported employment. Many mental health centers have a director of vocational rehabilitation who can refer individuals to an appropriate supported employment program. If possible, find a supported employment program that is closely integrated with the provision of mental health services.

Supported employment services may not be available in some places, or the distance needed to travel to a program may make it impractical or impossible. In these situations family members can help a loved one who wants to work find meaningful employment and support him in maintaining that work. The table on the facing page provides suggestions for how you can help your relative find work, based on the principles of supported employment.

Vince lived with his mother, Pauline, in a small town 60 miles away from the nearest major city and the local community mental health center. Pauline read about supported employment and thought Vince might be interested in working. She gently broached the topic by asking him whether he ever had any thoughts about working; was it something he might like to do? At first Vince was rather pessimistic, saying that he didn't know what difference it would make and that he probably wouldn't be able to work anyway. Over the next few weeks, Pauline encouraged Vince to think about what he might like to do with the extra money he could earn and the things that he might enjoy doing as part of a job.

Vince began to warm up to the idea of working and started to think about buying a music system and CDs. Pauline boosted Vince's confidence by telling him that she thought it was possible for him to work as long as he took it one small step at a time. She also promised to help him find and keep a job. Vince agreed that it might be worth a try, so they began to talk about jobs he might like, such as working in a store, as long as he didn't have to run the cash register. Pauline and Vince began to look around for possible jobs. When Pauline attended the monthly local NAMI support group, she mentioned her son's interest in work. One of the group members had a brother who owned a hardware store who was looking for someone to help in the store. Pauline and Vince went to meet with the store owner, who agreed to give Vince a try. Vince wanted to start slowly, so they settled on

Helping Your Loved One Find Work

Explore the possibility of work with your relative:
- Ask if your relative has thought about work or is interested in working.
- Explore with your relative some of the possible benefits of work (e.g., more money, something to do, social opportunities, feeling good about oneself).
- Explore possible concerns your relative might have about work (e.g., stress, meeting expectations, loss of disability income).
- Help your relative determine whether he/she needs more information about work before deciding whether to pursue it.
- Help your relative weigh the advantages and disadvantages of work and decide whether or not to pursue work (you can adapt Worksheet 22.3 to list the pros and cons of working).
- Avoid pressuring your relative to work.

If your relative is interested in work, explore his/her job interests and preferences:
- Talk about your relative's past work experiences (if any).
- Discuss the types of work he/she would like to do.
- Consider special skills, training, or degrees your relative has that may help in landing a job, such as computer programming, secretarial skills, mechanical ability, bookkeeping/accounting expertise, artistic ability, or cooking.
- Talk about the setting in which your relative would like to work (e.g., outdoors, office, store, restaurant, janitorial).
- If your relative has difficulty identifying job interests, talk about his/her other interests (e.g., hobbies, sports, theater, music, cooking) to discern possible job ideas.
- Identify a few possible job types to help focus your job search.

Find a job:
- Look in the classified ads in the newspaper with your relative.
- Walk around the business district of your town and look for help wanted signs.
- Let other family members and friends know about your relative's interest in working to elicit possible job leads.
- Attend meetings of your local chapter of the National Alliance on Mental Illness (NAMI) and let people know about your relative's interest in work.
- Explore possible job-finding resources on the Internet.
- Encourage your relative to elicit possible job leads at a local peer support program.
- Ask members of your relative's treatment team if they have any suggestions or leads for possible jobs.

Land the job:
- Talk over with your relative how you can help him/her get a job.
- Consider practicing job interviewing skills with your relative.
- Talk over whether it would help for you to speak directly with a prospective employer.
- Explore whether there is another person who could speak to a prospective employer on your relative's behalf.

Help your relative succeed on the job:
- Talk over ways you can help your relative succeed on the job.
- Be available to help with problem solving about difficulties encountered at work.
- Check in regularly with your relative about how work is going.
- Offer to meet with your relative's employer to iron out work-related difficulties.
- If your relative loses a job or quits, don't give up!
- Learn from job setbacks and work together to find a new job.

2 hours a day, 3 days a week. He learned how to stock the shelves and how to help customers find merchandise, and he discovered that he enjoyed it. After a month he increased his hours to 12 a week, and by the next year he was working 20 hours a week. Vince told his mother that he liked the work, that it made him feel good about himself, and that it gave him something to look forward to. He also saved enough money to buy a stereo system.

Legal Rights and the Americans with Disabilities Act

Discrimination against people with mental illness in the workplace and other avenues of daily life is a major difficulty that can have a scarring effect on those who suffer from it. For example, one individual said:

> I haven't bridged the gap between myself and other people because of the way I have been treated in the past. I have been discriminated against and my rights have been trodden on at different places I have worked because of my illness and others not understanding it. (quoted in Provencher et al.)

Discrimination against people with mental illness used to be very common, and until recently, it was not against the law. However, all of this changed in 1990 with the passage of the Americans with Disabilities Act (ADA) by the U.S. Congress. For the first time in American history, it was illegal to discriminate against individuals with disabilities, including major psychiatric disorders such as schizophrenia, in employment, housing, education, or medical care. Thus, the ADA provides some legal protection against discrimination in the workplace based on mental illness.

According to the ADA, employers cannot discriminate against prospective employees because they have a mental illness. Although this law is stated clearly, in practice it is difficult to know when an individual is being discriminated against because of her mental illness. However, the ADA also states that people who have disabilities are entitled to receive "reasonable accommodations" for their disability at the workplace. The definition of "reasonable accommodations" is flexible, but in general it means that the employer is obliged to make some modifications in the work environment (if possible), the individual's work schedule, or the specific duties of the job if such modifications would enable the person to do the required job and if the modifications do not place an undue burden on the employer. To formally arrange for a "reasonable accommodation," the employer must know that the individual has a psychiatric disability. Informal accommodations may be arranged without such knowledge and can be worked out individually with the employer.

Most employers are aware of the ADA and the rights it affords to persons with disabilities. However, violations of the ADA are possible, and if they can be proven, legal recourse is available to the person whose rights were violated. If you or your relative are concerned that his legal rights have been, or are being, violated, you should contact a legal agency that has experience with disability rights or your local mental health center. At the end of this chapter are some possible resources for obtaining help regarding violations of the ADA.

Supported Education

As the symptoms of schizophrenia gradually develop in late adolescence or early adulthood, people often have trouble focusing their attention on schoolwork. As a result, many people drop out of school early, before they've achieved their educational goals. Once people have stopped school, it is often hard to start again, partly because of the social difficulties inherent in explaining one's absence when returning to school and partly because of persistent symptoms or cognitive difficulties related to the illness.

A variety of programs is available to help your relative pursue her educational goals. Many supported employment specialists/teams also provide supported education services. Mental health centers often have arrangements with local schools to help individuals complete the necessary course work for a general equivalency diploma (GED) for high school. You can also find out about specific GED requirements from your local school system, and you can help your relative identify GED tutors or other instructional opportunities in your community. Internet courses that provide instruction for GED-related material are also available.

A variety of opportunities is also available for individuals who have graduated from high school and are interested in pursuing or resuming studies in college. Many colleges, especially community colleges, allow people to enroll as part-time students, enabling them to take one or two classes at a time. This format can be very helpful for people with schizophrenia, who often need to build up their study skills gradually by taking only one or two classes at a time. In addition, many colleges have special programs designed to accommodate the needs of people with psychiatric disorders; accommodations may include help with developing study skills, strategies for managing psychiatric symptoms, and tips on adjusting socially to the college environment. Furthermore, self-help organizations are available at many colleges for students with psychiatric disabilities who want support in dealing with common problems at school. Lastly, most colleges make tutoring services available to all of their students.

Another option for many people is to pursue training for a specific career. For example, your relative may have an interest in working as a cook, a word processor, an auto mechanic, or a cosmetologist. Specialty schools exist for many different fields; helping your relative find an appropriate program may be the most valuable step you can take to encourage him to pursue a career goal.

Your relative also has her rights protected by the ADA in educational settings. For example, depending on the nature of your relative's symptoms, she may be entitled to more time to take tests or to write papers. If your relative has difficulty meeting her course obligations because of symptoms or cognitive difficulties, you should explore whether requesting a reasonable accommodation from the instructor (or educational institution) would help address these problems. Tips for helping your relative pursue her education are provided in table below.

Yolanda developed schizophrenia at the age of 27 and 2 years later she married Keith. They had been married for 5 years when Keith began to sense some dissatisfaction in Yolanda about her life. They had two children, and Keith helped Yolanda by sharing many of the parenting responsibilities. Keith began to talk to Yolanda about how she felt about her family and her role as a stay-at-home mother. It took a while for Yolanda to open up, but eventually she was able to explain that although she loved being a mother, she wanted something else to do outside her home, like Keith, who worked as a carpenter. As they talked about it more, Yolanda revealed that she had always been interested in makeup, hairstyling, and fashion. As they explored the area further, Yolanda realized that she wanted to go back to school to become a cosmetologist. Keith supported Yolanda in pursuing this goal and, after some searching, found a cosmetology school where Yolanda could begin as a part-time student.

Tips for Helping Your Relative Pursue His/Her Education

Explore with your relative whether he/she would like to return to school:
- Discuss the possible advantages of getting a high school diploma, a college degree, or participating in a specialty training course, such as in a trade school.
- Explore possible career ideas.
- Consider the steps necessary to take to achieve career goals, including more education.

Identify possible educational programs:
- Consider possible programs through local mental health centers, colleges, trade schools.
- Consider suggestions from other family members, friends, and mental health or educational professionals.
- Review the possible options with your relative and consider the advantages and disadvantages of each.

Make a plan with your relative to enroll in an educational program:
- Get all the information you need about the program.
- Encourage your relative to start slowly by taking only one or two classes at a time.
- Anticipate possible problems that might come up and brainstorm solutions.

Support your relative's return to school:
- Show interest in your relative's progress in school.
- Help identify trouble spots and problem-solve with him/her about them.
- Explore options for supplementary tutoring, if necessary.
- Encourage your relative to look at setbacks when returning to school (e.g., a poor score on a test) as "learning experiences" that can help him/her do better next time.
- Keep your relative's long-term goal alive by bringing it up and praising his/her progress toward it.

Recognizing Your Relative's Abilities

Work plays an important role in defining who we are, both to ourselves and to others. Although it was once believed that people with schizophrenia were incapable of working, there is now overwhelming evidence that people who want to work can get meaningful jobs, contribute to society, and be rewarded for their efforts. The rewards of working are many: increased self-esteem, increased financial resources, something interesting to do, and greater integration into the community. But to help your relative pursue work (or related goals, such as school, volunteering, or other meaningful activities), you must first believe that he is capable of achieving this goal.

As outlined in this chapter, there are many ways of helping your relative find work or return to school. Programs may be available in your area to help your relative achieve these goals, or you may need to improvise by working together with your relative and tapping other resources available to you, such as family members and friends. Above all, believing in your relative and becoming aware of her personal strengths are the most important ingredients to helping her succeed at work or school.

Resources

Active Minds is a self-help organization of individuals with mental illness who are enrolled in colleges throughout the country. Their website is *www.activemindsoncampus.org*.

Becker, D. R., & Drake, R. E. (2003). *A working life for people with severe mental illness.* New York: Oxford University Press. This book describes the individual placement and support model of supported employment.

Provencher, H. P., Gregg, R., Mead, S., & Mueser, K. T. (2002). The role of work in recovery of persons with psychiatric disabilities. *Psychiatric Rehabilitation Journal, 26,* 132–144. This article, based on in-depth interviews with 14 individuals, describes the different roles of work in recovery from severe mental illness.

CHAPTER 27

Independent Living
and Self-Care Skills

W here your relative lives and her relationships with people in that set-ting can have an important bearing on the quality of her life. For some people with schizophrenia, living with parents or siblings is best because of the social support they receive and their ability to fit in with the fam-ily routine. For others, living elsewhere is preferable for a variety of reasons, such as greater privacy and independence, more structure or assistance, or lower lev-els of tension. Ultimately, the best living arrangement is one that balances the needs of your relative and those of the rest of your family.

Independent living is an important goal for many people with schizophre-nia—and one that you may already support for your relative. However, regardless of where your relative lives, improvement in his self-care and independent living skills can reduce dependence on others and improve self-esteem, health, social relationships, and vocational options. This chapter helps you and your relative determine the best living arrangement for all by assessing your relative's self-care and independent living skills (such as personal hygiene, meal preparation, and use of transportation) and learning strategies for helping your loved one develop these skills.

Evaluating Your Relative's Living Situation

If you're the parent of an adult child with schizophrenia who lives with you, you know it's not easy to determine whether it's best for her to continue living at home or to live elsewhere. Your adult child may feel that she is ready for more in-dependence and that moving out would be a logical step toward taking more control over, and responsibility for, her life. Sometimes family members feel a great deal of stress when a close family member with schizophrenia lives at home, and they may prefer that their relative move to a living situation that decreases the burden of responsibility on them. Some of the reasons that families commonly consider alternatives to their relative's living at home include extremely disruptive or violent behavior, severe substance abuse, substantial conflict between other family members, and inability or unwillingness to follow basic household rules.

Even when living elsewhere is best for both the person and his family, parents often feel guilty and worry that they are "abandoning" their child when he moves out. However, if and when you contemplate this decision, you may find it helpful to think of your relative's relocation as a positive step toward greater independence, not a setback. Furthermore, just because your relative lives away from home doesn't mean that you can't continue to support him and maintain a close relationship. In fact, many family members find their relationship with their relative *improves* after he leaves home, because everyone feels less tension.

Housing Options

People with schizophrenia vary widely in how much assistance and structure they need in their living arrangements. Some are very independent and need little or no assistance from treatment providers or their family. Others, however, require some supervision or assistance to meet their daily living needs and benefit from a daily structure when they move away from home. In our experience, many people with schizophrenia have difficulty moving directly away from home into a completely independent, unsupervised apartment. Independent living is a viable goal, but it may be better to pursue this goal through a gradual series of steps that involves living in progressively less supervised residences.

Because most people with schizophrenia want to live as independently as possible, *supported housing* has emerged in recent years as a common living arrangement. People live in their own apartment but have access to professional staff who assist them in meeting daily living and treatment needs. Such assistance may cover a wide range of activities involved in daily living, such as food shopping and meal preparation, money and medication management, accessing community resources, laundry, and maintaining an apartment. The extent of staff availability ranges from one setting to another and can include daytime or 24-hour availability. Supported housing and other types of living arrangements, such as community rehabilitation residences and group homes, are described in Chapter 5. When considering different housing options, it's important to determine the level of structure and supervision available, the cost of the housing, and whether or not your relative is eligible for financial assistance.

Deciding whether your relative should continue to live at home can be a difficult and emotional process. Keep in mind the goal of balancing the needs of your relative with those of the rest of your family. Start by identifying both the

Possible Advantages of Living at Home versus Living in Supervised or Supported Housing

Perspective	Advantages of living at home	Advantages of living in supervised or supported housing
Family members	• Easier to monitor illness • Many opportunities to provide support • Less expensive for my relative • Certain that my relative receives good meals and has a clean environment • My relative helps us do things around the house • Enjoy my relative's company	• Less tension and conflict at home • More time to ourselves • Could take a vacation without worry • Less responsibility on a daily basis • Fewer disruptions in the household • Might improve our relationship
Person with schizophrenia	• More living space • Fewer household responsibilities • Someone often around for company or help • Familiar environment • Income goes further • Feeling understood	• More privacy • Feeling more independent, self-reliant • Meeting new people • Having more to do • Fewer arguments with parents, siblings • Able to do more things on own timetable

advantages and disadvantages of your relative's living at home, from your perspective as well as your relative's. The table above compares some of the advantages of living at home to the advantages of living elsewhere, such as a community residence, group home, or supported housing.

Skills for Independent Living

If your relative moves away from home, she must be able to complete specific tasks required for living more independently, depending on what is provided in her new housing. Many people with schizophrenia who live with relatives already do chores regularly and contribute to the running of the household (see Chapter 16 for more information on developing household rules about chores). For example, Rudy lives with his sister and routinely does his own laundry and helps with preparing meals. He is very knowledgeable about the public transportation system and goes everywhere on the bus. Other people with schizophrenia who live at home lack some important skills for independent living, however. Eugene, for example, lives with his parents and is responsible only for making his bed and preparing his own snacks while watching television. He depends on his parents to manage his money and for shopping, cleaning, preparing meals, laundry, and transportation. Worksheet 27.1 at the end of the chapter will help you and your relative evaluate how much assistance she currently needs in performing tasks. Completing the checklist will give your relative useful information for selecting skills to work on so that she can be more self-sufficient in the future.

The more self-sufficient your relative is, the more housing options he will have. Just as important, improving independent living skills will help increase your relative's confidence and self-esteem and will often lead to improvements in relationships and work opportunities. Feeling independent in as many areas as possible is important to your relative's quality of life, whether he lives at home or elsewhere.

Breaking Down Skills into Steps

Once you and your relative have identified the skills that she needs to strengthen, focus on one or two at a time. Tackling everything at once can be overwhelming, not to mention frustrating. By breaking down each skill into smaller steps, you can help your relative learn many skills. The table on pages 412–413 lists common independent living skills and the core steps of each.

Broaching the Subject of Improving Living and Self-Care Skills

Some families are hesitant to talk with their relative about his living skills. You may be concerned that your relative will be embarrassed or angered by the topic and will resist your efforts. When broaching the subject, avoid being judgmental or critical. Instead, let your relative know that you understand how difficult it can be to perform particular tasks on a regular basis. Then point out how attending to a specific skill can be important to achieving some of his personal goals, such as living more independently, making friends, or having a girlfriend. Finally, offer to help your relative make a plan to work on a particular skill. The following vignette shows how one mother approached her son about his personal hygiene.

MOTHER: Mike, I've noticed that sometimes it seems to be a little hard for you to brush your teeth and take a shower.

MIKE: Yeah. Sometimes I forget.

MOTHER: I can understand that it might be hard to remember to do some of those things.

MIKE: Sometimes I just don't want to do it.

MOTHER: I can see how that might be tough. On the other hand, taking care of your hygiene can be important for making friends.

MIKE: I guess so.

MOTHER: You've told me that you'd like to have closer friends. How about if I give you a hand in helping you improve some of these areas of personal hygiene? It might help you in making friends.

MIKE: Okay, I'll give it a try.

Steps of Independent Living and Self-Care Skills

Preparing meals

- Using microwave to heat meals
- Preparing breakfast
- Preparing sandwiches and other cold entrees
- Using stovetop for boiling and frying
- Using oven for baking
- Knowing how to prepare some "stand-by" meals, such as macaroni and cheese, hot dogs, beans and rice, etc.

Cleaning the kitchen

- Washing dishes
- Wiping off the stove and counters
- Sweeping floor
- Washing the floor
- Scrubbing the sink
- Taking out the garbage

Cleaning the living and sleeping areas

- Straightening up
- Changing the sheets
- Vacuuming
- Dusting

Laundry

- Keeping dirty laundry in a hamper/laundry bag/basket
- Going to the laundromat (if no washing machine in apartment)
- Loading the washing machine and adding detergent
- Operating washing machine (choosing the correct temperature and cycle)
- Operating dryer (cleaning the lint trap, choosing the correct temperature)
- Folding and putting away clean clothes

Shopping for clothing

- Deciding which clothing should be purchased for the season
- Selecting stores appropriate for one's budget
- Going to the store
- Trying on items to make sure they fit
- Staying within budget

Cleaning the bathroom

- Scrubbing sink
- Scrubbing the bathtub/shower
- Cleaning the toilet
- Washing the floor

Using transportation

- Reading a road map and/or public transportation schedule
- Locating bus stops or subway stations
- For drivers, maintaining a driver's license and car insurance, practicing defensive driving, keeping car in good repair

Taking medication

- Filling prescriptions at the pharmacy
- Storing medications where they can be located easily
- Taking medications as prescribed (i.e., correct dose, correct number of times per day, same time every day)
- Developing a method to make sure that medications are taken regularly (e.g., setting up a pill box, using a checklist, marking a calendar)
- Using cues to remind oneself to take medications at the proper times
- Getting prescriptions refilled prior to using up the medication   *(cont.)*

Steps of Independent Living and Self-Care Skills (*cont.*)

Managing money

- Keeping track of income
- Keeping track of expenses
- Paying bills on time
- Making a budget and spending money accordingly
- Writing checks and balancing a checkbook
- Paying for basic living expenses before spending money on nonessentials

Making and keeping appointments

- Calling the doctor's office
- Identifying self and the reason for appointment
- Finding out if a referral or an insurance card is required at the appointment
- Writing down the appointment on a calendar or in an appointment book
- Checking a calendar or book regularly for dates of appointments
- Planning transportation
- Writing down a list of concerns or questions to raise at the visit
- Going to the appointment

Meaningful activities (see Chapter 28 for more details)

- Participating in activities or hobbies that one can enjoy by oneself (e.g., reading, puzzles, running, knitting)
- Participating in work or activities that one can enjoy with others (e.g., drop-in center, clubs, sports)
- Participating in employment or volunteer work

Grooming and hygiene

- Bathing or showering
- Washing hair
- Applying deodorant
- Brushing and flossing teeth
- Combing hair
- Wearing clean clothes appropriate to the season
- Trimming nails
- For men, shaving or trimming beard

Shopping for groceries

- Making a list
- Going to the store
- Locating grocery items
- Staying within budget
- Comparison shopping to get the most economical products
- Putting groceries away

Safety at home and on the streets

- Recognizing and avoiding potentially dangerous situations (e.g., walking alone on a deserted, unlighted street)
- Recognizing and avoiding potentially dangerous individuals
- Responding effectively to panhandling and other requests made on the street
- Responding effectively to offers of drugs
- Refusing unwanted sexual advances
- Avoiding having one's money stolen (e.g., placing wallet in front pocket, not displaying cash)
- Locking one's door, not opening the door unless one knows who it is

Time management

- Using an alarm clock
- Keeping a regular daily schedule of meals, going to bed, etc.
- Using a calendar to write down appointments and important events
- Scheduling time to fulfill responsibilities and complete chores
- Scheduling time for leisure

Guidelines for Improving Independent Living and Self–Care Skills

1. *Discuss the reasons a specific skill area is important.* Although pointing out advantages of learning particular skills can be useful, it is usually more effective to ask your relative questions to get her to consider how learning a skill could be helpful in attaining a goal. For example, if your relative wants to lose weight, you could ask questions about whether learning basic cooking skills could help her gain more control over the calorie and nutritional content of her meals. You could also ask questions about the effects of not being able to cook, such as having to spend more money eating out, and explore the major, longer-term consequences of not learning the skill. For example, you could mention that lacking basic cooking skills would limit her options for more independent living.

2. *Agree on specific steps of the skill to work on.* Help your relative identify the steps of the skill that are the biggest problem. Decide together which areas are most important to work on. For example, if your relative has difficulties with time management, ask what he thinks is most important in managing his time: Using an alarm clock to get up on time? Keeping to a regular schedule? Writing down appointments and important events? Making a schedule for tasks that need to be done daily?

3. *Set goals and plan follow-up.* Aim for attainable goals and avoid being overly ambitious at first. Be as specific as possible when setting goals. How many times a day or week should the steps of a skill be performed? If a daily goal is set, at approximately what time should it be done every day? If a weekly goal is set, on what day should the skill be performed? For example, if your relative has the goal of improving her personal hygiene, a realistic goal might be showering on Tuesdays and Fridays before breakfast and brushing her teeth every morning and night.

Planning for follow-up should include a specific date and time. For example, you and your relative could plan to meet on Saturday mornings at 10 A.M. As part of planning follow-up meetings, it may be helpful to set up a record sheet that your relative can use to record the skills he performs each day. Make the record sheet easy to use, with spaces to check off whether the skill was performed. Encourage your relative to post the record sheet where he will see it and be prompted to complete it regularly.

4. *Demonstrate how to perform the skill.* If your relative does not know how to perform the skill or has very little experience doing it, she may find it helpful to see you demonstrate it. For example, if your relative's goal is to keep the bathroom clean but she doesn't know how to scrub the sink and clean the toilet, you can show her how you do these chores. You should also make sure your relative has the necessary supplies. Without a sponge and a cleanser, for example, she could not scrub the bathroom sink.

5. *Ask your relative to practice the skill with you.* After your relative has had a chance to observe you performing the skill, he can practice it and get feedback

from you. For example, to improve his skills at making appointments on the phone, your relative could role-play it with you. You could then give your relative feedback on how well he performed the steps of the skill (e.g., including identifying himself and giving a brief reason for requesting the appointment).

6. *Agree on a plan for your relative to try the skill on her own.* After your relative has practiced the skill with you and feels more confident, figure out a time when she can try it alone. For example, if your relative is working on the skill of using public transportation and has practiced taking the bus with you, she could plan to take the bus independently to the library twice the next week, on Tuesday morning and Friday afternoon.

7. *Meet regularly to follow up on the plan.* At first, meeting at least weekly to follow up on your relative's plan to practice skills is wise. When you meet, praise your relative for any positive steps, even small ones. For example, if your relative is working on the skill of shopping for groceries and is able to purchase three out of the five items on his list, start by praising that accomplishment. You can then help him make a plan to increase the number of items purchased. At times you may need to modify the plan, either to work toward larger goals or to set smaller ones. When setting new goals after your relative has had success with a previous goal, try taking very small steps to avoid overwhelming him. For example, if your relative succeeds in picking up all five grocery items, you can suggest adding a few more to the list—but don't double the number.

Some people with schizophrenia master many or all independent living skills. Others continue to need help even after concerted efforts to learn the skills. For example, your relative may improve significantly in most of the independent living skills, but may continue to need some assistance with transportation or managing money. Keep in mind that your relative can still live away from home even if she is not completely independent. As mentioned earlier in this chapter and in Chapter 5, housing programs provide a range of assistance and support, including supported housing, group homes, and community rehabilitation residences. Your relative might also get some of the assistance she needs from other sources, such as family members, mental health agencies, religious groups, and community volunteer organizations.

Representative Payee Programs

Money management is a skill that bears additional discussion here. Many people with schizophrenia continue to have difficulty with managing their finances even when they make progress on other independent living skills. Running out of money before the end of the month is a common problem for many. If your relative has difficulties managing money, he may benefit from having someone, such as a representative payee, help him make a budget to ensure that basic needs are covered. A representative payee can be a private individual, a professional, or an agency that is designated to receive Social Security or Veterans Administration benefits on behalf of the person. The representative payee helps the person budget the money and disburses the funds to pay for current needs, including housing, groceries, utilities, medical expenses, and clothing. Keeping records of how the person's money is spent and reporting them to the Social Security or Veterans Administration is also part of the representative payee's responsibilities. Although it's possible for a family member to be someone's representative payee, many families prefer an independent person to play that role to minimize possible conflict. You can get more information about the representative payee program at your local community mental health center or at the office of the Social Security Administration.

Deciding to Move

The decision to seek other living arrangements can be initiated by the person with schizophrenia, her family, or both. Sometimes the person with the illness feels it's time to move on and raises the issue.

Estelline was 35 when she started talking with her parents about moving away from home because of tension and arguments. "I love my parents," she said, "but we get on each other's nerves being around each other all these years. I think we'd get along better if there was a little distance between us." Because Estelline needed help with various aspects of independent living, such as cooking, her parents were initially reluctant to consider her ideas about moving. However, she was persistent, asking her mother to give her cooking lessons and showing a strong motivation to become more independent.

Sometimes it's the family that initiates the discussion about whether it might be better for their relative to live away from home.

Francis, an only child, had lived with his mother for over 20 years after developing schizophrenia. His mother had provided everything for Francis over the years, including money management, cleaning, cooking, and overseeing his medication regimen. He stayed at home except for going to his doctor's appointments. As his mother developed health problems, she began to reevaluate whether it was best for Francis to live at home. Because Francis had no other social contacts and was not used to taking care of himself, she worried that he would be at a significant disadvantage if her health declined or if she passed away. She decided to talk to her son about her concerns.

Although it can be either the family or the person with the illness who initiates the idea of moving out, the actual decision to move on is usually consensual. Family members usually talk together about why the present living arrangement is not working, consider the various options, and decide what would be best for all concerned. Deciding to move away is generally a process that involves several conversations and the weighing of possible options. It may also involve a lengthy period while the person continues to live at home but learns and practices more independent living skills, or while the person waits for his choice of housing to become available.

Usually the person and her family come to a mutual agreement about the new living situation, but occasionally there may be lingering disagreements. The person with the illness may want to move out, but the family may not feel comfortable with this. Or the family may want their relative to live elsewhere, and she may be reluctant to do so or may even refuse. This last situation, though not common, is particularly difficult for parents.

Discussing Moving Out with Your Relative

Talking about moving out can be an emotional topic for you and your relative. However, advance preparation may allay some of your concerns and make it easier for your relative. The first issue you need to resolve before discussing alternative living arrangements with your relative is whether leaving is still an open question or whether you've already decided that you want your relative to leave home. Knowing whether the question is still open has direct bearing on how you present the situation to your relative. If you haven't decided whether you want your relative to leave, the primary purpose of the discussion is to exchange views and find out whether he would like to move. On the other hand, if you've already decided you want your relative to leave, it's best to be clear about it at the beginning, to avoid misleading him.

If you live with other family members who share the role of caregiver with you, try to come to an agreement before discussing the matter with your relative. Settling disagreements among family members will free you to support each other when presenting this issue to your relative. You'll also be able to anticipate and plan for different possible responses your relative might give.

If you firmly decide that you want your relative to move, you can present this decision to her in a family meeting. Arrange a time for this meeting when everyone is calm and select a place that is free of distractions. Present the decision to your relative in an honest, straightforward, unapologetic manner. Provide an explanation for your decision, but avoid justifying it. Also make it clear that your decision is not negotiable, while listening sympathetically to your relative's concerns and letting her know of your continued support.

Try to involve your relative as much as possible in planning the move to another living arrangement. Don't try to make all the necessary plans in a single meeting; give your relative some time to adjust to the idea of moving out.

MOTHER: Antonio, your dad and I have been doing a lot of talking recently, and we've come to the decision that it would be best for you to live somewhere else. We feel quite a lot of tension around the house, and we both think that all of us would be better off if you had a different living situation.

ANTONIO: What? You're kicking me out of my home?

MOTHER: We don't look at it that way. We still love you and want to support you, but we also feel that the time has come for you to move on. Moving away from home can be a positive step toward greater independence.

ANTONIO: But I don't want to go! This is my home and I like it here!

FATHER: I can understand your feelings. You've lived here your whole life, and you feel comfortable here. However, your mother and I think it's best now for you to live somewhere other than home. We think it's a step in the right direction, and we want to support you in taking that step.

ANTONIO: So now you're going to make me live in one of those group homes?

MOTHER: We don't know yet what the best living arrangement would be. We would like you to be involved in making some of these decisions. I understand that this is hard for you now, and we'll need to talk more about this over the next few days and weeks.

ANTONIO: I don't like the whole idea.

FATHER: I can see how this is upsetting to you, Antonio. We wanted you to know that this is a decision your mother and I have made, but we also want you involved in it as much as possible. Why don't we stop here, and we can pick up talking about it a little later. Okay?

ANTONIO: Okay.

In most cases gentle persistence, a unified front, and the involvement of your relative in all stages of this major change will produce a smooth transition for your relative from living at home to living elsewhere. Sometimes, however, your relative may adamantly refuse to leave, and his lack of cooperation becomes a major obstacle. When this occurs, your choices naturally become more restricted.

Some families initiate changes in their relative's living situation while she is temporarily in the hospital for treatment of a relapse. If your relative has recently been violent or has threatened violence, it may be necessary to petition to have her hospitalized. When your relative is in the hospital, you can inform the inpatient treatment team that she cannot return home after the hospitalization. The team must then assume responsibility for finding a suitable placement for her. If you take this route, you will need to be firm in presenting your position to the inpatient team (as well as to your relative), who may try to persuade you to allow her to return home. If your relative steadfastly refuses placements that the inpatient treatment team recommends, there is a small risk that she could be discharged with no living arrangement. More often, people eventually agree to a placement.

If your relative refuses to leave home but is not in a state in which he must be hospitalized, there are fewer recourses available to you. Legally, if you own your home, you can have him evicted. Most families do not see eviction as a viable option because of the level of confrontation involved. However, in very severe situations, it may merit consideration. If you're in this difficult predicament, you must work together with other family members toward evaluating strategies for encouraging your relative to leave. It may also be helpful to be in touch with your relative's treatment providers, who may be able to offer suggestions or support your decision during their interactions with your relative. Finally, the support and advice from other families who have been through the same experience are invaluable; help can be obtained through local chapters of organizations such as the National Alliance on Mental Illness (NAMI).

Supporting Your Relative's Independence

Becoming more independent is a natural progression in life. Developing schizophrenia can interfere with that process and may delay the development of the skills needed for living independently. If your relative has recently developed the illness, it's important to foster a vision of recovery from the start and to encourage her to do things for herself. However, even if your relative has had schizophrenia for many years, it's never too late to help her become more independent. Supporting your relative in taking steps toward independence both increases her options in life and, by decreasing dependence on you and the family, promotes self-confidence and self-esteem.

Resources

www.mmaci.org. The Money Management Advocacy Council Icon recruits nonprofit agencies and individuals interested in becoming representative payees. It sponsors workshops on effective and respectful methods to manage the money of beneficiaries.

www.ssa.gov/payee. This Social Security website includes detailed guides for individual payees and organizational payees. Both guides describe the responsibilities of payees.

Independent Living and Self–Care Skills Checklist

Instructions: With your relative, rate how independently he/she performs each activity.

Activity	Independently	With prompting	With help	Done by someone else
Managing money				
Shopping for groceries				
Meal preparation				
Shopping for clothing				
Cleaning				
Laundry				
Taking medication				
Making and keeping appointments				
Using public or private transportation				
Grooming and hygiene				
Leisure and recreation				
Time management				
Maintaining safety at home and on the street				

CHAPTER 28

Leisure and Recreation

School, work, and relationships make life meaningful for those with schizophrenia, as they do for all of us. But leisure time is just as important. Doing things we enjoy during our spare time gives us something to look forward to and something positive to reflect back on. Yet many people with schizophrenia have difficulty finding satisfying and enjoyable activities to pursue in their free time, and improving how they spend that time is a common goal. This chapter focuses on how you can help your relative develop rewarding leisure and recreational activities.

Reasons for Lack of Leisure and Recreational Activities

People with schizophrenia often have limited outlets for leisure and recreation and may enjoy these activities less than other people, for reasons related both to the symptoms and associated difficulties of the illness, and to the circumstances in which schizophrenia occurs.

Negative Symptoms

The negative symptoms of schizophrenia (described in Chapter 18) frequently interfere with leisure and recreation. *Apathy* (not caring about or being interested in things) makes it difficult to identify and seek out activities that might be enjoyable. For example, one person said, "I'd like to have a hobby, but it's hard to find something I'm interested in. Unless I'm interested, it doesn't seem worth the energy." *Anhedonia* (not being able to feel pleasure) makes it hard for the person to enjoy activities, even if it's something he used to enjoy. When a person derives no pleasure from an activity, it's only natural for him to resist participating in it.

Cognitive Difficulties

As described in Chapter 19, many people with schizophrenia have problems in their cognition (thinking), which includes the *executive functions* of the brain that encompass the ability to make decisions, to plan, and to solve problems. Problems in executive functions can lead to difficulties in planning and following through with leisure activities. For example, poor decision making can make it hard for people to decide which leisure activity to try, poor planning ability can lead to problems with carrying out their decision, and trouble with solving problems can turn small obstacles encountered along the way into insurmountable barriers.

In addition, people with schizophrenia often have difficulty paying attention and concentrating on a particular task. Being distracted easily can make it difficult to get involved in and enjoy leisure activities. For example, after Manuel developed schizophrenia, he found it difficult to play chess (a game he had loved previously) because he couldn't maintain his focus. Lastly, people with schizophrenia often have memory problems, which can make it difficult to remember times when they engaged in and enjoyed a leisure activity.

Age When Schizophrenia Develops

Schizophrenia usually develops during late adolescence or early adulthood (between the ages of 16 and 25). This is the time when most people are establishing the kinds of leisure and recreational activities they will enjoy as adults. The onset of schizophrenia can interrupt this natural process, and as a result, many people have not developed hobbies and activities that they can enjoy in their spare time. "My brother and his friends are always ready for a pick-up game of basketball," said Nate. "I would like to be able to join in, but I can't keep up with them on the court."

Lack of Economic Resources

Many people with schizophrenia have a low income, which can limit their participation in some leisure and recreational activities. For example, skiing involves buying or renting equipment, purchasing warm clothing, paying for transportation to ski slopes, and buying lift tickets. Although some activities are less expensive by nature (such as reading, drawing, and running) and other activities cost less when they are sponsored or subsidized by community agencies, the lack of financial resources remains an important factor that can discourage people from pursuing recreational activities.

Benefits of Leisure and Recreation

The significant benefits that can result from taking part in enjoyable and satisfying activities make it well worth the effort to help your relative incorporate leisure activities into her life.

Feeling Good

Participating in leisure and recreational activities usually improves mood and self-esteem. It's in our nature to want to enjoy ourselves and to have fun. If your relative spends all of his time on work and/or managing his illness, he may feel oppressed by life. Having hobbies and other things to do for fun can lighten his load. As one person said, "If I didn't have the fun of doing my artwork, things would look pretty grim to me. I don't think about my problems when I'm drawing, and it gives me a fresh perspective."

Structuring Time

Most people with schizophrenia benefit from structure in their lives. A lack of structure can lead to boredom, anxiety, and "off" sleeping habits (such as sleeping all day and being up all night), which can interfere with a person's ability to fit in socially with others. It can even contribute to a worsening of symptoms, including the psychotic symptoms of hallucinations and delusions. Participating in leisure and recreational activities can help structure your relative's time because it often involves setting up a schedule to participate in the selected activities and may also require arranging time to obtain materials, learn new skills, and seek out additional information. For example, when Celeste became interested in knitting, she set up times with her aunt to learn how to do specific stitches, went to a specialty shop to select yarns, checked out knitting books from the library, and joined a knitting club that met once a week at the local YWCA.

Decrease in Psychotic Symptoms

Research shows that when people with schizophrenia engage in recreational activities, their psychotic symptoms are less severe. Scientists believe that being involved in something that is fun and rewarding helps to distract people from their symptoms. For example, when Darnell was sitting at home with nothing to do, his parents noticed that he talked back to the voices he was hearing. However, when his friend came over to play checkers, Darnell focused on the game and did not respond to auditory hallucinations. See Chapter 17 for more strategies on coping with psychotic symptoms.

Social Involvement

Many recreation and leisure activities provide opportunities to meet others with similar interests and develop social relationships. Some leisure and recreational activities are more intrinsically social than others, such as sports teams or classes, but almost all can lead to contact with other people. For example, reading is one of the more solitary leisure activities, but an interest in reading can lead to interactions with librarians or bookstore salespeople, encounters with other people at the library or bookstore, attending an author's lecture, or joining a book discussion group. Furthermore, participating in leisure and recreational activities can play a key role in improving social relationships by providing interesting topics for conversations—often a difficult area for people with schizophrenia. As noted in Chapter 25, having something to talk about is critical to meeting new people and developing closer relationships.

Something to Work For and Save For

When people are involved in leisure and recreational activities, they often develop goals related to these activities. For example, a person who becomes interested in exploring nature may want to hike up a particular mountain trail. To do so, she may set up intermediate goals, such as increasing the number of miles she can hike, reading books and studying maps of the area, researching the plants and animals she might encounter, and talking to other people who have completed the hike. Developing leisure and recreational activities often gives people something for which they want to save their money—which, in turn, can increase their interest in managing their money effectively and motivate them to decrease spending on junk food, drugs, or alcohol. For example, when Peter became interested in saving money to buy a special fishing rod for fly-fishing, he planned to set aside a certain amount every week. He found that by cutting down on smoking and doing more comparison shopping at the grocery store, he could meet this goal more quickly.

A Model for Understanding the Experience of Enjoyment

In recent years psychologists have shown an increased interest in understanding what helps people enjoy life and feel a sense of well-being. For example, Fred Bryant, PhD, at Loyola University in Chicago has studied the factors involved in people's experience of enjoyment and pleasure. His research indicates that there are three stages of experiencing pleasure or having fun: *anticipation*, *savoring*, and *reminiscing*. By understanding the three stages of fun, you can help your relative get the most enjoyment out of leisure and recreational activities.

Anticipation

People usually look forward to activities they enjoy. You might think about specific aspects of the event that you expect to enjoy and imagine yourself involved. For example, if you were anticipating a trip to the zoo as being a fun experience, you might think about the interesting animals you'll see, walking outdoors in pleasant weather, eating a hot dog, and watching people go by.

If your relative has difficulty anticipating pleasant events, you can help by talking to him in a lighthearted, casual way about the upcoming event, highlighting aspects that you expect to be positive. Ask him questions that will prompt him to think of pleasant elements of the experience. Use language that reflects positive expectation, such as "That sounds like fun" or "That could be interesting." If you're going to participate in the event with your relative, use "I" statements to show your own positive anticipation. For example, prior to their visit to a museum, one father made comments such as "I'm really looking forward to visiting the museum again; I like the grand scale of the architecture." He also asked his daughter questions such as "What's your favorite part of the museum?" to pique her anticipatory interest.

Savoring the Experience

When you're experiencing a pleasant event, you can intensify or prolong the pleasure by "savoring the moment." Try identifying which parts of the experience you enjoy the most and focus on them more intensely. You can pay attention to the details and take a mental snapshot of what you're enjoying. You can tell others what you are enjoying at the time or make a mental note to describe the experience to others later.

Your relative may need help developing his savoring skills. For example, if you participate in an activity with your relative, you can talk out loud about what you're enjoying and encourage him to identify things he is enjoying in the moment. Appreciating what one is experiencing in the moment has much in common with a form of meditation called *mindfulness*, which helps people be more aware of their perceptions and sensations in the moment—what they are seeing, hearing, smelling, and feeling.

Angelique, whose son has schizophrenia, had helped him plan a leisure activity of dining out. At the restaurant, while they were eating their appetizers, she commented on how much she enjoyed the decor of the restaurant and the unusual spices in the food. When she asked her son what he liked about the restaurant, he said he liked the friendly staff and the dessert selection. Together they decided to order smaller main courses to save room for dessert. They ordered two different desserts to share and discussed what they liked about the flavor, the texture, and the appearance of each one.

If you don't accompany your relative, you can tell her you're interested in hearing what she enjoyed about the experience. It may help to ask your relative to look for specific things. For example, if your relative is going to the gym, you could say you're interested in hearing about the different exercise machines she uses at the facility and which ones she thinks are most beneficial. If your relative is going on a hike in a wooded area, you might say you're interested in whether she sees any unusual flowers or birds while hiking.

Reminiscing

After a pleasant event is over, you can look back on it in ways that prolong or rekindle your enjoyment of the experience. You may remember specific aspects of the experience that you especially enjoyed and may even visualize yourself going through the experience again. For example, a person who enjoyed swimming at the beach might recall the hot sun, the cool water, the invigorating feeling of plunging into the waves, and the good taste of the food he ate after swimming. Later he might recall a mental snapshot of the beach.

You can help your relative improve her ability to reminisce about pleasant events by practicing the act of conjuring up memories about the experience and focusing together on the most enjoyable parts. To help your relative develop this skill, start by asking her to recall memories soon after the event has ended, while the memories are fresh. The same memories can then be kindled at later times, making them easier to access. For example, you can ask your relative questions about specific events, highlighting aspects that she has indicated were positive. You could also look at photos or souvenirs together.

One father, whose daughter enjoyed attending a cooking class, asked for her help in preparing a recipe that had been demonstrated in the class that week.

On the way home from attending a dance class together, one woman talked to her partner about how she had enjoyed the music and the swaying motion of the dance. The next night she played a CD and asked her partner to practice the steps they had learned.

Steps for Helping Your Relative Improve Leisure and Recreation

Understanding and attending to the three stages of fun described above is a good foundation for helping your relative improve his enjoyment of leisure and recreation. Many people with schizophrenia also benefit from help in identifying and following through on developing new leisure and recreational activities. You and your relative may find the following steps useful.

1. *Talk about leisure and recreation and identify the benefits.* The first step is to raise the subject of leisure and recreational activities with your relative. What does she think about the amount and quality of her current leisure and recreational activities? Is she interested in finding more things to do in her spare time? How does she think her life might be different if she had more pleasurable activities to engage in? During your discussion, it's important to avoid pushing your relative to do more with her spare time than she is doing. It's also critical not to choose an activity for her. Almost no one is receptive to suggestions that begin "What you should do for fun is. . . ." Give your relative time to think about

the subject and what *she* would like to do. The process of developing more activities may be a slow one. Nevertheless, it's more effective to have several short, pleasant conversations than to push your relative into something she does not believe will be interesting or fun.

2. *Explore possible activities your relative might enjoy.* If your relative is interested in improving his leisure and recreational activities, it's helpful to brainstorm a list of possibilities with him. What does your relative enjoy doing now in his spare time? What did he enjoy doing in the past? What things do your relative's friends do for fun? Input from other family members, who may be aware of things your relative enjoys now or used to enjoy in the past, is often helpful. During brainstorming, don't evaluate or criticize any activities identified.

The table at the bottom of the page provides a list of possible leisure and recreational activities that people commonly enjoy. You and your relative might find it useful to review this list as you brainstorm possible activities.

3. *Select an activity and make a plan with your relative to try it out.* Review the list of possible activities with your relative. One activity on the list may clearly stand out to your relative as the best, but it may still be helpful to briefly review together the advantages and disadvantages of each activity, consider how much your relative is attracted to it, and how easily it could be pursued. After you've identified a few promising activities, you can help your relative make plans to try them out. Consider the necessary resources, such as information, equipment, skills, transportation, and money. Keep in mind that leisure and recreational activities are often sponsored or subsidized by a variety of community agencies, such as those listed in the table on page 428, and that sports equipment can be purchased secondhand.

When making a plan, help your relative determine the specific steps for try-

---

Examples of Leisure and Recreational Activities

- Attending adult education classes
- Participating in a sport
- Going out to eat
- Reading
- Visiting museums (art, history, science)
- Listening to music
- Taking an aerobics class
- Playing board games
- Taking dancing classes
- Taking a yoga class
- Making crafts
- Doing crossword puzzles
- Stargazing
- Drawing, painting, or pottery
- Knitting or crocheting
- Doing volunteer work
- Going to the movies
- Taking a martial arts class
- Taking a writing class
- Playing an instrument
- Hiking in nature
- Participating in weight training
- Playing card games
- Visiting the zoo or volunteering at the SPCA
- Pursuing a hobby
- Learning a skill
- Cooking
- Studying history, visiting historical sites
- Playing computer games

ing out the new activity and set a timetable for completing each step. It is often preferable to plan activities that involve other people, such as yourself, other relatives, friends, etc. Doing things together is a natural way of helping your relative identify and try new activities. Also, involving others in trying out a new activity improves the likelihood of completion and increases opportunities for helping your relative with all three steps of having fun (anticipating, savoring, and reminiscing). The last step of planning an activity should include a date for follow-up.

4. *Follow up on how the plan went.* Follow-up involves determining which steps of the plan were carried out, how successful each step was, and how your relative feels about participating in the activity so far. Follow-up meetings are also a good opportunity to help your relative look back on aspects of the experience that she enjoyed (*reminiscing*) and to look forward to doing the activity again in the future (*anticipation*).

First discuss the steps that were accomplished and praise all efforts. Then talk about steps that were not completed and troubleshoot obstacles. Ask your relative if he enjoyed the activity, keeping in mind that pleasure increases with experience in the activity. If your relative has not been enjoying the activity so far, brainstorm ways that the activity could be more rewarding, such as involving other people.

5. *Make another plan to do the activity again (or try a new one).* The next step usually involves making a plan to do the activity again, taking into account what you and your relative learned in following up the first plan. Examples of second plans include (a) completing steps that were not accomplished during the first plan, (b) involving more people in carrying out the plan, (c) revising the plan to be more practical, (d) repeating the steps of the first plan to get more experience, and (e) going to the next level. It's usually best to try an activity several times before your relative decides whether she likes it, because the more a person participates in something, the more likely she will find it enjoyable. However, in some instances, the next plan may be to try out a new activity. You and your

---

Agencies That Often Sponsor or Subsidize Leisure and Recreational Activities

- Psychosocial clubhouses
- Drop-in centers
- YMCA/YWCA
- Senior citizen centers
- Churches, synagogues, mosques, schools, community centers
- Community mental health centers
- Community colleges
- Chapters of the National Alliance on Mental Illness
- Organizations that sponsor involvement of persons with disabilities in sports (e.g., skiing)
- Museums

relative may find it helpful to refer back to the list of activities you completed at the beginning of this process or to take a new look at the table on page 427.

6. *When an enjoyable activity has been found, develop a regular routine.* When your relative has participated in an activity that he likes, help him make plans for doing it regularly, such as one to three times per week. To facilitate this shift into a regular routine, it might be helpful to reflect back with your relative about his positive experiences with the activity so far (*reminiscing*) and to help him think ahead about what it would be like to participate in the activity on a regular basis (*anticipation*).

Rodney, age 28, was working three afternoons a week as a sales clerk but spent most of his spare time sleeping or watching television. When his parents asked him how he felt about how he spent his spare time, he said he was bored but couldn't think of anything he wanted to do. He was receptive to the idea of his parents helping him come up with some ideas for activities, especially because he thought it would help him with his goal of meeting more people. When he met with his parents and brother Tony on a Saturday to talk about what kinds of things he liked doing, he came up with the following activities, many of which he used to enjoy: camping, renting videos, bicycling, and taking tae kwon do classes. He decided he preferred to try bicycling first, because it didn't require much equipment, he already knew how, and he could do it either on his own or with other people. His brother offered to help him fix up his bike.

With the help of his family, Rodney came up with a plan to repair his bicycle (starting on Sunday), purchase a bike helmet (within 1 week), and take a 45-minute bike ride the following Saturday. When they met on Sunday for follow-up, Rodney said he had started off on a bike ride on Saturday using the repaired bike and new helmet, but that after 15 minutes he was tired and felt the bicycle seat was very uncomfortable. He reported that he had enjoyed other parts of the ride, such as being outdoors and feeling the fresh air rush past him as he cycled. With input from his family, Rodney planned to purchase a cushioned cover for his bicycle seat on Monday, to go for two shorter rides (15 minutes) on Wednesday and Friday, and a 20-minute ride on Saturday.

When Rodney met with his family the next Sunday for follow-up, he said his seat was more comfortable and he was able to ride on Wednesday and Saturday as planned, although he skipped Friday because of fatigue. He reported enjoying the ride somewhat but thought it would be more fun to have someone to ride with him. Tony said he'd like to join Rodney for his next weekend ride, which they planned for Saturday. The next week Rodney reported that he was feeling stronger on his bike rides and that he especially enjoyed riding with Tony and talking about what they were seeing. Gradually, over the course of 6 weeks of riding alone during the week and with Tony on the weekend, Rodney built up his strength and self-confidence. When he noticed a poster for a biking club in the window of the local sporting goods store, he decided to join. He then worked on increasing the length of his rides during the week to 40 minutes each and his weekend ride with Tony to an hour, with the goal of being able to participate in the rides sponsored by the bicycle club.

The Rewards of Recreation

Helping your relative find recreational and leisure activities that she enjoys may take time and effort, but it can be extremely rewarding, both for you and your relative. Participating in activities together and talking about what you're enjoying can bring you closer and make you more optimistic about the future. Having schizophrenia does not mean that your relative cannot enjoy life.

Resources

Compeer at *www.compeer.org* offers programs and services that promote volunteering as a friend to someone with a mental illness.

Hahn, T. N. (1987). *The miracle of mindfulness: A manual on meditation* (M. Ho, Trans., rev. ed.). Boston: Beacon Press. This book is written by a well-known poet and Zen master and describes an approach to meditation, concentration, and relaxation in practical, accessible language.

Liberman, R. P. "Recreation for Leisure Module" of *Social and Independent Living Skills* (SILS). Available at *www.psychrehab.com/module_recreation.html*. This module contains a trainers manual, client workbook, and video focusing on helping people improve their enjoyment of recreation and leisure.

Seligman, M. E. P. (2002). *Authentic happiness: Using the new positive psychology to realize your potential for lasting fulfillment.* New York: Free Press. This book emphasizes the importance of identifying one's strengths, virtues, and abilities. Chapters 5, 6, and 7 ("Satisfaction about the Past," "Optimism about the Future," and "Happiness in the Present") are especially relevant to helping people find enjoyment in their lives.

Weiss, A. (2004). *Beginning mindfulness: Learning the way of awareness.* Novato, CA: New World Library. Mindfulness meditation encourages people to slow down and be aware of what they are experiencing in the present moment (e.g., thoughts, feelings, physical sensations, and perceptions).

CHAPTER 29

Dealing with Stigma

Practically everyone with a mental illness faces the problem of stigma at some time in life. Social attitudes, including beliefs about mental illness, are hard to change and can have a profound influence on people's opportunities and self-image. Although stigma is common and changing societal attitudes may seem overwhelming, there is much you can do to help your relative cope with and overcome the effects of stigma on his life. As people become more knowledgeable about schizophrenia, stigma naturally begins to diminish, albeit slowly. Furthermore, many of the efforts that you make to help your relative combat the effects of stigma and to address stigma directly where you see it help to gradually change social attitudes about mental illness. Many people change their point of view when they can see for themselves that mental illness is nothing to be afraid of and that individuals with these problems can make valuable contributions to their families and communities. This chapter is aimed at helping you minimize the effects of stigma on your relative and deal with common situations in which stigma may be a problem.

What Is Stigma?

Stigma refers to negative public attitudes or beliefs about individuals who belong to a particular group, such as individuals with a mental illness, a substance abuse problem, an infectious disease (such as the HIV virus), a neurological problem (such as epilepsy), or a history of problems with the criminal justice system (such as serving time in jail or prison). When stigma is present, any individual belonging to a particular category, such as schizophrenia, is assumed to possess all of the negative stereotypes associated with that category and is therefore feared, disliked, or avoided. As a result of this fear and avoidance, people in the general public often have little opportunity to change their stigmatizing beliefs about those individuals. This lack of opportunity only serves to perpetuate the negative stereotypes.

What Are the Effects of Stigma?

Stigma can have a wide range of effects on people with mental illness. People in this category are sometimes denied housing or jobs due to the stigma associated with their disorders. Socially, people may feel uncomfortable or hesitant to interact with someone they know has a psychiatric illness. People with mental illness may be more likely to be the victims of crime, yet they may be less likely to be taken seriously by law enforcement officials. Even within the helping professions, a certain degree of stigma may prevail: People with mental illness may have reduced credibility because they are falsely believed to make up or exaggerate their complaints.

In addition to the far-reaching effects of stigma on work, housing, and social opportunities, it can have an even more pernicious effect on the individual when she incorporates the negative beliefs about mental illness into her own self-image. When people come to believe that they are inferior, "damaged goods," or otherwise tarnished by having a mental illness, they stigmatize themselves. Although self-stigma can be problematic for anyone with a mental illness, it can be an even greater problem for a person with schizophrenia. There are so many misconceptions about schizophrenia that people with the illness very often harbor the same misunderstandings.

Self-stigma about having schizophrenia may affect your relative in many ways. He may refuse to acknowledge having schizophrenia because he feels that to accept the label would be tantamount to admitting he is crazy, worthless, or has nothing to contribute to society. As discussed in Chapter 24, the refusal to accept the diagnosis of schizophrenia may serve to avoid the self-stigma often present in people with schizophrenia.

The belief that she is inferior because she has a mental illness can contribute to your relative's feelings of hopelessness, helplessness, and grief. Most critically of all, your relative may give up trying to accomplish goals, avoid taking on the challenges of life, and resign herself to a passive acceptance of the status quo. An old saying goes, "If you think you can't do it, you can't." People who self-stigmatize often believe they can't do things; as a result they never try and therefore do not accomplish any desired changes.

What Causes Stigma?

There are many theories about the causes of stigma. Research has shown that stigmatizing attitudes toward people with mental illness are strongly related to beliefs that people with mental illness are often violent. Thus, the more the general public believes that people with mental illness are violent, the more likely they will avoid such individuals and deny them opportunities in the important life domains of work, housing, and social connections. Why do so many people believe that individuals with schizophrenia are prone to violence? Research on the relationship between schizophrenia and violence has shown that people with the disorder are somewhat more likely to be violent than people who don't have the disorder, although the vast majority of people with schizophrenia are not violent (see Chapter 23 for more discussion of the relationship between schizophrenia and aggression). Uninformed people in the general public, however, often have exaggerated perceptions of the link between violence and schizophrenia, believing that many, if not most, people with the disorder are violent.

One explanation for this misconception is the common negative portrayal of schizophrenia in the media. When people with schizophrenia are involved in a violent crime, their acts often receive a disproportionate amount of media coverage in the newspapers, TV, and radio. When someone who does not have a mental illness commits such a crime, the story has less sensationalism and is often not reported in the popular media. This slanted perception can be magnified further when the only information a person has about mental illness is what she learns from the media.

In addition to the tendency to sensationalize crimes committed by people with a mental illness, fictional portrayals of people with mental illness in movies, TV, and books also frequently portray these individuals as violent. In contrast, there are comparatively few portrayals of people with mental illness, especially schizophrenia, as compassionate, caring, strong, or accomplished individuals, either fictional or in real life, to counteract the negative portrayals. The net result is that people whose main source of information about mental illness is the popular media often inaccurately perceive individuals with schizophrenia and other mental illnesses as being prone to violence and criminality.

Research on stigma shows that the more familiar a person is with mental illness, such as having a friend or family member with a mental illness, the more accepting the person is of those individuals and the less likely she is to fear and avoid them. Knowing people who have schizophrenia provides accurate information that most people with this disorder are not dangerous and that they lead worthwhile lives with a sense of personal dignity. The more people get to know others who have mental illness, the less stigmatizing they tend to be in their attitudes and behaviors toward them.

Coping with Stigma

Although the pervasive effects of stigma are rooted in common social misconceptions about the nature of schizophrenia and other mental illnesses, there are a variety of ways you can help your relative deal with and even overcome these effects.

- *Develop a vision of recovery.* Perhaps the most important step you can take to deal with the effects of stigma is to become aware of your own attitudes and beliefs about schizophrenia and to challenge yourself to develop a vision that recovery from the illness is possible. In Chapter 3 we described a perspective on recovery from mental illness that focuses not on the presence of symptoms, impairments, or other types of pathology but rather on the ability of people to move forward in their lives by pursuing their dreams, aspirations, and goals. By developing a belief that recovery is possible, sharing your thoughts and hopes with your relative, and learning about his hopes, you'll be able to erase some of the more devastating effects of stigma on people with schizophrenia. Family members' belief that people with schizophrenia have a future can go far in improving the self-esteem and confidence of the person with the illness.

Developing a vision of recovery is not something you do alone; it involves your relative and other members of your family as well. Sharing the successful stories of other people with schizophrenia who have moved forward in their lives can help your family see that schizophrenia does not signify the end of opportunities but is, rather, just a twist in the road of life of the type that everyone faces. Talk to your family about individuals with schizophrenia who have achieved a variety of accomplishments, such as having rewarding relationships, returning to school or work, parenting their children, helping others in their communities, and contributing to society in areas such as the arts or sciences. For sources of success stories of people with schizophrenia, see the websites and videotapes listed as additional resources in Chapter 3. It's also helpful to learn about famous people who were diagnosed with schizophrenia, such as those listed in the table on the facing page.

A vision of recovery can also help people get past mourning the loss associated with schizophrenia and feeling sorry for themselves and their family. A vision of recovery involves the realization that people with schizophrenia are like other people in most ways, with the same needs, motivations, and desires. This vision can prevent or undo stigmatizing beliefs among relatives that schizophrenia is a unique curse or burden that sets the individual apart from family and society.

- *Educate yourself and others.* At the heart of combating stigma is educating yourself and your family, including your relative with schizophrenia, about the nature of the disorder and how to treat it. By reading this book, you've taken the most important step toward changing and undoing the effects of stigma: You are becoming an expert on the illness, learning how to treat it collaboratively with professionals, and moving forward with your life and your relative's. Although this book provides you with much information about schizophrenia, there are many other sources of information, and new things are being learned every day about this complex illness. Continuing the process of educating yourself and your family about schizophrenia can help you remain hopeful and informed about the disorder and provide you with ammunition to ward off the negative stereotypes of the disorder that are the cause of so much stigma.

Famous People with Schizophrenia

Tom Harrell (1947–present) is a musician who has been named jazz trumpeter of the year three times by *Downbeat Magazine* and was nominated for a Grammy Award. He is known for composing and performing intricate melodies and has recorded 20 CDs.

Meera Popkin (?–present) is an actress and singer who has starred in musicals in New York and London, such as *Cats* and *Miss Saigon*. She continues to act and has also written articles about her experience with schizophrenia.

John Nash (1928–present) is an American mathematician who made discoveries in math that had very important applications in the field of economics. He was awarded the Nobel Prize for Economics in 1994. His story is told in *A Beautiful Mind*, a book that has also been made into a movie.

William Chester Minor (1834–1920) was an American army surgeon who also had vast knowledge of the English language and literature. He made major contributions to the Oxford English Dictionary, the most comprehensive dictionary in the world.

Vaslav Nijinski (1890–1950) was a Russian dancer who is legendary because of his physical strength, light movements, and expressive body language. He is especially remembered for a dance piece called "Afternoon of a Faun."

• *Explore whether your relative is self-stigmatizing.* Talking with your relative about what she thinks of herself can help you determine whether your relative stigmatizes herself for having a mental illness. If your relative does self-stigmatize, you can explore her beliefs about the illness and what they mean for her future. These beliefs are often inaccurate and can be corrected by providing more accurate information, by gently encouraging your relative to consider the possibility of a brighter future, and by helping her participate in peer support programs (described later in this chapter). Beliefs about being a victim of an illness, having no future, and being a social outcast can also lead to self-pity and resentment toward an "unfair" and "unjust" world. Such an attitude, although understandable, may put off other people and limit your relative's efforts to improve her life. Helping your relative see that she is a worthwhile person and that life offers challenges to everyone can help her develop a new perspective that empowers her to take charge of her own future.

Eduardo was 22 years old, in his senior year at college, when he developed schizophrenia and had to drop out of school. Everyone in Eduardo's family felt sorry for him, especially his mother, who felt he deserved more in life. After learning more about schizophrenia and developing a vision of recovery, Eduardo's mother began speaking with him about his thoughts and beliefs about himself and his problems. Gradually Eduardo opened up to his mother and said that he felt defective and had no hope or future. Eduardo talked about how he had been forced to drop out of college and how his siblings had gone on to marry and raise families while he had been left with nothing. Eduardo's mother began to ask him about his strengths, which included his musical ability (he had taught himself guitar and piano), his kindness toward children and animals, and his mechanical skill (he had always enjoyed fixing things and was majoring in engineering in college when he developed schizophrenia). As they talked, Eduardo's mother helped him challenge his beliefs that he was defective and that he had nothing to offer others. By helping Eduardo focus on his strengths and realize that everyone faces problems and challenges, Eduardo's mother was able to help him develop a more positive way of looking at himself and to encourage him to begin taking charge of his life again. Eduardo's attitude toward himself and his world gradually began to change. Instead of feeling sorry for himself and resentful toward others, he realized that he had special gifts and that through hard work and the support of his family he could turn his life around and change the areas he really cared about.

• *Talk about disclosure with your relative.* The decision about whether and when to disclose a psychiatric illness is a highly personal one many people with mental illness actively struggle with. You can help your relative by talking with him about disclosure issues and trying to understand his concerns. Some people choose to be open with others about having a psychiatric illness, whereas others prefer to be more private. Many people with severe mental illness report that they cope with stigma by being extremely selective about whom they choose to disclose their illness to. Significant numbers of people lie about their disorder when applying for a driver's license, for example, or a job, entrance to a school, and when talking to casual friends or acquaintances. Although refusing to disclose can be effective, it also can have a downside: Fearful that people will find out the truth, the person avoids situations in which his "secret" might be uncovered by others. Empathizing with your relative about the difficult decision he has to make and helping him weigh the advantages and disadvantages of disclosure in different situations may be helpful.

One important factor that contributes to an individual's willingness to disclose mental illness is her family's attitudes toward, and beliefs about, mental illness. Families who are ashamed of having a member with a mental illness are less likely to share their experiences with others and tend to convey this negative attitude to their relative with schizophrenia. Your own willingness to be open about having a loved one with a mental illness may influence your relative's inclination to disclose her disorder. However, if your relative is not comfortable with your sharing information about her psychiatric illness with a wide range of people, you must respect her desire for privacy.

There are relatively few hard and fast rules about when and how to disclose that one has a mental illness. In general, it is preferable if some degree of relationship with the other person has been established before disclosure is made. For example, when meeting another person for the first time, before any personal connection has been established, disclosing one's mental illness may scare off the person. Having any kind of an illness, whether medical or psychiatric, is generally considered personal information that is not shared casually until people know each other better. Thus, premature disclosure of a mental illness can violate the social norm that implicitly dictates people gradually disclose more personal information about themselves as they get to know each other better.

In some circumstances, in contrast, disclosure may be very helpful and can prevent problems from developing later. For example, if a person with schizophrenia needs a reasonable accommodation for his job (such as taking more frequent, brief rest breaks because of difficulties sustaining attention over long periods of time), disclosing the psychiatric illness to the employer may be wise. Although it may be possible to work out an accommodation with the employer without disclosing this information, the employer is legally obligated to provide that accommodation only if he knows that the employee has a psychiatric disability and the accommodation does not impose a significant hardship on the employer (see following material and Chapter 26). Helping your relative weigh the pros and cons of disclosing in different situations may ease the difficulty of making these decisions.

• *Know your relative's rights.* As a person with a mental illness, your relative has rights that are protected by federal laws. The Americans with Disabilities Act specifically prohibits discrimination against people with a mental illness in housing, work, education, and medical care. You and your relative should be familiar with these rights and where you can take your concerns if you think these rights are being violated. Information on this issue is provided in the Resources section at the end of this chapter.

• *Join an anti-stigma campaign.* A growing number of campaigns have been developed in recent years aimed at addressing the problem of stigma and mental illness. These campaigns typically include a wide range of people concerned with stigma (such as professionals, individuals with mental illness, clergy, family members, interested people in the community) and involve a variety of activities (such as distributing educational materials, providing lectures and discussions in public forums, and confronting negative and inaccurate media portrayals of persons with psychiatric disorders). You might consider joining an anti-stigma campaign and encouraging your relative to participate with you. The social action involved in fighting against stigma may energize and empower you and your relative about your ability to deal with negative attitudes toward mental illness. Of course, the long-term goal of anti-stigma work is to foster acceptance of mental illness. See the Resources section at the end of the chapter, under "Anti-Stigma Campaigns," for specific contact information.

• *Help your relative explore peer support programs.* Many people with severe mental illnesses benefit tremendously from participation in peer support programs that exist either independently or in collaboration with local community mental health centers. Peer support programs provide people with opportunities to learn about the experiences of others with mental illness, to share different strategies for coping with symptoms, to support one another in pursuing recovery goals, and to discuss ways of handling the stigma of mental illness. Partici-

pants often feel better about themselves as their hopes and aspirations are supported, and as the challenges they have experienced in coping with mental
illness, both internally and socially, are validated by others who have had similar
experiences. In addition, some peer support programs specifically address the
problem of negative social attitudes by participating in anti-stigma campaigns,
which may involve activities such as speaking at public forums, talking at schools,
and confronting media outlets when negative and inaccurate (or distorted)
depictions of mental illness appear. Information about where to find peer support programs is provided in Chapter 5.

  • *Help your relative use self-enhancement.* One effective way many people fight
the effects of stigma is to identify positive aspects of themselves and to remind
themselves of these on a regular basis by making positive self-statements. One
woman said, "I rely on the fact that I know I'm just as good as anybody else, in
the eyes of God, in the eyes of myself." Another described the value of writing
positive self-statements in her journal: "I do things like affirmative statements
that I write in my journal every night. . . . I do lots and lots of things to reinforce
that I am a human being, that I have value" (both quoted in Wahl, 1999).

Overcoming Stigma by Keeping Hope Alive

The stigma associated with schizophrenia is real and can translate into lost
opportunities, rejection by the very people one wants acceptance from, and a
loss of self-esteem. Perhaps the most profound effect of stigma is its power to
damage or demolish a person's belief in herself and in the possibility and hope
of recovery from the disabling effects of mental illness. By being aware of the
social and personal effects of stigma and talking them over with your relative in a
loving and supportive way, you can create an environment that encourages her to
tackle these difficult issues.

  Supporting your relative, instilling hope that he can achieve personal goals
and live a worthwhile and satisfying life, and empathizing with his struggles while
avoiding getting sucked into pity/self-pity are your most powerful weapons
against the effects of stigma. By remaining upbeat and optimistic about your relative's future, you can help him move forward in recovery and avoid becoming
sidetracked by the public ignorance at the root of stigma.

  Public opinions have changed over the past several decades as people have
become more aware of how common mental illness is, and of the ability of individuals to cope with their illness and make contributions to society. Critically
important voices in changing social attitudes toward mental illness have been
those of relatives and people with mental illness. Being willing to speak openly
about mental illness and advocating for the rights and humanity of individuals
like your relative will contribute to this society's progress toward public acceptance and understanding of mental illness. Your willingness to confront and

work toward changing public attitudes is important not only to your relative but also to countless individuals like her who are striving to overcome mental illness and its social repercussions.

Resources

Publications

Clay, S., Schell, B., Corrigan, P. W., & Ralph, R. (Eds.). (2005). *On our own, together: Peer programs for people with mental illness*. Nashville, TN: Vanderbilt University Press. Meeting other people with mental illness who are positive role models is one of the many advantages of participating in peer programs, especially if your relative experiences self-stigmatization. This is an excellent book that provides a history of peer support, describes different types of peer support programs (such as drop-in centers, peer support and mentoring, and educational programs), and provides information about finding a local peer support program.

Corrigan, P. W. (2004a). *Beat the stigma and discrimination: Four lessons for mental health advocates*. Chicago: Chicago Consortium for Stigma Research. This manual for people with mental illness and their families can be downloaded at *www.casra.org*, click on "Advocacy" and look under "Other Resources."

Corrigan, P. W. (Ed.). (2004b). *On the stigma of mental illness: Practical strategies for research and social change*. Washington, DC: American Psychological Association. Summarizes the research of the Chicago Consortium for Stigma Research, providing an overview of the problem of stigma, different perspectives, and a variety of social change strategies.

Corrigan, P. W., & Lundin, R. (2001). *Don't call me nuts! Coping with the stigma of mental illness*. Chicago: Recovery Press. This excellent book, coauthored by a psychiatric rehabilitation expert and a person with severe mental illness, describes the effects of stigma on people's lives and strategies for coping with it.

Farina, A. (1998). Stigma. In K. T. Mueser & N. Tarrier (Eds.), *Handbook of social functioning in schizophrenia* (pp. 247–279). Boston: Allyn & Bacon. This chapter provides a comprehensive review of research on stigma in mental illness.

Penn, D. L., & Wykes, T. (2003). *Journal of Mental Health, 12*(3). This issue was devoted to the problem of stigma in severe mental illness.

Wahl, O. F. (1995). *Media madness: Public images of mental illness*. New Brunswick, NJ: Rutgers University Press. This book illustrates and discusses the negative portrayal of mental illness in the media.

Wahl, O. F. (1999). *Telling is risky business: Mental health consumers confront stigma*. New Brunswick, NJ: Rutgers University Press. This book describes the results of a nationwide survey of persons with mental illness to chronicle their experiences with stigma and discrimination and the strategies they have used to cope with both.

Beyond the label: An educational kit to promote awareness and understanding of the impact of stigma on people living with concurrent mental health and substance use problems. (2005). Centre for Addiction and Mental Health, 33 Russell Street, Toronto, Ontario, M5S 2S1, Canada. E-mail: *marketing@camh.net*. This educational kit provides information and resources for combating stigma due to mental illness and substance use problems, and includes group activities, information sheets, presentation tips, and suggestions for using the kit in the community (includes a CD-ROM).

Anti-Stigma Campaigns

The Center to Address Discrimination and Stigma helps people design, implement, and operate programs that reduce discrimination and stigma: *www.adscenter.org.*

The Chicago Consortium for Stigma Research (CCSR) is a multidisciplinary group of scientists who seek to advance research on stigma, including understanding the phenomenon of stigma, developing and testing models that explain why it occurs, and evaluating strategies that help to diminish its effects: *www.stigmaresearch.org.*

"In Our Own Voice" was developed through the National Alliance on Mental Illness (NAMI) for people with mental illness to educate others about recovery from mental illness and to reduce stigma. Information can be obtained at the organization's website: *www.nami.org.*

"StigmaBusters" is an anti-stigma campaign developed by NAMI. Information can be obtained at the organization's website: *www.nami.org.*

The Substance Abuse and Mental Health Services Administration (SAMHSA) campaign "Mental Health: It's Part of All Our Lives" includes advertisements that educate the public about mental illness. Educational materials can be obtained from SAMHSA's National Mental Health Information Center (800-789-2647) and from its websites in English (*www.allmentalhealth.samhsa.gov*) and Spanish (*www.nuestrasaludmental. samhsa.gov*).

The World Psychiatric Association campaign, "Reduction of Stigma and Discrimination Due to Schizophrenia," focuses its international campaign on building a network of individuals and organizations who are committed to fighting against stigma and discrimination and giving people with schizophrenia a chance to live worthwhile lives. Information about establishing an anti-stigma program and educational materials are available from:

> Norman Sartorius, MD
> H.U.G., Belle-Idée
> 2, chemin du Petit-Bel-Air
> 1225 Chêne-Bourg/Genève
> Switzerland
> E-mail: *Norman.sartorius@hcuge.ch*
> Phone: 41-22-305 57 41
> Fax: 41-22-305 57 49

www.openthedoors.com. This website contains a compendium of different campaigns devoted to fighting stigma throughout the world. It was assembled by the World Psychiatric Association campaign, in the preceding entry.

CHAPTER 30

Planning for the Future

Planning for the future of your relative with schizophrenia is a natural extension of your caring relationship. Some people with schizophrenia are very independent and need little or no assistance, whereas others rely on their family members for more assistance, such as providing a place to live, additional funds for expenses, and help with daily living needs. However, there are natural limitations on the duration of time that most families can continue to assist a relative, due to problems such as aging, the emergence of health problems, or financial difficulties. Parents are often painfully aware of their own mortality and the effects that their absence will have on their offspring.

This chapter helps you and your relative plan for the future so that you don't leave things to chance. We provide suggestions for assessing your relative's needs, establishing a dialogue with other family members, and planning for how specific needs will be addressed. The last section of the chapter discusses how your relative can optimize his independence to be as prepared as possible for the future. Planning now can be a relief to you, your relative, and other family members and can also increase everyone's ability to enjoy their time together.

Working Together with Your Relative

We recommend that you involve your relative in planning for the future from the very beginning. After all, it is your relative's future that is at stake, and she is the most important person in the planning process. To make the best plan, you need to know her goals, viewpoints, and preferences. Even if your relative chooses not to be involved in all of the planning discussions, your decisions and activities on her behalf don't have to be kept a secret. You should share with your relative the results of any planning discussions you have with other family members.

Your relative should not be pressured to attend every single planning discussion. He may decline to participate (especially in the early stages) for a variety of reasons, such as concentration difficulties, distraction caused by intrusive symptoms, or anxiety related to thinking about the future. However, encourage your relative to participate as soon as possible so that he can express his opinions and preferences about his future. His identification of preferences and specific requests is not a guarantee that you can provide them all. The planning process is similar to a negotiation, in that everyone's needs and abilities must be taken into consideration. For most families, compromises are necessary on everyone's part to come up with a workable plan. However, if your relative plays an active role in the planning process, the final plan is much more likely to be successful.

Assessing Your Relative's Needs

The first step in planning how your relative will manage in the future is to assess how her basic needs are being met now and how these needs can continue to be met. Although your relative's situation can change and she might need more or less help than is required now, the present and recent past are usually the best indicators of what will be needed in the future.

People with schizophrenia vary greatly when it comes to how independently they live and how much help they need.

Mitch lives independently, manages his own money, does his own shopping and cooking, and occasionally turns to his family members for social support and loans.

Rico lives with his parents, who do the cooking and laundry and take him to his mental health appointments.

Irene lives in a community residence where the staff members supervise her activities; she relies on her father to bring extra money and cigarettes every week. He also attends treatment planning meetings twice a year and helps Irene advocate for the services that are most beneficial.

Worksheet 30.1 at the end of the chapter will help you and your relative assess how much assistance he is currently receiving in six major areas: housing, activities of daily living, coordination/oversight of treatment, social support, money, and structured activities.

Involving Other Family Members in the Planning Process

Involving other family members in making plans for the future can have several advantages. Other family members may be able to provide new ideas or offer to help in ways that you cannot anticipate. Or they may have strong reservations about taking on responsibilities in the future. Meeting together to discuss the situation is the best way to understand all members' points of view and the degree to which they would like to contribute to the future care of your relative.

Raising the Subject of Planning Ahead

Some parents hesitate to bring up the subject of "what will happen when we're gone." They may feel that it is bad luck or pessimistic to think about when they will no longer be around. They may think they should figure out everything by themselves or other people don't want to be bothered. Or they may think everything will work out on its own and someone else (such as another adult child) will spontaneously step in to take over at the right time.

Although bringing up the subject of planning for the future can initially cause some anxiety, the costs of not planning ahead are far greater. Without a clear plan, your relative could be left in an insecure, unstable situation, and other members of your family could be left in a stressful, confusing position. Keeping family members involved and informed of the planning process will avoid the kind of "surprises" that can be so disruptive when primary caregivers are no longer available.

When it comes to talking about the future, bear in mind that other family members are probably already thinking about it. Even if they have not talked out loud about it, the subject is likely on their minds. Surveys have shown that most people with schizophrenia and their family members are quite concerned about the future. For example, in a study of educational needs conducted by one of us (KM), "What happens when parents are no longer available" was among the top 5 topics (out of 45) most requested by both family members and their relatives with schizophrenia. Therefore, raising the subject of planning ahead will probably not shock anyone; instead, it may be a relief to have the topic in the open.

James's father decided when he turned 60 that it was important to start planning for the future. Since James lived with his parents and they helped him in several ways, there were a number of issues to address. His father first approached James, saying "Your mother and I would like to get together with you to talk about the future. It's been on our minds a lot, and maybe it's been on yours, too. We're in good health, but we realize that we won't be around forever. So we'd like to talk together about your future and what would be best for you. We figure it will take a while to work out a good plan, so we think it's important to get started. What are your thoughts about this, James?" James said that the topic made him nervous, but he thought it was a good idea to talk about it. He was open to his parents' idea of starting the planning process by figuring out what he was currently doing for himself and what he needed help with. He and his parents completed Worksheet 30.1 the following night.

Initiating Family Meetings

It's helpful to think in advance about how to approach other family members regarding planning for the future. When raising this topic, be matter-of-fact and brief. Let other family members know your concerns and that you think it would be helpful to talk things over together. Suggest a day and time when as many people as possible can participate. Plan to keep the initial meetings relatively short and expect that it will take several meetings over the course of weeks or even months before satisfactory plans can be worked out. For some families, group meetings are not practical because of distance or differences in schedules. In such situations, you can talk with people individually, either in person or on the phone, or arrange a conference call.

After James and his parents completed Worksheet 30.1, his father approached James's three siblings (Laura, Frank, and Joan) in the following way: "Your mother and I would like to get together with you and the rest of the family to talk about James's future. We've been thinking about this a lot and figured that maybe you have, too. We've already spoken to James. It will probably take some time to figure out what's best for all concerned, so there's no time like the present to get started. We'd like to get together with you and James this Sunday after dinner around 7:00 for about an hour. Could you come then? We'd appreciate it." At James's request, his father also asked his uncle Paul to come to the family meeting, too, because they were very close.

Making a Plan

Six questions should be answered in making a plan for your relative's future:

1. Where will my relative live?
2. Who will assist with his activities of daily living?
3. Who will coordinate or oversee treatment for her mental and physical health?
4. Who will provide social support and linkage to the community?
5. How will money issues be handled?
6. What meaningful activities and structure will my relative have?

Some questions might be easy to answer. For example, if your relative is currently living in supported housing and is happy with that living arrangement, the issue of where she will live will probably not be complicated. If your relative and her brother have had a close relationship over the years and both have expressed a desire for the brother to help with managing her finances, the question of who will help with money management may require little discussion. If your relative is fully independent in activities of daily living, no planning will be needed in this area.

Some issues in planning for the future can be more difficult to resolve, however, and it may be helpful to use a step-by-step method of solving problems, as described in Chapter 15 and illustrated in the following example. Although the example shows how problem solving can be used in a family meeting, you can also use the steps of problem solving by yourself.

Step 1: Defining the Problem(s) and Establishing a Common Goal

In family meetings try to promote an atmosphere wherein everyone feels free to ask questions, share information, and express honest concerns. It's especially important to share information and ask questions to come to a common understanding of your relative's specific needs. In the initial meetings be sure to avoid putting people on the spot by asking them, for example, what they are going to do to help before they've had a chance to fully understand what they're getting into. It's usually better to hold off deciding who can do what until everyone involved knows the full range of what needs to be done.

Think of planning for your relative's future as a family problem—something that all family members have an investment in solving. This does not mean that all members have the same capabilities or willingness to be closely involved with providing care in the future, but it does suggest that all family members are invested in arriving at an adequate plan for their relative. When family members reflect on their mutual concern for their relative's welfare, they often see planning for the future as a common goal.

James and his family reviewed the areas in which he needed help (using Worksheet 30.1 as a guide) and noted that many areas were going well and did not require much planning. For example, he was independent in most activities of daily living and regularly participated in meaningful activities such as church, volunteering, reading, and attending the drop-in center. The family also recognized that if James's parents were no longer available to help, he would need a place to live, a regular source of social support, assistance with cooking, someone to oversee his treatment, and help with managing his money. The family began to think of their overall goal as "How can we help James continue to live a pleasant life in the future?" No single family member was pinpointed as being "the answer" to all of James's needs.

The family first addressed areas where James needed minor assistance and which were relatively easy to resolve: James's sister Laura would make sure he continued to have social support by checking on him weekly and hosting holiday and birthday dinners; his brother Frank would help James manage his money, which would include a trust fund to supplement his disability check; and Uncle Paul would provide the transportation needed for James to continue attending church, volunteering at the zoo, and going to the library. James wanted to continue taking the bus to the drop-in center once a week.

The family then focused on the questions they could not answer as readily: Where will James live? Who will help with meal preparation? Who will oversee his treatment and make sure he is getting the services he needs?

At this stage of planning for the future, it's important to know the overall extent of your relative's needs, but you need not try to solve everything at once. Instead, try to work on one or two problems at a time to make the overall task more manageable.

Step 2: Generating Options

Try to make early family discussions of options free and open, with as much brainstorming as possible. These discussions will be most effective when members avoid evaluating the options too quickly (e.g., saying, "That will never work") or pressuring family members to assume certain roles. In our example, James's brother Frank began the discussion of housing options by saying, "I think James should live with Joan because she has the biggest house." Their father reminded him that they were just talking about options now and that "no one really knows what's best until we know what all the possibilities are."

To come up with solutions, you need to investigate the range of options, including community resources (see Chapter 5). For example, to determine the best place for your relative to live, investigate different types of living situations, such as supported housing, group homes, and housing that might be available through the local community mental health center or private agencies. During the brainstorming session, family members need to suggest as many options as possible, even if they don't think they would use each one. Regardless of what solution you end up choosing, knowing about a variety of possible solutions may be helpful in the future.

James and his family decided first to tackle the problem of needing someone (in addition to his case manager) to help monitor his treatment, because it would have a bearing on many of the other problems that they needed to solve. At their second family meeting, Joan offered to consult with James's counselor at the community mental health center. The information she acquired was used to generate the following options at the next meeting: (1) James's case manager could completely monitor his overall treatment, (2) the siblings could take turns monitoring, (3) his sister Joan could take primary responsibility for this task.

Step 3: Evaluating the Options

When it comes time to evaluate options, your relative must be involved if he isn't already participating in the planning process. After all, it is your relative's future and his well-being at stake. Each option has advantages and disadvantages and would have different effects on the people involved. In some instances, it may be necessary to find out more about some options in order to evaluate them adequately. For example, if your relative were interested in a supervised community residence, it would be important to know the admission criteria, the waiting period, the cost, what the residence looks like, and where it is located.

When evaluating the three different options regarding who would oversee James's treatment, the family came up with the following advantages and disadvantages:

- Case manager alone. *Advantage = professional who knows a great deal about the mental health system. Disadvantage = James had three different case managers in the past 2 years and said it was difficult for each new person to understand all of his history.*
- Siblings taking turns. *Advantage = the responsibility would be shared evenly. Disadvantage = James said that he would find it confusing.*
- Joan. *Advantage = Joan is very close to her brother and said she felt good about doing something active to help him. James said that it was an advantage that Joan had attended several appointments with him in the past and already knew his doctor. Disadvantage = Joan had 2-year-old twin sons and a 6-year-old daughter and was quite busy with her own family responsibilities.*

Step 4: Choosing the Best Option or Combination of Options

There is no one right solution to the problems involved in planning for the future. The best you can do is to choose an option that has the strongest chance of meeting the needs of your relative and that has the least chance of being a burden to another family member. In general, the solutions that seem to work best are those that attempt to balance the needs of everyone involved.

In discussions about the advantages and disadvantages of the options regarding who would oversee James's treatment, everyone felt most comfortable with Joan taking this role but were concerned about putting too much pressure on her. Laura said she would like to babysit for Joan's children one morning a week to free up some of her time. Frank commented that he worked at home 2 days a week and could serve as a backup if Joan needed help on those days and on weekends.

Everyone was happy with the solution of Joan's taking primary responsibility for overseeing James's treatment, with assistance from her siblings, as needed.

Step 5: Planning How to Carry Out Options

Once a decision has been made, it's important to make a plan to implement it. Some decisions require very intensive planning, especially tasks such as changing your relative's living situation, working out the financial terms of a will, and improving her independence. In such instances it's helpful for family members to divide the responsibility for completing various tasks. It's also important to set a realistic time frame for each task and to schedule a follow-up meeting to determine whether the steps are being accomplished. Some parts of the plan can be done immediately, whereas others take more time.

James and his family made the following plan:

1. *James will meet with Joan and review with her the members of his treatment team and what is included in his current treatment (within 1 week).*
2. *James will call his counselor and case manager to let them know about the decision to have Joan help oversee his treatment. (Call to be made within 2 weeks.)*
3. *Joan will call James's case manager to introduce herself and ask to set up a meeting. In addition, she will ask to be included in the next treatment planning meeting. (Call to be made within 3 weeks.)*
4. *Laura will babysit for Joan's children when she attends the meeting with the case manager.*
5. *Uncle Paul will start taking John to church every other week (starting next Sunday).*
6. *James's parents will call a friend from NAMI to get the name of an attorney who is experienced in making wills and setting up trust funds (within 2 weeks).*
7. *Frank will meet with James and his parents to start learning about his finances (within 3 weeks).*
8. *Family will meet to follow up (in 4 weeks, Sunday, at 7:00 P.M.).*

Step 6: Evaluating How the Solution Is Being Carried Out

It's critical to know that your plans are being followed and are accomplishing what you hoped. For example, if you decide to establish a trust fund for your relative, the lawyer needs to be contacted and the papers must be drawn up appropriately. If this task is delayed, the financial security you planned for your relative may not exist at the critical time. Similarly, in James's situation, if his sister Joan did not develop a relationship with his treatment team, the smooth transition that James and his family envisioned would not be possible.

James and his family started their follow-up meeting by reviewing the plan they had made the previous month and what they had been able to accomplish. James had gone over his treatment with Joan and had called both his counselor and case manager. Joan called the case manager and scheduled an appointment for Wednesday, 2 days after the family's follow-up meeting. The treatment team meeting was scheduled in 4 months. Uncle Paul had taken James to church one Sunday but was unable to do so on the other Sunday because of illness. James's parents had gotten the name of an attorney, but had not called her yet. Frank had had one meeting with James and his parents about finances, but the financial records were not well organized and he could not accomplish all that he had hoped. The following plan was made:

1. *Joan will attend the meeting with the case manager, with Laura providing babysitting (Wednesday of next week).*
2. *Uncle Paul will plan to take James to church every other Sunday and will call Frank if he is sick and cannot drive; if Frank is unavailable, he will call Laura.*
3. *James's parents will call the attorney and set up an appointment. (Call will be made within 2 weeks.)*
4. *James and his parents will organize his financial records (within 2 weeks).*
5. *Frank will meet with James and his parents to talk about finances (within 3 weeks).*
6. *Family will meet to follow up (in 4 weeks, Sunday, at 7:00 P.M.).*

James's parents told the family how pleased they were with how things were going so far and that it had been a big weight off their minds. James said he felt "okay" about the plans being made but was nervous about the changes they implied. He also said he wondered most about where he was going to live, and the family agreed they should begin to address the housing issue at the next meeting, after Joan had met with the case manager.

We suggest that you reevaluate plans for your relative at least every year to determine whether he has the same needs and whether the same resources are available. For example, in James's situation, it would be necessary to modify the plans if Joan decided to return to full-time employment or if James became more independent by increasing his cooking skills.

Long-Term Planning for Needs
Related to Finances and Ongoing Assistance

Although many of the problems encountered in planning for the future can be solved by following the steps described in the preceding material, some topics require special information and preparation. Such topics include estate planning and evaluating whether to use organizations designed specifically to provide life-time assistance to individuals with mental illness.

Estate Planning

When planning for your relative's financial security, keep in mind that she may be receiving benefits based on financial need, such as Supplemental Security Income (SSI) and public assistance (sometimes referred to as "welfare"), as described in Chapter 5. If a person receiving such benefits has an inheritance that is not legally safeguarded, the federal or state officials can claim that the person no longer needs financial assistance and is no longer eligible to receive them. Furthermore, SSI and public assistance are tied to health care benefits, such as Medicaid, which helps to pay for inpatient and outpatient medical and mental health expenses. Keep in mind that even if your relative no longer needs the financial benefits, she will almost invariably continue to need health care benefits. The costs of necessary doctor's visits and medications are very high and beyond the means of most individuals to pay privately.

If you wish to leave money or property to your relative after you die and maintain his eligibility for benefits, consult a lawyer who is knowledgeable about wills and trust funds for persons with mental illness. The lawyer can help you protect your relative's inheritance from government agencies and, if necessary, from your relative's own inability to manage funds. The lawyer can help you understand the state and federal laws as they relate to your individual situation. Chapters of the National Alliance on Mental Illness (NAMI) often maintain a list of lawyers with the kind of expertise you need. Some lawyers may even have a reduced rate if you have limited financial resources.

Although each family's situation is different and each state has its own laws regarding inheritances, it may be helpful to review some estate planning options:

- *Full inheritance* means you leave funds and assets directly to your relative. This option is rarely chosen by families because it jeopardizes governmental benefits. You must also exercise extreme caution in using this option because the person receiving such an inheritance would be put under the stress of managing the assets and investments. Given that the course of schizophrenia can be variable over time, even if your relative is functioning independently now, a recurrence of symptoms could alter her judgment and ability to handle finances.

- *Disinheritance* means you're not leaving anything directly to your relative with schizophrenia. You can leave your assets to another family member with the understanding that he will care for your relative. If the expectations of this family member are informal, this option will not jeopardize your relative's eligibility for government programs. For some families this works very well, especially if there is a relative who has an ongoing and close relationship with your family member. However, many families hesitate to use this option because their relative may perceive it as a sign of lack of affection. Also, the assets left to the other family member are vulnerable to his judgment and creditors. For example, if the other family member divorces, the assets would be a factor in the divorce settlement. In rare circumstances, the other family member may have a change of heart and decide that he has more need of the money than your relative with schizophrenia. Finally, if you disinherit your relative, another relative is not legally obligated to care for him.

- *Trusts* involve placing your assets in a special fund for your relative: in the form of an *inter vivos trust* (during lifetime) or a *testamentary trust* (in a will). A *supplemental needs trust* can appoint a trustee to distribute the funds on behalf of your relative and can stipulate that the funds are meant to pay for costs that are not covered by governmental programs such as Medicaid or SSI. For example, such a trust can stipulate that income or principal cannot be used for food, clothing, or shelter. If drafted properly, such a trust would mean that neither the income nor the principal would be considered an available resource by government agencies determining eligibility for their programs.

The *trustee* is the person who will distribute assets based on the specific provisions of the trust you establish. It is important to choose someone whose judgment you trust and who will have your relative's best interests at heart. It is also important to spell out your wishes as specifically as possible when you draft the trust, so that the trustee can carry them out. For example, specify if you want the funds of the trust used for recreation, special services, trips, musical equipment, classes, and so on. Keep in mind that the trustee will not have authority over your relative, only over the funds.

Organizations That Provide Lifetime Assistance

In recent years several organizations have been founded to provide services for adults with disabilities whose relatives are either deceased or no longer able to care for them. These organizations usually hire staff members to monitor the needs of the person, obtain financial and health care benefits, preserve or improve the quality of the client's life, and respond to crises. The staff members generally develop individual care plans and schedule regular appointments to meet with their clients. One example of such an organization is the Planned Lifetime Assistance Network (PLAN), which is currently available in over 20 states. Naturally, PLAN and other organizations that provide long-term assistance must charge fees. To locate PLAN in your state, contact the National PLAN Alliance, which is listed in the Resources section at the end of this chapter. It is important to remember that PLAN programs are not substitutes for the services provided in the public domain; rather they are designed to do what families have been doing for their relatives.

Any organization that provides lifetime or long-term care needs to be evaluated carefully. Basic questions to ask include:

"How long has the organization been in existence?"
"How many clients have you provided services to?"
"How is your money invested?"
"How financially secure is your organization?"
"May I talk to someone who has used your services?"
"What exactly is provided in return for the fees you require?"

For some families, lifetime care organizations may be a good solution to planning for the future; for others, they may not be suitable.

Optimizing Your Relative's Independence

In planning for the future, family members may find that their relative's options are limited by how much she can do independently. For example, in James's situation, he was not able to prepare meals. If he had more daily living skills, perhaps he would be able to live alone or in supported independent housing.

Many times family members underestimate what their relative can do or they find it simpler to do things for him. In the short run, it may feel good to provide a needed service for your relative. However, in the long run, you may not really be doing him a favor. If your relative relies on you too much, he will not be prepared for the future when you will no longer be able to do these tasks.

In contrast, taking steps to increase your relative's independence can be one of the best ways you can help. Even small improvements in independence can lead to a better quality of life. Chapter 27 provides ideas for improving your relative's abilities in a variety of skills related to independent living. In addition, you may find the following suggestions helpful as you plan for the future.

- *Choose a specific area to work on.* Carefully assess the areas where your relative needs the most help. Reviewing Worksheet 30.1 at the end of the chapter can be a good start to identifying specific skills on which to focus. It is usually best to concentrate on improving your relative's skills in one area at a time, starting with an area where it is likely that improvement can be made more readily.

James is able to serve himself cold cereal for breakfast and to microwave prepared meals but does not do any food preparation beyond that. James said he would like to be more independent in the kitchen. His mother offered to help him increase the number of meals he can prepare, such as making sandwiches, scrambling eggs, making salads, and cooking pasta dishes.

- *Set a series of modest, attainable goals.* It is unrealistic to expect dramatic improvement in a short time. Instead, start small and build your relative's confidence and willingness to keep trying.

James's mother began by praising how well he prepared his breakfast and asking him to help her fix sandwiches for lunch. The first day she explained where the supplies for ham sandwiches were kept (in the refrigerator and the pantry) and asked him to lay out the ingredients (loaf of bread, ham, and mustard) on the counter. She thanked him for his help and proceeded to make the ham sandwiches.

The next day she asked him to lay out the supplies and to take out the appropriate number of slices of bread. Two days later, she demonstrated the steps of putting on the ham and mustard. Each time he accomplished a step, she thanked him. If he missed a step, she let him know what the step should have been. Within a few weeks, James was able to make sandwiches for himself and his parents.

Over the next several months, James's mother slowly added salads and scrambled eggs to his repertoire in the kitchen. She only proceeded to teach how to prepare a new dish when James showed confidence in the previous one. The next goal that she and James set was increasing his ability to budget his money.

- *Expect that the process will not always be smooth.* If your relative is accustomed to having another person do certain tasks for her, she may resist change. It's helpful to reassure your relative of your affection and to explain that asking her to do more is a sign that you care about her independence and well-being. Let your relative know that you appreciate her efforts, and praise even small steps she takes toward improving her independence.

• *Initiate difficult transitions as soon as possible.* Some plans for the future involve making major changes, such as moving to a new living situation. It is usually best if you're available to help your relative make such a transition, even if doing so means making a change before it's absolutely necessary. A gradual transition is usually easier and gentler, although some people are not able to follow through on changes until they have no other choice. Your relative will benefit, however, from whatever support you can give while he is moving toward more independence.

James had lived at home his entire life. If he decided that the best option for his future was to move to a supported apartment, it would be best to begin the process while he was still living with his parents. If he found a supported apartment that he liked, he could move there, spend some time with his parents on weekends, and invite his family to visit him at his new home.

The Value of Planning Ahead

Making plans for your relative's future can be a complex and emotional process. However, by talking openly with her and other relevant family members, making decisions with your relative that are practical and satisfy her basic needs, and seeking legal advice when needed, you can decrease the amount of stress that will result when you are no longer available to provide care. You can further prepare your relative by helping her to become as independent as possible. Planning for the future is an ongoing expression of your love and concern for your relative, and everyone in the family will benefit from your efforts.

Resources

Russell, L. M., Grant, A. E., Joseph, S. M., & Fee, R. W. (1993). *Planning for the future: Providing a meaningful life for a child with a disability after your death.* Evanston, IL: American Publishing. This thoughtful book contains important information about developing an overall plan for the well-being of your loved one, including suggestions about wills, trusts, and maintaining government benefits (such as SSI).

National PLAN Alliance. 203 Woodlawn Avenue, Saratoga Springs, NY 12866. Phone: 518-587-3372; e-mail: npa@nycap.rr.com. This organization will help you locate PLAN programs throughout the United States; in addition, its "Life Planning Workbook" helps families plan for the future of adult relatives with a developmental disability or a mental illness.

Assistance Currently Being Provided (p. 1 of 2)

Area of life	No assistance in this area	Some assistance in this area (specify)
Housing		
• At home?		
• Own apartment?		
• Supported housing?		
• Group home?		
• Other?		
Daily Living		
• Meal preparation		
• Shopping for groceries and clothing		
• Cleaning		
• Laundry		
• Taking medication		
• Making and keeping appointments		
• Transportation		
• Grooming and hygiene		
• Time management		
Coordination/Oversight of Treatment (mental and physical health)		
• Coordination of services		
• Setting up and attending regular psychiatric appointments		
• Monitoring early warning signs		
• Monitoring effectiveness of medication and presence of side effects		
• Resolving mental health crises		
• Setting up and attending regular medical appointments		

Area of life	No assistance in this area	Some assistance in this area (specify)
• Following up with specialists, additional services		
• Advocating for needed services		
Social Support and Linkage to the Community		
• Companionship		
• Support		
• Celebrating birthdays		
• Celebrating holidays		
• Going to religious services or attending other community activities		
• Going out for meals		
• Checking in on a regular basis		
Money		
• Keeping track of income and expenses		
• Ensuring bills are paid on time		
• Helping to prepare a budget		
• Serving as representative payee		
• Providing supplemental funds		
Structure and Meaningful Activities		
• Routine in everyday life		
• Activities to enjoy alone		
• Activities to enjoy with others		
• Regular involvement in at least one of the following: school, work, volunteering, recreation/leisure activities, hobbies, community activities		

Resources

United States

Information, Self-Help, and Advocacy Organizations

Active Minds on Campus

www.activemindsoncampus.org

— A student-run organization that uses peer outreach to increase students' awareness of mental health issues and encourage students to seek help as soon as it is needed.

Bazelon Center for Mental Health Law

www.bazelon.org

— Focuses on legal issues pertaining to mental illness and developmental disabilities, including involuntary admissions and advance psychiatric directives.

Center for Mental Health Services (CMHS)

www.mentalhealth.org

— Provides information on a variety of services and programs for people with mental illnesses, including information about the illnesses, housing assistance, and anti-stigma campaigns.

Center for Reintegration

201-869-2333

www.reintegration.com

— The Center provides information on finding meaningful work, restoring relationships, and moving toward independent living. The website offers helpful information about schizophrenia, healthy lifestyles, and being involved in work and the community. It also contains information about ordering its free magazine, *Reintegration Today*.

Compeer, Inc.

www.compeer.org

— An international, not-for-profit organization with volunteer-based programs and services that provide supportive friendships for people receiving mental health treatment. Headquartered in Rochester, NY, the organization has nearly 100 affiliate locations across the country and around the world, including Canada and Australia.

Consumer Organization and Networking Technical Assistance Center (CONTAC)

800-598-8847

www.contac.org

— A resource center for consumers and consumer-run organizations across the United States. Available services and products include informational materials, on-site training, skill-building curricula, communication capabilities, networking, and customized activities promoting self-help, recovery, leadership, business management, and empowerment.

GROW

888-741-4769 (toll-free) or 217-352-6989

— A self-help organization that encourages people to share their experiences and strengthen each other in support groups. Most GROW groups are located in Illinois and New Jersey, but additional groups are planned in other states.

Mental Health Recovery

802-254-2092

www.mentalhealthrecovery.com

— Mary Ellen Copeland has written several books and developed a variety of programs for helping people in the recovery process, including the Wellness Recovery Action Plan (WRAP). Her website offers helpful information, a free newsletter, and a list of publications and workshops that can be purchased.

Mental Illness Education Project (MIEP)

800-343-5540

www.miepvideos.org

— Seeks to improve understanding of mental illness through the production of videotapes for people with psychiatric disorders, their families, mental health practitioners, administrators, educators, and the general public.

NARSAD (National Association for Research on Schizophrenia and Depression) Artworks

www.narsadartworks.org

— Supports and promotes artwork by individuals with mental illness; its website offers high-quality art products for sale by artists with mental illness, including holiday cards, posters, T-shirts, and paintings.

National Alliance on Mental Illness (NAMI)

800-950-NAMI (helpline)

www.nami.org

— The largest organization in the United States providing support, education, and advocacy for consumers, families, and friends of people with mental illness. NAMI offers educational and support groups for families and consumers, supports increased funding for research, and advocates for adequate health insurance, housing, rehabilitation, and jobs for people with psychiatric disabilities. Each state has a chapter and many communities have their own chapters. Many chapters offer, among their programs, "Family-to-Family," a series of classes where families can learn more about mental illness and strategies for coping. The NAMI website has numerous helpful educational handouts on mental illness and treatment.

National Empowerment Center (NEC)

www.power2u.org

— Provides information, programs, and materials focused on recovery from mental illness; refers people to local support groups; provides guidance for setting up new groups; provides newsletter and audiovisual materials.

National GAINS Center

www.gainsctr.com

— Funded by the Substance Abuse and Mental Health Services Administration (SAMHSA), this center is dedicated to preventing those with major mental illness from getting involved in the criminal justice system and improving the treatment of those already involved. It promotes activities that further the principles of *G*athering information, *A*ssessing what works, *I*nterpreting/integrating the facts, *N*etworking, and *S*timulating change.

National Mental Health Association (NMHA)

www.nmha.org

— Provides information and referral services for people in the process of recovery.

National Mental Health Consumers' Self-Help Clearinghouse

www.mhselfhelp.org

— Provides information about psychiatric disorders, technical support for self-help groups, and a free quarterly newsletter for consumers. It sponsors an annual conference. Spanish language services are available.

National Mental Health Information Center

800-789-2647

www.mentalhealth.samhsa.gov

— Part of the Substance Abuse and Mental Health Services Administration (SAMHSA), this clearinghouse formerly known as the Knowledge Exchange Network (KEN) offers free information about mental health, including publications, references, and referrals to local and national resources and organizations. Click on "Publications" and select "Online Publications" for helpful handouts, booklets, and information.

National Schizophrenia Foundation (NSF)

www.nsfoundation.org

— Develops and maintains Schizophrenics Anonymous support groups, which can be found in many states. Its website has several first-person accounts, educational materials, and information about public awareness programs.

schizophrenia.com

www.schizophrenia.com

— A nonprofit Web community providing in-depth information, support, education, and lists of articles, books, audiotapes, and videotapes related to schizophrenia. Janssen Pharmaceutica helps to sponsor the website.

Substance Abuse and Mental Health Services Administration (SAMHSA)

www.samhsa.gov

— SAMHSA is an agency of the U.S. Department of Health and Human Services that was created to focus attention, programs, and funding on improving the lives of people with, or at risk for, mental and substance abuse disorders. One of its recent projects has been to develop and disseminate toolkits of evidence-based practices for severe mental disorders. The website provides information about mental illnesses and substance abuse and current projects related to treatment and recovery.

United States Psychiatric Rehabilitation Association (USPRA)

410-789-7054

www.uspra.org

— A nonprofit organization for professionals, families, and persons with psychiatric illnesses committed to promoting, supporting, and strengthening community-based psychosocial rehabilitation services and resources. It also publishes a journal, newsletters, and a resource catalog.

Research Organizations

National Alliance for Research on Schizophrenia and Depression (NARSAD)

800-829-8289 or 516-829-0091

www.narsad.org

— A private, not-for-profit organization that raises funds for scientific research into the causes, cures, treatments, and prevention of brain disorders such as schizophrenia and depression.

National Institute of Mental Health (NIMH)

www.nimh.nih.gov

— Engages in research on the causes and treatment of mental disorders. Its website provides educational materials and an extensive list of free publications on psychiatric disorders, including a comprehensive listing of helpful resources.

Stanley Medical Research Institute (SMRI)
301-571-0760
www.stanleyresearch.org
— A nonprofit organization that supports research on the causes and treatment of schizophrenia and bipolar disorder through work carried out in its own laboratories and
through support of researchers worldwide.

Books about Schizophrenia and Other Mental Illnesses

Amador, X., & Johanson, A. (2000). *I'm not sick, I don't need help*. Petonic, NY: Vida Press.

Andreasen, N. C. (2001). *Brave new brain: Conquering mental illness in the era of the genome*.
New York: Oxford University Press.

Beard, J. & Gillespie, P. N. (2002). *Nothing to hide: Mental illness in the family*. New York:
New Press. First-person accounts.

Burke, R. D. (1995). *When the music's over: My journey into schizophrenia*. New York: Basic
Books. First-person account.

Chuei, C. C., Verma, S., & Ann, C. (Eds.). (2003). *Delusions, possession or imagination? Experiencing and recovering from psychosis*. Singapore: SNP Editions (*www.snpcorp.com/
webshop/int_pub.asp*).

Deveson, A. (1991). *Tell me I'm here: One family's experience of schizophrenia*. New York: Penguin Books. First-person account.

Green, M. F. (2001). *Schizophrenia revealed*. New York: Norton.

Holly, T. E. & Holly, J. (1997). *My mother's keeper: A daughter's memoir of growing up in the
shadow of mental illness*. New York: Avon Grove. First-person account.

Jenkins, J. H., & Barrett, R. J. (Eds.). (2004). *Schizophrenia, culture, and subjectivity: The
edge of experience*. Cambridge, UK: Cambridge University Press.

Kaplan, B. (Ed.). (1964). *The inner world of mental illness*. New York: Harper & Row.

Kawanishi, Y. (2005). *Families coping with mental illness: Stories in the U.S. and Japan*. New
York: Routledge. *Note*: The similarities in how families in both cultures are affected
by mental illness is most striking.

Keefe, R. S. E., & Harvey, P. D. (1994). *Understanding schizophrenia: A guide to the new
research on causes and treatment*. New York: Free Press.

Kytle, E. (1987). *The voices of Robby Wilde*. Washington, DC: Seven Locks Press.

Marsh, D. T., & Dickens, R. (1998). *How to cope with mental illness in your family: A self-care
guide for siblings, offspring and parents*. New York: Jeremy P. Tarcher/Putnam.

McLean, R. (2003). *Recovered, not cured: A journey through schizophrenia*. Crows Nest, New
South Wales, Australia: Allen & Unwin. Available from *www.allenandunwin.com*.
First-person account.

Mercato, S. (1992). *The shell people: My story of schizophrenia*. Brampton, Ontario, Canada:
Ashlar House Publishing and Promotions. First-person account.

Miller, R., & Mason, S. (2002). *Diagnosis: Schizophrenia*. New York: Columbia University
Press.

Nasar, S. (1998). *A beautiful mind: The life of mathematical genius and Nobel laureate John
Nash*. New York: Simon & Schuster.

Neugeboren, J. (1998). *Imagining Robert: My brother, madness and survival.* New York: Holt. First-person account.

Neugeboren, J. (1999). *Transforming madness: New lives for people living with mental illness.* New York: Morrow.

Schiller, L., & Bennett, A. (1994). *The quiet room: A journey out of the torment of madness.* New York: Warner Books. First-person account.

Secunda, V. (1998). *When madness comes home: Help and hope for children, siblings, and partners of the mentally ill.* New York: Hyperion.

Steele, K., & Berman, C. (2001). *The day the voices stopped: A memoir of madness and hope.* New York: Basic Books. First-person account.

Swados, E. (1991). *The four of us: A family memoir.* New York: Farrar, Straus, & Giroux. First-person account.

Torrey, E. F. (2001). *Surviving schizophrenia: A manual for families, consumers and providers* (4th ed.). New York: HarperTrade.

Woolis, R. (2003). *When someone you love has a mental illness* (rev. ed.). New York: Jeremy P. Tarcher/Penguin Books.

Wyden, P. (1998). *Conquering schizophrenia: A father, his son, and a medical breakthrough.* New York: Knopf. First-person account.

Videotapes

A Beautiful Mind. (2002). Universal Studios. Movie adaptation of the book by Sylvia Nasar, based on the life of Nobel Prize laureate John Nash, provides a good idea of the confusion of experiencing schizophrenia and the difficulty distinguishing between what is real and what is not. Available in videotape or DVD format.

The Bonnie Tapes. (1997). Mental Illness Education Project (*miepvideos.org* or 800-343-5540). In a series of three videotapes ("Mental Illness in the Family," "Recovery from Mental Illness," and "My Sister Is Mentally Ill"), 27-year-old Bonnie and her family talk together about schizophrenia and how it has affected them.

I'm Still Here. (1996). Wheeler Communications Productions. Available from Direct Cinema Limited (*www.directcinema.com* or 310-636-8200). A poignant collection of stories of several individuals and their families living with schizophrenia, with some coping very well and others experiencing significant challenges.

Living with Schizophrenia. (2002). New York: Guilford Press and Monkey See Productions (*www.guilford.com*). Four individuals with schizophrenia share their personal recovery journeys.

A Love Story: Living with Someone with Schizophrenia. (1991). Penny Frese. Available from Wellness Reproductions (800-669-9208).

Nurseminars Videos. (1989–1995). Mary Moller. This series of videotapes includes topics relevant to professionals and families, such as "Understanding Relapse," "Understanding and Communicating with a Person Who Is Hallucinating," and "Understanding and Communicating with a Person Who Has Delusions." Available from Nurseminars (509-468-9848) or Wellness Reproductions (800-669-9208).

Out of the Shadow. (2004). Vine Street Pictures. Susan Smiley filmed this documentary about growing up with a mother with schizophrenia. The website *www.*

outoftheshadow.com has information on how to purchase copies of the film, or you can call 310-636-0116.

Schizophrenia: Surviving in the world of normals. (1991). Fred Frese. Available from Wellness Reproductions (800-669-9208).

Magazines and Journals

American Journal of Psychiatric Rehabilitation. Published three times a year by Taylor and Francis, this journal is written for providers of rehabilitation services and for persons with psychiatric disorders and their families. It features original research articles as well as theoretical papers, reviews, commentaries, and first-person accounts that reflect on the rehabilitation process and recovery.

Community Mental Health Journal. Published six times a year by Springer Publications, this journal focuses on articles related to improving services for people with psychiatric disorders.

Journal of the World Psychiatry Association. Available free online, this journal contains articles on a variety of psychiatric illnesses, including schizophrenia.

Psychiatric Rehabilitation Journal. Published quarterly by Boston University in collaboration with the U.S. Psychiatric Rehabilitation Association (USPRA), this journal publishes articles relevant to the rehabilitation of people with severe psychiatric disability and is intended for readers with a professional and personal interest in the field of psychiatric rehabilitation.

Psychiatric Services. Published monthly by the American Psychiatric Association, this journal contains research articles related to treatment and services for persons with mental illnesses.

Reintegration Today. Published quarterly by the Center for Reintegration and made possible by an unrestricted educational grant from Eli Lily, this is a free magazine for consumers, family members, and practitioners. You can subscribe to the magazine at *www.reintegration.com* or by calling 800-809-8202.

Schizophrenia Bulletin. Published quarterly by Oxford University Press, this journal contains research and review articles about recent developments and empirically based hypotheses regarding the etiology and treatment of schizophrenia.

Schizophrenia Digest. Published quarterly by Magpie Publications (*www.schizophreniadigest. com*), this magazine is intended for consumers, family members, and practitioners.

Schizophrenia Research. Published bimonthly by Elsevier Press, this journal emphasizes new research that contributes to the understanding and treatment of schizophrenia disorders.

Canada

Organizations

Alliance pour les malades mentaux, Inc. (Alliance for the Mentally Ill)
www.amiquebec.org
— Provides support, education, guidance, and advocacy. Many helpful fact sheets are available in English and French.

Canadian Health Network (CHN)

www.canadian-health-network.ca

— A national, nonprofit, bilingual Web-based health information service, including educational materials about physical and mental health. The site provides extensive links to sources of information about a variety of mental illnesses, as well as how to stay physically healthy (e.g., tips for nutritious meals, exercise plans, avoiding skin cancer).

Canadian Mental Health Association

www.cmha.ca/

— A nationwide charitable organization that promotes mental health and supports the resilience and recovery of people experiencing mental illness. Its website has helpful information sheets on various diagnoses and aspects of treatment and a special program for practicing "mind and body fitness." A wide range of specialized programs and services are offered at centers throughout Canada.

Early Psychosis Intervention Program (EPI), South Fraser, British Columbia

www.psychosissucks.ca

— The site offers easily accessible information on psychosis, treatment, associated problems, substance use, and recovery. Downloadable PDF files include fifteen excellent handouts on a wide range of topics, including "What Is Psychosis?" "Goal Setting," and "Problem Solving."

Fédération des Familles et Amis de la Personne Atteinte de Maladie Mentale (FFAPAMM)

www.ffapamm.qc.ca

— Provides information and support for families and friends of individuals with mental illness (its website is in French).

Prevention and Early Intervention Program for Psychoses (PEPP)

www.pepp.ca

— Website describes PEPP's treatment program for early intervention of psychosis and includes information about a well-established family support group, family stories, and helpful links to other websites.

Schizophrenia Society of Canada

www.schizophrenia.ca

— Provides support, education, and advocacy for people with schizophrenia and their relatives. It has numerous branches, including the following:

> Alberta (*www.schizophrenia.ab.ca*)
> British Columbia (*www.bcss.org*)
> Manitoba (*www.mss.mb.ca*)
> New Brunswick (*www.schizophrenia.ca/nbprov.html*)
> Newfoundland and Labrador (*www.ssnl.org*)
> Nova Scotia (*www.nsnet.org/valleyssns*)
> Ontario (*www.schizophrenia.on.ca*)

Prince Edward Island (*www.schizophrenia.ca/peiprov.html*)

Quebec: AMI Quebec: Alliance for the Mentally Ill (*www.amiquebec.org*) and Societe Quebecoise de la Schizophrenie (*www.schizophrenie.qc.ca*)

Saskatchewan (*www.schizophrenia.sk.ca*)

Self-Help Resource Centre, Toronto, Ontario

www.selfhelp.on.ca

— Promoting self-help, this site offers information about how to start and maintain a self-help group.

World Fellowship for Schizophrenia and Allied Disorders (WFSAD)

416-961-2855

www.world-schizophrenia.org

— WFSAD has its headquarters in Canada but is an international organization dedicated to lessening the problems faced by people with serious mental illness and their families. Its website and members' newsletter includes educational materials about mental illnesses, reports of current research, and personal stories from around the world.

Books, Newsletters, and Videotapes

Family to Family: A Newsletter for First-Episode Psychosis Families. Developed and produced by first-episode psychosis families, this newsletter provides a venue for sharing information and support. Three issues available annually as PDF downloads at *www.cmha.ca.*

A Map of the Mind Fields: Managing Adolescent Psychosis. National Film Board of Canada. In this video three young people and their families share their personal stories. The film offers practical tools for understanding the problems and finding the solutions to mental health problems among children and youth. To order on-line: *www.nfb.ca*; or phone: 1-800-542-2164—*identification #: 113C9104260*

One Day at a Time. Canadian Mental Health Association, National Office. In this videotape, several members of a first-episode psychosis parent support group describe their experiences as parents of young people with psychosis. Order at *www.cmha.ca.*

Rays of Hope. A 268-page reference manual for families and caregivers from the Schizophrenia Society of Canada. Available for download at *www.schizophrenia.ca*, click on "Support & Education."

The Secret of the Brain Chip: A Self-Help Guide for People Suffering from Psychosis. (2000). DeHert, M., Magiels, G., & Thys, E. English version in collaboration with McKenzie, K. This book is primarily in the form of a graphic novel (comic book).

Your Education—Your Future: A Guide to College and University for Students with Psychiatric Disabilities. A comprehensive resource for Canadian students that provides information on all aspects of postsecondary education. It includes checklists to help students make decisions and also features the experiences and advice of students with psychiatric disorders from across the country. Available at *www.cmha.ca*, click on "Understanding Mental Illness" then "Education and Mental Illness."

Australia and New Zealand

Association of Relatives and Friends of the Mentally Ill (ARAFMI)

— Offers a range of services for caregivers of people experiencing mental illness, including support groups, information, and telephone counselling. The Queensland branch sells a number of helpful publications, CDs, and videotapes on the following topics, some of which are packaged into kits: "Coping with Mental Health Problems: A Handbook for Family Carers," "Dual Diagnosis: Mental Illness and Substance Use," and "Supporting People with Psychiatric Disabilities." Branches in Australia include:

New South Wales (*www.arafmi.org/*)
Northern Territory (*www.depressionet.com.au/famfr/arafmi_nt.html*)
Queensland (*www.arafmiqld.org/*)
South Australia (*www.users.senet.com.au/~panangga/mhrc/*)
Tasmania (*www.depressionet.com.au/famfr/arafmi_tas.html*)
Victoria (*www.arafemi.org.au/*)
Western Australia (*www.arafmi.asn.au/*)

International Early Psychosis Association (IEPA)

www.iepa.org.au

— IEPA is an international network for people involved in the study and treatment of early psychosis. They host an international conference on early intervention every 2 years.

It's All Right

www.itsallright.org

— A website for teenagers who have a mental illness or who have a relative with mental illness, it offers information and suggestions specifically aimed at young people.

Mental Health Council of Australia (MHCA)

www.mhca.org.au/

— A nongovernment organization representing and promoting the interests of the Australian mental health sector, committed to achieving better mental health for all Australians.

Mental Health Foundation of Australia (Victoria)

www.mhf.org.au and *www.mentalhealthvic.org.au*

— The oldest mental health association in Australia, it is an organization of professionals, consumers, and families concerned with mental health issues and provides referrals and education.

Mental Health Foundation of New Zealand

www.mentalhealth.org.nz/

— Provides information, resources, and advocacy for mental health consumers and their families in New Zealand.

Mental Health Resource Centre

www.users.senet.com.au/~panangga/mhrc/

— A nongovernment umbrella organization of mental health support organizations for the people of South Australia.

Neuroscience Institute of Schizophrenia and Allied Disorders (NISAD)

www.nisad.org.au

— A nonprofit, independent Australian medical research organization that studies the causes of schizophrenia. The website contains links to support systems in Australia and to current and past research.

ORYGEN Youth Health

www.orygen.org.au

— Previously known as "Early Psychosis Prevention and Intervention Centre" or "EPPIC," this organization is composed of a specialist youth mental health service, a research center, and a range of educational, advocacy, and health-promotion activities. Its website contains numerous helpful handouts on psychotic disorders, and it conveys an optimistic attitude about the outcome of mental illnesses such as schizophrenia, especially when early intervention is provided. ORYGEN has influenced the delivery of services in many countries.

Royal Australian and New Zealand College of Psychiatrists (RANZCP)

www.ranzcp.org

— This website describes the role of psychiatrists in treating mental health and contains guidelines for professionals, including how to work collaboratively with families and other caregivers.

SANE Australia

www.sane.org

— A national charity that helps people affected by mental illness through campaigns, education, and research. Its website contains fact sheets about schizophrenia in English, Greek, Italian, and Vietnamese. A special website is provided for teenagers with a mental illness or a relative with mental illness (*www.itsallright.org*). SANE also provides a helpful newsletter and sells several practical written guides, videos, and CDs about schizophrenia, including the following:

- *SANE Guide to Schizophrenia*
  Helps people diagnosed with schizophrenia, their family, and their friends by explaining what it means to have this diagnosis, examining effective treatments, and exploring what family and friends can do to help.

- *SANE Guide to Psychosis*
  Helps people who have had a psychotic episode and their family and friends understand what it means to have this diagnosis, how it is treated, and what family and friends can do to help.

- *Schizophrenia—Let's Talk about It* (video)
  Bill Kelly in conversation with writer, journalist, and filmmaker Anne Deveson and others about how mental illness has affected their lives.

- *SANE CD-ROM Guide to Psychosis*
Sounds and images are used to explain what psychosis means, how it feels for those who experience it and their families and friends, and what treatments help.

- *Voices: The Auditory Hallucinations Project* (interactive CD)
Explains how it feels to hear voices and what can be done to help.

To order, visit the SANE Bookshop at *www.sane.org* or call 03 9682 5933.

Schizophrenia Fellowship of Australia
— A membership-based not-for-profit organization that works with people with mental illness and their families and friends to improve their well-being and provide a voice for change. Many branches offer a program called "Well Ways: A Traveler's Guide to Wellbeing for Families and Friends of People with Mental Illness," which consists of a series of workshops involving group discussions, videos, and practical demonstrations aimed at increasing the capacity of families, caregivers, and friends to care effectively for themselves, other family members, and their relative living with mental illness. The Schizophrenia Fellowship has branches in various Australian states, including the following:

Mental Illness Fellowship of Victoria (*www.mifellowship.org*)
Schizophrenia Fellowship of New South Wales (*www.sfnsw.org.au/*)
Schizophrenia Fellowship of South Queensland (*www.sfsq.org.au/*)
Mental Illness Fellowship of South Australia (*www.mifsa.org.au*)

Schizophrenia Fellowship of New Zealand (SFNZ)
www.sfnat.org.nz/
— All branches offer support, education, advocacy, and information, and some offer additional services.

Great Britain

Organizations

Carers' Website of the Department of Health
www.carers.gov.uk
— Offers fact sheets about mental illness and advice on practical matters such as entitlements to benefits and respite.

Making Space
www.makingspace.co.uk
— A charity that helps all those affected by schizophrenia and other forms of serious and enduring mental illness, including the person, caregivers, and family members. It is run by people who have a direct and personal experience. The organization conducts self-help groups in northern England and employs support staff who are trained to help family members in a variety of ways, including providing behavioral family therapy.

Mental Health Care

www.mentalhealthcare.org.uk

— Contains information about mental health and illness, research findings from the Institute of Psychiatry and South London and Maudsley Trust, and personal stories written by caregivers.

Mind

www.mind.org.uk

— A large mental health charity in England and Wales that has a national phone helpline and local associations that offer a variety of services, including supported housing, crisis helplines, drop-in centers, counseling, befriending, advocacy, and employment programs. It has published a number of fact sheets and pamphlets, which can also be viewed on its website.

Mental Health Foundation

www.mentalhealth.org.uk

— This leading charity is designed to support people with mental illness and learning disabilities, providing information on specific mental health problems, where to get help, treatment, and rights.

National Institute for Mental Health in England (NIMHE)

www.nimhe.org.uk

— To improve the quality of life for people of all ages who experience mental distress, this organization has identified three strategic priorities: system transformation to ensure efficient and effective care and treatment, work force development, and changes in practice to ensure rapid access to the best possible care.

The Princess Royal Trust for Carers

www.carers.org

— Offers useful information and support for all unpaid caregivers throughout the UK. Its website includes information about a wide variety of illnesses (mental illnesses, dementia, physical illnesses, etc.) and sponsors discussion boards. It has a separate website (*www.youngcarers.net*) for young people who are caring for relatives with mental illnesses.

Rethink (formerly the National Schizophrenia Fellowship)

www.rethink.org

— A widespread organization that provides practical support in the form of information, housing, community services, caregiver services, employment, advocacy, and other services throughout England and Northern Ireland. It also provides a range of useful leaflets, booklets, and other materials to help people deal with severe mental illness.

Revolving Doors Agency

www.revolving-doors.co.uk

— The U.K.'s leading charity concerned with mental health and the criminal justice system runs programs at police stations, courts, and prisons to support people with mental illness who have "fallen through the net" of mainstream psychiatric services.

The Royal College of Psychiatrists

www.rcpsych.ac.uk

— The website contains several helpful leaflets on a wide variety of mental health problems, from schizophrenia to alcohol abuse to posttraumatic stress disorders. It also provides links to the schizophrenia guideline of the National Institute for Health and Clinical Excellence (NICE guideline, *www.nice.org.uk*) and to the Partners in Care campaign (*www.rcpsych.ac.uk/campaigns/pinc/index.htm*), which focuses on caregivers, professionals, and individuals with mental illness working together in partnership. Their checklists for caregivers, people with mental illness, and psychiatrists contain contain excellent questions.

SANE

www.sane.org.uk

— SANE (originally an acronym for Schizophrenia—A National Emergency) was founded to raise public awareness about mental illness and to offer support to those who are affected by it. Its helpline, SANELINE (*www.sane.org.uk/public_html/SANE_Services/SANELINE.shtm*), provides practical information, crisis care, and emotional support to callers affected by mental health problems in themselves or relatives. Its newsletter, SANETALK, is provided to members (back issues can be purchased), and it also publishes several educational pamphlets about mental illness and its treatment.

Turning Point

www.turning-point.co.uk

— The UK's leading social care charity provides services for people with complex needs across a range of health and disability issues, including mental illness and substance abuse. It offers residential and community-based services in 200 locations in England and Wales.

UK Council for Psychotherapy

www.psychotherapy.org.uk

— Promoting psychotherapy for the public benefit, the council publishes the annual National Register of Psychotherapists, including only psychotherapists who meet the training requirements and abide by its ethical guidelines.

Books

Birchwood, M., & Jackson, C. (2001). *Schizophrenia*. London: Psychology Press. *Note.* This book is part of a series called "Clinical Psychology: A Modular Course," primarily aimed at undergraduates and graduate students, but families may also find it helpful.

Chadwick, P. (1997). *Schizophrenia, the positive perspective: In search of dignity for schizophrenic people*. London: Routledge. *Note.* The author, who has experienced schizophrenia himself, examines an alternative point of view, suggesting that schizophrenia gives people valuable qualities such as extra perceptions, empathy, and sensitivity.

Gopfert, M., Webster, J., & Seeman, M. V. (Eds.). (2004). *Parental psychiatric disorder: Distressed parents and their families*. Cambridge, UK: Cambridge University Press.

Jones, S., & Hayward, P. (2004). *Coping with schizophrenia: A guide for patients, families and caregivers*. Oxford, UK: Oneworld Publications.

Kuipers, E., & Bebbington, P. (2005). *Living with mental illness: A book for relatives and friends* (3rd ed.). London: Souvenir Press.

Ramsay, R., Gerada, C., Mars, S., & Szmukler, G. *Mental illness: A handbook for carers*. (2001). London: Jessica Kingsley.

Turner, T. (2003). *Schizophrenia: Your questions answered.* London: Churchill-Livingstone Press.

Warner, R. (2000). *The environment of schizophrenia: Innovations in practice, policy and communications*. London: Brunner-Routledge.

Singapore

Action Group for Mental Illness

www.agmi.org.sg

— This organization comprises health care providers, caregivers, and individuals who are interested in improving the lives of people with mental illness.

Singapore Association for Mental Health

www.samhealth.org.sg

— SAMH is a voluntary welfare organization (nongovermental and nonprofit) that seeks to promote the social and mental well-being of the people of Singapore, including the care and rehabilitation of the mentally ill, and to reduce the stigma of mental illness.

Index

About the Authors

Kim T. Mueser, PhD, is a clinical psychologist and professor in the Departments of Psychiatry and Community and Family Medicine at Dartmouth Medical School in Hanover, New Hampshire. A renowned expert in the field of schizophrenia and other severe mental illnesses, his research has been supported by the National Institute of Mental Health, the National Institute on Drug Abuse, and the Substance Abuse and Mental Health Services Administration. In 2003 he received a Distinguished Investigator Award from the National Alliance for Research on Schizophrenia and Depression. Dr. Mueser has coauthored seven prior books and published over 200 articles in peer-reviewed journals; his work is widely cited in the field.

In addition to working with individuals, groups, and families, Dr. Mueser conducts workshops nationally and internationally aimed at teaching clinicians effective treatment and rehabilitation methods for people with schizophrenia and other serious mental illnesses. Dr. Mueser's personal experience with a family member with schizophrenia has enhanced his understanding of the effects of the illness on the family.

Susan Gingerich, MSW, is a clinician and consultant with over 20 years of research and clinical experience working with people with mental illness and their families. Based in Philadelphia, she has provided effective and caring treatment to individuals, groups, and families in a diversity of settings, including inpatient units, outpatient clinics, residential treatment centers, state hospitals, as well as home visits.

Dr. Mueser and Ms. Gingerich have collaborated for over two decades on the treatment of schizophrenia. Working together as cotherapists in family therapy and group therapy for individuals with schizophrenia, they have coauthored four books, including *Coping with Schizophrenia* and *Social Skills Training for Schizophrenia*.